PRAISE FOR
Best Practices for a Healthy Heart

"Dr. Samaan attacks the myths and hype around cardiovascular health and lays out the fundamentals in an easy-to-digest format. Her seven steps are clear, straightforward, and supported by scientific data, as well as her own personal experiences as a cardiologist. This book provides the best up-to-date information on cardiovascular disease prevention."

—MICHAEL CRAWFORD, MD, FACC, Chief of Clinical Cardiology, University of California, San Francisco

"As a fellow physician, I see too often that many people neither heed subtle warning signs of pending heart disease nor realize they can take a proactive role toward improving heart health. In a reader-friendly, clear, concise, and comprehensive narrative, Dr. Samaan lays out a simple, lifelong approach to effectively preventing heart disease that will also improve overall health."

—JEFF BALSER, MD, PHD, Vice Chancellor for Health Affairs, Vanderbilt University, and Dean of the Vanderbilt University School of Medicine

"Wonderfully comprehensive . . . Dr. Samaan's achievement in terms of the detail and scope of her book is very impressive. While this book touches on all aspects of cardiovascular disease, it does so in an easily readable and understandable style for the lay person, and yet it has value for the professional."

—GERALD C. TIMMIS, MD, Professor of Internal Medicine, William Beaumont School of Medicine, Oakland University

THE EXPERIMENT

Best Practices

for a

HEALTHY HEART

HOW TO STOP HEART DISEASE
BEFORE *OR AFTER* IT STARTS

SARAH SAMAAN, MD, FACC

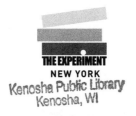

THE EXPERIMENT
NEW YORK

The Experiment
260 Fifth Avenue, Suite 3 South
New York, NY 10001-6408
www.theexperimentpublishing.com

To preserve patient confidentiality, patients' names and identifying characteristics have been changed. Any resemblance to actual persons is coincidental.

The information in this book is not intended to take the place of medical advice from the reader's personal physician. Please consult with your physician or other health care professional before beginning any diet or health program. The author and publisher expressly disclaim responsibility for any adverse effects arising from the use or application of the information presented in this book.

The Experiment's books are available at special discounts when purchased in bulk for premiums and sales promotions as well as for fundraising or educational use. For details, contact us at info@theexperimentpublishing.com.

Many of the designations used by manufacturers and sellers to distinguish their products are claimed as trademarks. Where those designations appear in this book and The Experiment was aware of a trademark claim, the designations have been capitalized.

Cover design by Alison Forner
Author photograph © Jesse Hornbuckle
Text design by Pauline Neuwirth, Neuwirth & Associates, Inc.

Library of Congress Cataloging-in-Publication Data
Samaan, Sarah.
Best practices for a healthy heart : how to stop heart disease before or after it starts / Sarah Samaan.
p. cm.
Summary: "This book acts as a guide to the 'best practices' for optimal heart health, serving as a resource for patients diagnosed with or aiming to prevent heart disease. In it, Dr. Samaan provides advice on diet, supplements and alternative medicine, the effects of caffeine and alcohol, stress management, and more"—Provided by publisher.
Includes index.
ISBN-13: 978-1-61519-047-8 (pbk.)
ISBN-13: 978-1-61519-147-5 (electronic) 1. Heart—Diseases—Prevention—Popular works. 2. Heart—Diseases—Diet therapy—Popular works. 3. Heart—Diseases—Nutritional aspects—Popular works. I. Title.
RC684.D5S26 2011
616.1'205—dc23
2011035691

ISBN 978-1-61519-047-8
Ebook ISBN 978-1-61519-147-5

Manufactured in the United States of America

Distributed by Workman Publishing Company, Inc.
Distributed simultaneously in Canada by Thomas Allen and Son Ltd.
First published May 2012

10 9 8 7 6 5 4 3 2 1

Dedicated with love and gratitude to my mother,
Dr. Jean Moffatt Samaan

And to the memory of my father,
Dr. Naguib Samaan

CONTENTS

PREFACE
WHY I WROTE THIS BOOK

WHEN I ENTERED medical school in 1984, the ink barely dry on my liberal arts degree, my future was as much of a mystery to me as the complicated anatomical illustrations in my textbook on gross anatomy. As my studies progressed, the intricate connections of nerve, muscle, and bone gradually came together into a comprehensible but utterly miraculous whole. Nurtured by inspired professors and powered by my will to thrive in the challenging profession I had chosen, I came to understand the human body not only as an organism of myriad chemical, molecular, and structural functions, but also as a singular, individual being.

My choice to pursue cardiology was truly an organic one. I enjoyed the immediacy of intensive care, but I realized that it was also important for me to know my patients as individuals in order to help them regain as independent and unencumbered a life as possible. Cardiology was a perfect fit.

My father, who was a physician, and his family also inspired my decision to pursue cardiology. Their sad legacy of cardiovascular disease impressed upon me the consequences of genetics and life choices. My grandmother died of a heart attack at age 48. She was obese and no doubt suffered from many associated health problems, most of which would have gone unrecognized in her time. When she died, she left eight children behind.

My spry and lean grandfather lived to the ripe old age of 90, but his children must have inherited their mother's genes. As a child, I dreaded the emotionally charged long-distance phone calls my father received as heart disease picked off his siblings, one by one. A favorite uncle died on the way to my sister's wedding. A devastating heart attack took the life of another uncle, a heart surgeon, shortly after he left the hospital against his cardiologist's advice. All told, six out of my seven beloved aunts and uncles have died—several before the age of 60. Most were obese, and, unlike my father, they chose a sedentary lifestyle, too busy or disinclined to exercise.

My dad was just a little overweight. He ate fairly well, and he was always physically active. Despite his reasonably healthy lifestyle, he had dangerously high blood pressure, but he would never take medicine for more than a few months or go for checkups. He believed that he had everything under control. When he was 64, he suffered a stroke. The stroke was debilitating, and he never found much joy in life afterward. With his stroke came a diagnosis of diabetes, a condition that had probably gone undetected for years. He lived a sad and frustrating life for seven more years before succumbing to heart and kidney failure.

My father's active lifestyle is probably what bought him more years of health than his siblings had. What he lacked was preventive medicine, which could have made an enormous difference. As a doctor, he knew better, but as a human being, he did not want to admit to being anything less than invincible. My dad's case is particularly poignant for me because so much of what happened to him was preventable and treatable. His death was a natural event, but one that I believe could have happened many years later. He might have been able to enjoy the retirement he worked so hard for, share his children's achievements, and revel in knowing his grandchildren.

My father became ill and died during my medical training, which gave me a deep appreciation of the power of prevention and the terrible consequences of denying the vulnerability of our bodies.

I would be remiss if I did not mention my mother and her powerful influence upon my life. She is a British woman, now in her 70s, who grew up at a time when higher education was considered a luxury for a girl, and not worth the expense. Of my grandmother's five children, my mother was the only girl, and my grandmother was determined that her daughter would have the independence and opportunities that she hadn't. To my grandmother, that meant an education.

As fate would have it, my mother, an avid reader, was greatly influenced by what she read of physician, medical missionary, and musical scholar Albert Schweitzer, the 1952 recipient of the Nobel Peace Prize. Her father and his cronies teased and ridiculed my mother, but she persevered and became the first in her family to attend a university. She graduated from medical school in 1957, intent on heading to Africa to follow in Dr. Schweitzer's footsteps as a medical missionary. Along the way, she met my father, a darkly handsome and brilliant but decidedly foreign physician. Their mixed marriage alienated her family for years, but she was in love and determined to make it work.

One thing led to another and, before she knew it, she was a mother of five, living in Houston, and practicing family medicine. Although our family was highly unconventional, responsibility for child raising fell squarely on my mother's shoulders. It is a tribute to her love, devotion, and high expectations that we, her children, have all had the opportunity to pursue our unique dreams in our own ways.

During my father's long illness, my mom continued to work, but she devoted the remaining time in her day to his care and comfort. After his death, she moved to the country ranch they had purchased together years before.

She now lives with a menagerie of ponies, donkeys, cows, dogs, cats, chickens, peacocks, and any other creatures who decide to call her place home. For many years into her retirement, she volunteered at a medical clinic for the homeless and underserved, teaching her brand of care and compassion to newly minted doctors-in-training.

I am profoundly grateful for the lessons my parents taught me. Although my father, like many doctors of his generation, didn't accept the frailties of his own body until it was too late, he treated his patients with great care and respect. Years after his death, I am still deeply touched by the remembrances of his former patients.

My mother is truly a healer; she has touched thousands of lives and continues to make a difference for people who might otherwise go unnoticed. From both of my parents, I have learned that there is so much we can do to enrich our lives with good health. We must live life with love and zest, and care for the bodies that carry us through this ever-changing, unpredictable world.

Thanks in large part to my parents' legacy, I have always embraced a healthy lifestyle. In college, I quickly realized that eating well and making time for exercise helped keep my mind clear and sharp and my life balanced. An avid equestrian, hiker, and yoga enthusiast, I have learned that good health must be nurtured and never taken for granted. That is a philosophy I try to share with my patients.

Over the years, my cardiology practice evolved, and I became a strong advocate for preventive cardiology. Fully 85 percent of heart disease can be prevented, and yet it remains our leading cause of death and a major cause of disability and misery. Thanks in part to my work as a spokesperson for the American Heart Association, I've had the opportunity to bring this message to a wide range of people. In the process, I have learned to keep an open mind in my search for answers to the questions that my patients and listeners have raised. Many times, these searches have opened my own eyes to new and unexpected discoveries.

More than anything, this book is an expression of gratitude to my family, patients, and mentors for the lessons they have taught me. I hope it will inspire you to seek a healthier, more joyful way of life and to nurture your own heart, and, in the process, the hearts of those you love.

INTRODUCTION

AS A CARDIOLOGIST, I consider the prevention of heart disease to be my most important and most difficult duty. During a heart attack, when the heart muscle is abruptly cut off from vital blood flow and oxygen, my responsibility is clear and well defined: Restore blood flow to preserve life. If you're my patient, your role in this situation is essentially passive. Usually, your only voice in the matter is to give me consent to treat your condition. While a heart attack may get my adrenaline flowing as I hop out of bed at 3 AM for another run to the hospital, I know that, with appropriate and timely attention, my medical teammates and I can usually care for the problem. Prevention, however, takes more dedication and hard work—and it must come from you.

Cardiovascular disease (CVD), which includes heart attacks, high blood pressure, abnormal heart rhythms, stroke, atherosclerosis (cholesterol buildup in the blood vessels), and congestive heart failure, is our leading cause of death, claiming the lives of one in three of us, yet in most cases it is preventable. Heart attacks are far from being a malady of the elderly—nearly half of all heart attack victims are younger than 65. Thanks to modern medical research, we can easily identify the major factors that contribute to heart disease: high blood pressure, diabetes, high cholesterol, smoking, a sedentary lifestyle, obesity, and genetics. But knowing our risk is not enough. Preventing heart disease must become a way of life—a commitment to an active lifestyle, an investment in a healthy diet, and a resolution to live mindfully, aware that all of our choices carry consequences.

HONORING THE GIFT OF LIFE BY LEARNING TO CARE FOR YOURSELF

An important part of caring for yourself is to enlist a partner in health—a supportive and skillful physician who can discuss your concerns with genuine interest in you as a person, as well as provide up-to-date medical knowledge, treat conditions you can't control with healthy living alone, and ensure your efforts to achieve good health are successful.

Caring for yourself also means listening closely to the messages your body is sending. Outside of medicine, my passion is horses. For all their beauty and strength, these noble animals depend utterly on humans for their comfort and health; they must trust that their owners will make the right choices for them. When an owner overlooks the signs that a horse is in distress or lacks the knowledge to give appropriate care, the outcome can be tragic. We must learn to listen to our own complex and wonderful bodies, just as we would to such a magnificent creature entrusted to our care. That is how we honor the remarkable gift of life. It is not enough to make promises to do better. Caring for yourself requires conscious action and daily commitment.

A DOCTOR'S JOURNEY

I began working on this book in 2001. My initial idea was to write a diet book for people interested in losing weight while improving their heart health. However, as the book evolved, I realized that a healthy heart requires more than diet alone. I needed to address the questions my patients were asking about stress, exercise, hormones, alternative therapies, and supplements. When I couldn't find a resource that covered these and other preventive measures in a scientifically rigorous yet easily accessible fashion, I decided to take matters into my own hands. This book is the result.

In the medical field, we use the term *best practices* to refer to the most up-to-date, evidence-based information available that will help us provide our patients with the best possible care. I applied those principles as I explored a wealth of research on nutrition, supplements, stress, hormones, and other important aspects of heart health. Most of the resources I used are well respected, peer-reviewed scientific journals that are readily available but outside the sphere of the typical physician. All told, I spent well over three thousand hours researching and synthesizing the scientific literature to create a book that addressed the issues my patients were eager to learn about.

While I have always preached the mantra of "diet and exercise," only while writing this book did I realize just how deeply our small habits and daily choices are connected to our health and well-being. I know that writing this book for you has made me a better doctor, and I hope that you are able to put these "best practices" to work in your own life. You truly hold your heart in your own hands. Treat it with love and care.

Take Charge of Your Numbers

NONE OF US is typical. We come in an endless variety of shapes, sizes, and colors, each of us with our own rich spectrum of passions, obsessions, and talents. But one thing we all share is a dependence on our marvelous body to take us through this life in good health.

Being heart smart means understanding that there is more to life than calculations and statistics, while realizing that there are some numbers we can control. The first step to a heart-loving lifestyle is to get a handle on body size, waist circumference, cholesterol, triglycerides, and other important measurements of heart health. These figures can add or subtract years of well-being, but it's up to us to do the math.

1

What You Need to Know and Why You Should Care

TWENTY-FOUR HOURS a day, seven days a week, every thirty seconds in the United States, someone will die of a heart attack—the number one killer and the most important health risk that all of us, men and women, face today.

We fear cancer, and rightly so, but heart disease takes a far greater toll. Cardiovascular disease (CVD) kills more than 750,000 Americans each year. That's nearly 200,000 more people than die from cancer, our next most common killer. For simplicity's sake, the terms *CVD* (which includes heart attacks, strokes, heart failure, hypertension, and other diseases related to the heart and blood vessels) and *heart disease* will be used interchangeably throughout this book.

In addition to its human toll, heart disease is a tremendous financial drain. The American Heart Association estimated that its cost to the U.S. economy in 2010, including treatment, maintenance, disability, and loss of work productivity, was over $300 billion. If we continue on our current track, health-care costs related to CVD are expected to triple by 2030, seriously straining our already struggling economy.

PREVENTION: IT'S A PERSONAL THING

It doesn't have to be this way. Imagine a revolutionary medical breakthrough that could reduce the chances of having a heart attack by 60 to 75 percent.

This new therapy is guaranteed to boost your mood; make you appear more attractive; help you lose weight; liven up your sex life; lower your chances of developing other diseases, such as diabetes and certain forms of cancer; and reduce your risk of dementia and stroke. Moreover, it's all natural, nearly 100 percent safe, and basically free.

Who would refuse such an amazing treatment that would transform health care and save billions of dollars every year? The answer: most people in this country and maybe even you.

I'm not talking about complicated laboratory science or another fruitless search for the fabled fountain of youth. The secret to combating heart disease is available right now. It's called prevention. And the key is your lifestyle.

Cardiovascular disease starts its silent assault on the arteries of the heart and other organs decades before it shows up as a heart attack or stroke. Atherosclerosis, or buildup of cholesterol plaques in the arteries, begins as early as childhood. Small cholesterol plaques in the coronary arteries, which feed the heart its vital blood supply, can be found in more than 15 percent of "normal" American teenagers and in 85 percent of people over the age of 50.

A heart attack occurs when one or more of these arteries get blocked and blood can't reach the heart muscle. The blockage is usually due to an unstable cholesterol plaque within a heart artery that ruptures or cracks. The body treats this as an injury and sends blood platelets to the damaged area to seal it off. This process results in a blood clot forming inside the artery, abruptly blocking blood flow. Without blood and oxygen, the heart tissue literally begins to die and can no longer function normally.

A heart attack generally occurs in a segment of the heart artery that is already damaged by years of slow, progressive cholesterol buildup.

In most cases, a heart attack does not just "happen" at age 45, 60, or 75. It is a process, and it has been building for many years.

CALCULATING THE ROLE AND RISKS OF LIFESTYLE

A healthy lifestyle, including a heart-friendly diet, daily exercise, not smoking, and maintaining an optimum weight, will reduce your cardiovascular risk by more than 70 percent and extend your life span by nearly fifteen years.

We know more about heart disease prevention than ever before, but the lifestyles Americans choose are increasingly toxic. Less than one in six, regardless of gender, choose to practice a healthful way of life.

Most people in this country are overweight, and more than one in three is obese. Since the 1960s, the prevalence of obesity has nearly tripled. As a major contributor to high blood pressure, high cholesterol, and diabetes, weight is far more than a cosmetic issue. Sadly, men and women all too often sacrifice their health and financial well-being for fast food and sedentary entertainment.

Smoking virtually guarantees that our lives will be shorter and our health-care costs greater. Despite the well-known dangers of tobacco, it continues to ensnare nearly 21 percent of men and 18 percent of women in the United States, dramatically increasing their chances of heart disease, stroke, cancer, and a myriad of other miseries, and stealing health and vitality.

INHERITED RISK AND LIFESAVING MEDICINES

Whereas heart disease is often preventable with lifestyle alone, many of the risk factors that lead to heart disease are impacted by inherited conditions. I have learned in my practice as a cardiologist that bad luck is an unfortunate fact of life, and high cholesterol, high blood pressure, diabetes, and other serious health problems can develop in people who are absolutely committed to a healthy way of life. These conditions become more prevalent as we age, despite our best efforts.

We are fortunate to live in a time in which a wide array of lifesaving medications is available to help treat these and so many other problems. By starting medical therapy early, we can often prevent heart disease and other long-term complications such as kidney failure and stroke. Most of the drugs commonly used are unlikely to cause serious side effects, although careful monitoring and regular follow-up are important. Although taking pills and going for checkups may seem a bit cumbersome, when you add necessary medical therapy to a healthy lifestyle, you may reduce your cardiovascular risk by as much as 85 percent.

CLEARING THE WAY: EXPOSING THE DANGEROUS MYTHS OF HEART DISEASE

Your road to heart power begins with blowing the roof off some of the most common heart disease myths, half-truths, and fallacies.

MYTH NO. 1:
HEART DISEASE IS A MAN'S PROBLEM.

FACT: Heart disease is far and away the leading cause of death of American women. Although women tend to develop it about ten years later in life than do men, two out of every five women will die of disease of the cardiovascular system. Too many others will suffer serious disability or a lower quality of life.

MYTH NO. 2:
HEART DISEASE IS FOR OLD PEOPLE.

FACT: Heart disease is not an old-age malady. Fully 45 percent of all heart attacks occur before the age of 65, and each year, more than twenty-five thousand American men and eight thousand American women under the age of 45 will die from a heart attack. Medical science has made tremendous progress, and heart attacks are not always the death sentence they once were. But although death rates from heart disease are declining overall, they are on the rise for women under 45. At the same time, we are seeing a slower decline in death rates for younger men, when compared to those for older folks, likely due to dangerously unhealthy lifestyle choices.

MYTH NO. 3:
HEART DISEASE SYMPTOMS ARE THE SAME FOR WOMEN AND MEN.

FACT: Women's symptoms may be very different. When a heart attack strikes, women younger than 50 are more than twice as likely to die as are men of the same age, in large part because they ignore their symptoms until it's too late.

The classic, textbook warning signs of heart disease can occur in both men and women: chest pain that sometimes radiates to the left arm or neck, clamminess, nausea, and shortness of breath. Usually the pain, known as *angina*, is brought on by exertion or stress, and relieved in five to ten minutes with rest.

In the month leading up to a heart attack, many people will experience angina, but all too often the pain is ignored or brushed off as indigestion. Women are more likely to notice extreme fatigue, insomnia, back pain, and shortness of breath, without chest pain. Whatever the symptom, anything that comes on with physical (or emotional) stress and resolves with rest deserves an urgent evaluation.

During a heart attack, men will typically feel severe chest pain, but not everyone will experience heart pain the same way. Forty percent of women suffering from a heart attack report no chest pain at all. Women are more likely than men to complain of nausea, fatigue, neck and jaw pain, shoulder pain, and back pain, and are less likely to break out in a cold sweat. Shortness of breath and a sense of overwhelming weakness are also more common in women. However, men may also experience symptoms of this nature. Whatever form they may take, the symptoms of a heart attack may wax and wane, but are generally relentless. Immediate medical attention is critical, as we are often able to prevent or minimize any permanent damage if we can treat the problem in time.

These are not complicated differences, but you can't ignore the less-than-classic symptoms just because they are not what you might consider typical.

MYTH NO. 4:
HEART DISEASE IS USUALLY INHERITED.

FACT: Up to 85 percent of heart attacks are preventable. Obesity, smoking, lack of exercise, poor eating habits, and other unhealthy choices are major, but preventable, risk factors.

It's easy to blame your parents for our health woes, but the truth is that though your genes may interact with other risk factors, only about 15 percent of heart disease can be blamed on genetics alone. You might inherit high blood pressure or high cholesterol, or a susceptibility to diabetes, but those are problems that can be managed with a combination of a healthy diet, regular exercise, and, when needed, medication. On the other hand, it's important to know your family history. If your mom had a heart attack before age 65, or your dad before 55, then your risk may be up to two times greater than the average person's. In that case, it's especially important to choose a heart-smart lifestyle and to get regular medical checkups.

THE AMERICAN HEART ASSOCIATION'S GUIDELINES

THE AMERICAN HEART ASSOCIATION (AHA) has issued guidelines help physicians make appropriate recommendations for every individual, regardless of gender, age, or risk profile. You will learn about the ways that these principles can transform your life for the better in later chapters of this book, and I will explain what these terms mean in language that you can understand. To get a jump start, here are the basic best practices to ensure a healthy heart:

* Get 30 minutes of exercise most days of the week.
* Limit dietary saturated fat to less than 10% of daily calories.
* Limit trans fats to less than 1% of total calories.
* Consume less than 300 mg of cholesterol daily.
* Increase omega-3 fatty acids, especially if you are at high risk for cardiac disease.
* Follow a heart-healthy diet high in fruits, vegetables, grains, low-fat dairy, fish, and legumes.
* Maintain a body mass index between 18.5 and 24.9.
* Keep a waist circumference of less than 35 inches.
* Strive for a blood pressure of less than 120/80.
* Set a goal of LDL cholesterol less than 100, and HDL greater than 50.
* Do not smoke or use any form of tobacco, and avoid secondhand smoke.

These straightforward guidelines will help you understand the profound effects of the many simple choices you make every day. Understanding is the first step to achieving balance and control of your own health and well-being. The more you know, the more power you hold in your own hands. Through *Best Practices for a Healthy Heart,* you will discover the tools of prevention and learn how you can alter the course of your own life, regardless of where you stand on the heart disease continuum.

A DAY IN THE LIFE OF HEART DISEASE

As a cardiologist, I see the results of an unhealthy lifestyle and untreated risk factors each day. We are fortunate to live in an era of sophisticated cardiac interventions and surgeries, but despite all our modern technology and lifesaving skills, the responsibility for prevention is yours.

To illustrate how prevention can save your life and the path that poor lifestyle habits can take you down, let me share with you a typical day in my life as a cardiologist.

At 7:15 AM I begin my rounds with 57-year-old Jim, who was hospitalized the night before with a severe heart attack in progress. Fortunately, Jim got to the hospital in time, and my on-call partner opened up a critical blockage in one of his major coronary arteries before any permanent damage was done. Jim smokes two packs of cigarettes a day, doesn't exercise, and could stand to lose about 30 pounds.

Jim's father died of a heart attack at the age of 58, but Jim says he never thought it could happen to him. What he doesn't yet realize is that the process of atherosclerosis has been underway for the past thirty-five years, churning along as a consequence of innumerable unhealthy daily choices, combined with his unfortunate genetic makeup.

My next patient is a 48-year-old woman whose weathered face betrays her years of smoking. Sherry rides her bike regularly with her boyfriend, but recently noticed more shortness of breath and a strange ache in her back and arms. She tried not to worry, but when her symptoms got worse, she headed to the hospital for a checkup. Unfortunately, Sherry has already suffered a heart attack, probably a few days before she came to the hospital. Her heart muscle is working at about half its normal capacity. She swears to me that she will never smoke again. That's good, because another heart attack would probably kill her. She will need open-heart surgery before she leaves the hospital.

Later in the day, I see a 39-year-old gentleman who weighs more than 300 pounds. Jesse, an insurance broker, is diabetic, has high blood pressure and high cholesterol, and worries about the breathlessness he feels when he climbs the stairs to his third-floor apartment. We will schedule a stress test and hope that the results are good. However, I fear that Jesse is already well on his way to developing heart disease. Even if the stress test is normal, I will urge him to work on prevention, and he will certainly need medication. Jesse expresses qualms about the cost and possible side effects of these prescriptions. While I am sympathetic, the fact remains that, if his conditions are left untreated, he is likely to suffer irreversible damage to his heart, brain, kidneys, and other vital organs. I explain to Jesse that his high blood pressure, high cholesterol, and diabetes may even disappear if he loses weight, improves his diet, and commits to exercising regularly.

In the office, Hank, one of my favorite patients, arrives for a routine visit. He is a charming 85-year-old gentleman who has endured two bypass operations and the loss of his beloved wife. With the help of a careful selection of medications and an active and optimistic outlook, he lives life to its fullest. In fact, his exercise stress test time is better than those of many seemingly healthy people half his age.

Carmella comes to see me about her blood pressure. She is 35 years old, pregnant with her third child, and never lost the 60 pounds she gained with her first two pregnancies. We have worked hard to control her hypertension, but she needs two drugs to keep it down and is seeing a high-risk obstetric specialist to help her and her baby get through the pregnancy safely.

The last patient of the day is 30-year-old Kharim, who has seen the ravages of heart disease in his own family. Prompted by the recent death of his father at the age of 53, Kharim has started working out regularly. When I first met him, his cholesterol was dangerously high—too high to treat with diet and exercise alone. Kharim has responded beautifully to a low dose of cholesterol-lowering medicine and a heart-smart diet.

Just one day brings a wide array of opportunities for preventive care to make a tangible difference in so many lives.

HERE'S THE GREAT NEWS

Eighty-five percent of heart disease is preventable. That means living a heart-smart lifestyle and seeking medical care for the risk factors that you cannot control. You have the power to make the difference in your own life and in the life of those you love. The choices you make and the chances you take each day are what give you the power to live a longer, stronger, healthier, and happier life.

2

Overweight:
What's the Big Deal?

WEIGHT LOSS IS a $40 billion industry, but just how people become overweight is no great mystery. If your dietary intake and your energy output are not in balance, you will gain weight. It's as simple as that. Nutrition and exercise are the keys to your heart, your mind, and your well-being. Although it is possible to be overweight and physically fit, there is no question that excessive weight will literally drag you down, affecting your health, your job, and your relationships.

Like many people, you may notice your scale creeping up a pound or two every few months. Perhaps you shrug it off, hoping the weight will leave as mysteriously as it came. Unfortunately, time has a way of growing those few unwanted extra pounds into a serious health problem.

Five pounds of weight gain each year may hardly seem worth worrying about, but fast-forward five years, and now you're stuck with 25 pounds of unwanted and unhealthy fat and a closet full of clothes that don't fit.

THE STATS ON FAT

If you're overweight, you're not alone. Two out of every three American adults are overweight. Nearly half of those who are overweight meet the criterion for obesity, meaning they are at least 20 percent above the recommended weight for their height. All told, that translates to 65 million obese Americans, and the number continues to grow. This is a dramatic change from the 1960s, when only about 13 percent of adults were obese. If the current trends in weight gain continue, it is estimated that the lifetime risk of obesity will be close to 40 percent for women and 50 percent for men.

WHY IS OBESITY SUCH A BIG DEAL?

If you carry some extra weight, as most people do, it might come as a surprise to learn that you may in fact be obese by medical standards. The body mass index (BMI), which is now considered a vital sign on par with blood pressure and pulse, uses height and weight measurements to calculate where your weight falls on the healthy-weight continuum. Take a look at the "Obese or Overweight: How to Find Out" chart on page 19 and learn to calculate your body-mass index, or turn to the appendix (page 346) for more detailed information.

Why does it matter? It's not a question of aesthetics. In the United States, obese girls are less likely to attend college than are girls of normal weight, limiting their social and financial opportunities. Fair or not, studies on the subject have found that people of both genders who are obese are more likely to be socioeconomically disadvantaged, to be poorly treated by supervisors and coworkers, and to be passed over for a promotion. Obese women are especially hard hit. They are often viewed as less successful, less energetic, and less in control.

However, the problems go much deeper than that. Being overweight is associated with a higher risk of diabetes, high blood pressure, elevated cholesterol, and depression—all of which significantly increase the chances of cardiovascular disease. In fact, even without those particular health complications, the risk of a heart attack is at least doubled in an obese person as compared to that in a person of medically appropriate weight (see "Know Your Risk Factors," page 349).

People who carry most of their fat in the abdominal area (known as abdominal adiposity, or visceral fat) have an even higher risk for heart disease and other health problems, because they are prone to diabetes and high cholesterol. (Sometimes this shape is referred to as an "apple," whereas people who carry most of their weight in their hips and thighs are known as "pears.") Although the American Heart Association guidelines recommend that women maintain a waist size of no more than 35 inches, the risk for heart disease actually begins to rise when the belly bulges beyond 33 inches; for men 35 inches appears to be the safe upper limit.

Fat that collects around the waist can churn out a toxic mix of hormones and inflammatory substances that have been strongly linked to a higher risk of heart attacks, blood clots, and other health problems.

Not only does obesity expose the heart and other organs to these dangerous chemicals, it also requires the heart to work overtime, pumping blood through literally miles of extra capillaries, and may result in measurable changes in the heart's ability to do its work efficiently. The heart may become thicker and less elastic. These two factors have been associated with congestive heart failure, a condition that is twice as common in obese individuals as in those of normal weight.

Although most commonly associated with older folks, heart abnormalities of this type have been reported in obese teens and young adults. Because congestive heart failure causes fluid retention and shortness of breath, it has a major impact on quality of life and mortality. The good news is that in many cases, weight loss can reverse the damage done to the heart.

People who suffer from obesity are also more likely to develop serious heart rhythm disturbances such as atrial fibrillation, a rapid and irregular heart rhythm that increases the risk for stroke by 50 percent.

Obesity intensifies your risk of a frightening range of diseases and ailments. Most people don't realize it, but obesity increases the probability of developing many different types of cancers, including breast, colon, esophageal, uterine, pancreatic, liver, and prostate cancers. It has been estimated that one in seven cancer deaths in men and one of every five in women can be directly attributed to obesity.

The brains of obese patients appear to age much more quickly, according to UCLA research scientists, ratcheting up the risk for Alzheimer's dementia. And a host of other health problems, including liver disease, gallstones, sleep apnea, gastric reflux, stroke, blood clots in the legs and lungs, and arthritis, can be directly attributed to obesity. Obesity even raises the risk of miscarriage.

People who are obese have a death rate twice that of their slim counterparts. On average, obesity will shorten life span by ten to twenty years, thanks to the diseases and disorders it spawns.

Obesity also strikes the pocketbook. People who are obese spend 36 percent more on health care and 77 percent more on medications than does the general population. A 2010 study from George Washington University estimated that the annual personal cost of obesity, including medical bills, lost productivity, insurance, and even higher gasoline usage, is about $4,900 for women and $2,600 for men. The Centers for Disease Control calculates that, nationally, the medical cost of obesity exceeds a staggering $147 billion each year.

OBESITY AND OVERWEIGHT: WHY WORRY?

* Obesity kills 112,000 people every year.
* Overweight and obesity cost the United States $147 billion annually for health care and lost productivity.
* Obese people spend 36% more on health care and 77% more on medications.
* At least half of the medical costs of overweight and obesity are funded by taxpayers through Medicare and Medicaid.
* Sixty-six percent of Americans are overweight; by 2015, the number will reach 75% unless we change our lifestyles.
* Approximately 32% of Americans are obese; that number may reach 40% by 2015.
* Childhood obesity has tripled since 1976.

HOW DID WE GET THIS WAY?

The easy explanation for these alarming statistics is that we are eating more and exercising less. Our average daily calorie consumption has increased by 300 to 500 calories during the past thirty years. How this has come to be is more complicated.

The Rise of Fast Food

Although many people become overweight without the assistance of fast food, the explosion of fast-food restaurants tempting us with high-fat, superfast, and super-sized meals is doubtless an important piece of the puzzle. In 1970, about 10 percent of the average family's food budget was spent on meals out. By 2000, it had risen to 50 percent. As our national spending on restaurant meals surged by nearly 50 percent between 2000 and 2008, that figure has surely risen. Currently about half of our daily calories are eaten out. What's worse, one in three kids now eats fast food every day.

This fast-food mania has hit us right in the gut. Although commercials for fast-food joints typically feature energetically slim and happy characters, people who eat fast food just twice a week are over 50 percent more likely to become obese than are those who eat their meals at home, and may be more likely to suffer from depression.

We are a nation of overachievers when it comes to eating. A recent study from the University of North Carolina found a dramatic increase in portion sizes over the past twenty years, particularly in fast-food restaurants, but also in meals eaten at home. Researchers at New York University found that portion sizes at most restaurants are at least two times that of a "standard" serving, and often as much as eightfold larger. Furthermore, studies have shown that both children and adults will eat more when offered more and that many of us underestimate the amount of food we eat. The wider the selection of foods we have access to, the more likely we are to overeat.

Snacking

Absentminded between-meal and late-night snacking, often on highly processed junk food, is a major source of gratuitous calories. Giving in to those daily snack attacks will boost our daily calorie count by an average of 30 percent each day, and often substantially more. Although snack calories, including soft drinks, carry every bit as much weight as meal calories, it's easy to follow the "out of sight, out of mind" philosophy and forget to take these extra calories into account at mealtime.

Sometimes people who are trying to lose weight are counseled to eat five to six meals daily, with the idea that somehow this will help control the appetite. This is more urban legend than actual fact. A 2009 Canadian study comparing the two strategies, with identical caloric restriction, found absolutely no difference in weight loss between groups given six small meals compared to those who consumed three normal meals daily.

TV: The Couch Magnet

Snacking while planted in front of the television is practically an American institution. Numerous studies have found that the more TV you watch, the more likely you are to become obese, diabetic, or both. Someone who watches TV just one or two hours daily is 60 percent more likely to be obese than is the next-door neighbor who watches less than an hour a day. Watch even more, and the numbers get worse. A Scottish study found that watching four or more hours of TV or other screen-based entertainment (including video games) daily more than doubled the overall risk of death when compared to those with less than two hours of screen time each day.

CAN IT BE IN YOUR GENES?

I often hear the excuse, "My fat is genetic" or "My metabolism is slow." Before falling back on old defenses, take a step back and critically evaluate your eating habits. Studies have shown that more than half of us underestimate the amount of food that we eat, generally on the order of 20 percent. Ironically, men and women who are trying to lose weight tend to underestimate even more substantially than do those who are not on a weight-loss program. Most overweight people simply eat more, yet may honestly believe that they are eating less.

At the same time, we are inclined to overestimate the number of calories we burn. A study from the University of Texas found that that the more overweight a woman is, the more likely she is to overrate her physical exertion. For instance, walking for thirty minutes is very good aerobic exercise, but it uses fewer than 100 calories, or less than half of a small serving of fries. In fact, it is nearly impossible to lose weight by exercise alone, because most people with a weight problem eat far more extra calories than they are able to burn off at the gym.

To be fair, there do appear to be genetic and hormonal factors that predispose to obesity and binge eating in a relatively small number of people. However, a British report describing a newly discovered "fat gene" established that the gene accounted for only about 7 extra pounds of body weight in people unlucky enough to carry it. A study of nearly 3,500 Americans found that while 10 to 15 percent carried a gene that put them at risk for obesity, only those who ate at least 22 grams of saturated fat (typically from meat or dairy) each day were likely to become obese. Another study found that the gene only appears to cause trouble when the affected individual chooses a sedentary lifestyle. What this means is, even though the genes may influence your chances of becoming obese, the choices of how and what you eat and how much you exercise are still yours to make.

To help regulate appetite and feeding, your body manufactures a cornucopia of hormones that have powerful effects on the feeding centers of your brain. Perhaps 5 percent of obese people have a true chemical imbalance of these hormones. On the other hand, obesity itself can lead to hormonal changes that may affect a wide range of bodily functions, including appetite.

What about metabolism? Well, slimmer people tend to keep moving (you might call it fidgeting) even when they are doing sedentary tasks, and this may well explain some of the apparent differences in metabolism. A Mayo Clinic study suggested that fidgeters may burn upward of 350 extra calories a day. Even more telling, people who are obese sit for an average of two hours more per day than do people who are lean.

ARE YOU OBESE OR OVERWEIGHT? HOW TO FIND OUT

There are several techniques that can determine scientifically whether your weight is above the medically safe range. The simplest and most common tool is the body-mass index (BMI). Use the quick and easy table I've provided to help you see where you fall on the healthy-weight continuum. Go to the appendix (page 346) to get your exact number, or you can calculate your BMI yourself by dividing your weight in kilograms by the square of your height in meters.

A BMI between 18.5 and 24.9 is usually considered healthy, whereas 25 to 29.9 falls into the "overweight" category. In general if your BMI is 30 or more, you are considered, for medical purposes, obese. Morbid obesity is defined as a BMI over 40.

Asian people may be healthier with a BMI of 21 or less, as they tend to develop hypertension, elevated blood sugar, and high cholesterol at BMIs above this point. Also, exceptionally muscular people may be misclassified using this scale, but for most people, the ranges are accurate.

ARE YOU OVERWEIGHT?

HEIGHT (FEET) (INCHES)	WEIGHT (POUNDS) HEALTHY	WEIGHT (POUNDS) OVERWEIGHT	WEIGHT (POUNDS) OBESE
4 10	88 to 118	119 to 143	over 143
4 11	91 to 123	124 to 148	over 148
5 0	95 to 127	128 to 153	over 153
5 1	98 to 131	132 to 158	over 158
5 2	101 to 135	136 to 163	over 163
5 3	104 to 140	141 to 168	over 168
5 4	108 to 144	145 to 174	over 174
5 5	111 to 149	150 to 179	over 179
5 6	114 to 154	155 to 185	over 185
5 7	118 to 158	159 to 191	over 191
5 8	121 to 163	164 to 196	over 196
5 9	125 to 168	169 to 202	over 202
5 10	129 to 173	174 to 208	over 208
5 11	132 to 178	179 to 214	over 214
6 0	136 to 183	184 to 220	over 220
6 1	140 to 188	189 to 226	over 226
6 2	144 to 193	194 to 232	over 232

THE SKINNY ON WEIGHT LOSS

It is never too soon to tackle a weight problem. Obesity begins in childhood and young adulthood. What you do now bears serious implications for your future health and well-being, and for the health of those you love. Even if you are only a little overweight in your early 20s, you carry a high probability of developing obesity by the time you hit your mid-30s, regardless of gender. Furthermore, obese parents are more likely to raise obese children, continuing the cycle of obesity, poor health, and poor quality of life.

The good news is that you do not need to attain an "ideal" weight to begin to reap the benefits of weight loss. People who are already seriously overweight can significantly lower their chances of high blood pressure, diabetes, and elevated cholesterol by losing just 5 to 10 percent of their body weight. The more weight lost, the greater the rewards.

ACHIEVING A HEART-HEALTHY WEIGHT

There is no magic to losing weight. You simply must eat less than you burn.

Fight the Food Triggers

It is critical to identify the triggers and to begin to tame the urges that lead to overeating. For many people, eating while exposed to a simple distraction, such as a TV show or video game, blunts the normal sense of fullness, leading to a sort of oblivious overeating. This mindlessness accounts for the mysteriously empty bag of tortilla chips at the end of Monday night football. It also explains why moviegoers can eat massive tubs of popcorn without ever coming up for air.

Serving size can be a trigger, too, so portion control is critical for both food and drink. It takes a good fifteen to twenty minutes for your body to register a sense of fullness, but if you gulp down your food, you are finished well before you ever get the signal to stop. So slow down and really experience your food. Take your time to savor your meals, make every bite count, and you really will eat less.

MY PATIENT BEN had struggled with his weight for years, hoping that he could wish it away, but at the age of 45, he was still eating like a teenager. After I sent him home from the office with a third prescription for blood pressure medications and a diagnosis of high cholesterol, he resolved to get serious. By simply cutting out fast food, bringing healthy snacks to the office, keeping a food diary, and working out three days each week, Ben lost 20 pounds in just three months. He was thrilled when I told him that we could cut his blood pressure meds in half, and even happier to be sporting a pair of jeans he hadn't been able to zip up since his 30s.

Beware of Snacking

If you are truly hungry, choose a piece of fruit, such as an apple or some unsweetened dried fruit. The fiber will help fill you up and quiet your cravings. If you enjoy snacking and decide to indulge, factor it in with your daily calorie allowance, and cut back at mealtime. Choose a protein-rich snack, such as an ounce of low-fat cheese with a couple of whole wheat crackers or a small tub of plain yogurt with a little honey or jam. An ounce or less of nuts is another good choice.

Although a few brands of granola bars and protein bars offer a hearty dose of energy without excessive fat, most are highly caloric (more than 200 calories) and loaded with sugar and preservatives. Play it smart by keeping your snacks under 150 calories, and limit snacking to no more than twice a day.

Control Cravings

Keep an honest food diary (see page 49) and become aware of what you are eating. Studies show that using your smartphone to keep track of calories, fat, and nutrients can make a big difference by keeping you accountable to yourself and providing instant feedback.

Create a distraction. As simple as it sounds, it often helps to take a walk, brush your teeth, call a friend, or direct your attention to something that takes your mind off eating. A project that requires you to use your hands, such as woodworking, knitting, or scrapbooking, is another great option.

If you can find something better than food to use as a reward or a way of dealing with stress, over time, your cravings will diminish, your sense of accomplishment will surge, and you will glow with good health.

FRUSTRATED WITH HER reliance on comfort food, my patient Jenny turned to her dog, Scooter, for help. Now, any time she feels a snack attack coming on, she takes Scooter out for a walk or a game of fetch. If it's late at night or the weather is bad, Scooter is happy to be chased around the sofa or to lie on his back for a tummy rub. In the ten minutes it takes to play with her dog, Jenny's cravings have usually subsided. Scooter adores the extra attention, Jenny feels and looks better than ever, her heart is healthier, and her blood pressure has dropped a good ten points.

GET HELP IF YOU NEED IT

IF YOU SUFFER from uncontrollable binge eating or purging, or have anorexic tendencies, don't hesitate to ask your doctor or a competent mental health specialist for help. It is also important to seek medical attention if you believe your overeating is brought on by serious depression or obsessive behavior. Mental illness can be a powerful impediment to good physical health, and it cannot be overcome by willpower alone.

Medical and Surgical Options

If you are morbidly obese (100 pounds or more over your ideal weight, or have a BMI of 40 or greater), or if you are suffering the consequences of obesity, such as diabetes, high blood pressure, and other medical problems, a lap-band, gastric sleeve, or gastric bypass procedure may be something to consider. These operations reduce the amount of food you're able to put into your stomach and thereby increase the sense of satiety. I've seen these surgeries work for some people, although not everyone will achieve dramatic weight loss.

Any surgery carries potential risks, including a small but real risk of death. Life-threatening bleeding, blood clots, infections, and chronic diarrhea are potential complications of gastric procedures, particularly the gastric bypass. Many people will regain the weight lost, and in some cases, the bands will slip or erode. Unless you are truly unable to control the urge to overeat any other way, my advice is to steer clear of surgery.

Currently there are no really effective medications available to help you lose weight. Orlistat (marketed as Alli) helps prevent the absorption of fat through the intestine, but has the unfortunate side effect of sometimes uncontrollable grease-laden diarrhea, as well as intestinal gas with oily spotting. When it was sold only as a prescription medication, I quickly gave up prescribing it, because virtually everyone who took the drug had such mortifyingly unpleasant side effects, without enough weight loss to justify the humiliation. There have been several reports of liver damage, and with the average amount of weight lost running less than 10 pounds, I can't recommend this drug.

A dangerous revival of the HCG (human choriotropic gonadotropin) diet has taken hold in many communities, often led by stand-alone weight-loss clinics. This ostensible diet involves extreme caloric restriction, on the order of 500 calories daily, along with physician-prescribed injections of HCG. HCG is a hormone made by the placenta during pregnancy, and its only legitimate use is as a fertility aid. HCG carries a risk for serious blood clots that can trigger heart attacks, strokes, and blood clots in the leg veins that may travel to the lungs, causing a potentially fatal condition known as pulmonary embolus. What's more, the effectiveness of HCG was debunked way back in the 1970s in medical studies carried out in the United States, Germany, and South Africa. Not surprisingly, scientists determined that the calorie restriction was the only reason people lost weight on this plan.

There are other medications, and combinations of medications, that may help some people, but for the most part, weight loss is fairly paltry with any of these options, and none of them are good long-term solutions.

Achieving a healthy weight is part of the process of building a healthy and heart-loving lifestyle—a process that will enrich and sustain your life for years to come. It is not easy, but it is certainly not complicated. It is perhaps the most important opportunity you will ever have to change your life and the lives of those you love.

BEST PRACTICES:
YOUR WEIGHT

* Don't just look in the mirror or at the scale; calculate your BMI to determine whether you are the best weight for your height and frame.
* If you need to lose weight, start now. The more you procrastinate, the more your weight will increase.
* Take the time to enjoy a smaller portion size, without distractions such as television.
* Cut back on between-meal eating, particularly snacks consumed purely from habit, not hunger.
* When you do feel hungry for a snack, choose produce, nuts, or small portions of protein-rich foods, such as cheese or yogurt.
* Keep a food diary (see page 49) to track what triggers you to snack passively or overeat.
* Develop non-food-related strategies to relieve stress or

boredom, such as a hobby that keeps your hands busy; the less sedentary you are in the process, the better.

* Speak to your physician if it is difficult for you to maintain a heart-healthy weight on your own.

* Avoid quick-fix solutions such as diet drugs, which do not address the true issues behind excessive weight and can even be medically dangerous.

* Consider weight-loss surgery only as a last resort. It doesn't always work and may cause serious side effects and complications.

3

The Good, the Bad, and the Ugly: Understanding Cholesterol and Your Lipid Profile

C HOLESTEROL IS STRONGLY linked to heart disease, yet only one in three Americans is aware of his or her numbers. No matter how healthy we think we are, every one of us should know our lipid profile. A lipid profile is a measurement of total cholesterol, including a calculation of LDL ("bad") and HDL ("good") cholesterol, along with the amount of triglycerides circulating in the bloodstream. Not all cholesterol is harmful, and not everyone with a healthy lifestyle will have favorable levels. In this chapter, I'll explain what those numbers mean, describe what your optimal levels may be, and tell you about a range of less traditional blood tests that may complement the lipid profile and provide additional information about your risk for heart disease. The latest national guidelines recommend that all adults get a full lipid profile every five years; those with risk factors should do so more frequently. Medical treatment of lipids will be discussed in chapter 13 (see page 214).

* * *

CHOLESTEROL

A quick needle stick, a spin through the analyzer, and—voilà!—your cholesterol profile. One of the greatest advances in medical science over the last few decades has been the explosion of knowledge regarding cholesterol and its effect on our entire body, but most especially on our heart and brain.

Nothing can take the place of a healthy diet, but your cholesterol levels are only partially controlled by the food you eat, and you can't assume that by eating well you are home free. Sometimes your body simply makes too much of the bad stuff. Seemingly healthy people die every day from heart attacks brought on by high cholesterol that was undiagnosed, untreated, or both. Although choosing a heart-smart diet is the first step for most people, medical treatment can be lifesaving for those at high risk for heart disease and stroke.

Cholesterol is often made out to be the bad guy, but it also a plays a major role in maintaining good health. For example, cholesterol contributes to the protection of normal cell membranes and is required for the production of many of your hormones. But you only need a little cholesterol to get the job done, and an LDL cholesterol deficiency is virtually unheard of.

While cholesterol plays a critical role in heart disease, it is only a part of the puzzle. Blockages may build up even when levels are normal, and not everyone with high cholesterol will develop heart problems. That is because, to do damage, cholesterol has to get into the walls of the arteries, where it becomes atherosclerosis, or plaque. This process is sometimes referred to as "hardening of the arteries." Many different factors, including diet, exercise, lifestyle, blood pressure, other medical conditions, and genetics can affect the way your body handles cholesterol.

Even more important than the total amount of cholesterol circulating in your bloodstream are your levels of LDL and HDL cholesterol. Measurements of cholesterol levels are expressed as numbers that represent the amount of cholesterol present per deciliter of blood, abbreviated as mg/dL.

Lousy Cholesterol

LDL is shorthand for low-density lipoprotein. I tell my patients that the *L* stands for "lousy." LDL is responsible for ferrying cholesterol from the bloodstream into the arteries. Not surprisingly, high levels of LDL put us at greater risk for cholesterol buildup in the arteries of our heart, brain, other vital organs, and limbs.

For optimal health, your LDL should be under 100 mg/dL. Yet among American adults, the average LDL cholesterol is 130 mg/dL. More than one third have LDL cholesterol levels over 130 mg/dL, and nearly 20 percent have dangerously high levels exceeding 160 mg/dL.

If you have been diagnosed with atherosclerosis, whether in your heart, brain, or other blood vessels, your LDL cholesterol should be less than 70 mg/dL. At this level, the plaque can be stabilized, making it less likely to cause a heart attack or stroke. In some cases, the cholesterol buildup may even shrink slowly, although it rarely, if ever, disappears entirely.

Diabetic people (whose risk of cardiovascular disease is up to four times that of nondiabetics) and those with multiple risk factors should also aim for an LDL of less than 70 mg/dL. Conventional risk factors in addition to diabetes include high blood pressure, tobacco use, a family history of early heart disease (men before age 55, women before age 65), age, and gender. Being female and at least 55 years old (or male and at least 45 years old) starts you off with one risk factor (for more information, see "Know Your Risk Factors," page 349).

For many, achieving this goal of less than 70 mg/dL means medical therapy, but dietary changes have the potential to make a significant impact. An overall healthy lifestyle will limit the dose required to achieve an ideal cholesterol profile and consequently reduce the potential for drug side effects.

It is a common misperception that a low LDL can be dangerous. In fact, traditional human societies of hunter-gatherers around the world tend to run LDLs in the 50 to 70 mg/dL range. Healthy newborns may have cholesterol levels as low as 30 mg/dL. Because we don't have a lot of information about the health effects of such levels in adults, your doctor may start to ease off on your medication if your cholesterol level drops below 50 mg/dL.

If, like many people, you find yourself in a gray area—no heart disease, no diabetes, but at least two risk factors for coronary disease— then national guidelines dictate that your target LDL should be no greater than 130 mg/dL and preferably less than 100 mg/dL. Those with one or no major risk factors should have an LDL no greater than 160 mg/dL, although many cardiologists, including me, would argue that even this relatively low-risk group should strive for an LDL cholesterol reading of 100 mg/dL or less.

■ OTHER LDL TESTS MAY DIG DEEPER

If your cholesterol level or risk profile is borderline, your doctor may choose to check a more detailed cholesterol profile, in which subclasses of LDL cholesterol are measured. Although this is not a common test, it can be useful in certain situations. Smaller, denser LDL particles are more damaging than larger, "fluffier" ones, because they can more easily slip into the wall of the arteries and are also more vulnerable to harmful oxidation reactions that make the particles even more dangerous. Thus, all other factors being equal, someone with a borderline-normal total LDL cholesterol but a high level of small LDL particles may well be at greater risk for heart disease than is someone whose LDL particles are large. In this case, drug therapy in addition to diet and exercise may help reduce the chance of cardiovascular disease (see page 214). Nevertheless, both types of LDL are associated with cardiovascular risk.

This in-depth type of blood test, often referred to as advanced lipid testing, can be quite expensive. A simpler and less expensive blood test for apoprotein B provides similar information, because higher levels indirectly indicate that there are more of these harmful small LDL particles. That is because there is one apoprotein B unit attached to each LDL particle, so the more small dense LDL you have, the more apoprotein B will be detected. Apoprotein B is what helps the LDL to hook onto and "unlock" a cell, allowing it to enter and release its load of cholesterol inside the cell.

There is much debate on the usefulness and cost-effectiveness of advanced testing as, in most cases, careful interpretation of your standard lipid profile (with or without a measurement of apoprotein B) can give your doctor the information needed to create a treatment plan.

When assessing your cardiac risk, another test your doctor might suggest is a coronary calcium score. This involves taking a quick CT scan of the heart arteries to detect signs of cholesterol buildup. Cholesterol plaques generally become hardened and calcified over time, and the scan is able to detect this calcification, hence the term "calcium score." The score indicates whether there is plaque and, if so, how extensive it might be. A score can range from zero (indicating a very low likelihood of cholesterol buildup) to several thousand. The coronary calcium score is often used to help a physician decide whether to start cholesterol medication in someone who is at an intermediate level of risk. (People without heart disease or diabetes, but with two or more risk factors, are considered to fall into the intermediate risk category). The test does not say anything specific about blockages, although people with a very high score (meaning a great deal of calcium is in their arteries) are more likely to have significant disease. The presence of any calcification at all is an indication that the process of atherosclerosis has begun and that efforts to lower cholesterol must become more aggressive. Although reassuring, a lack of calcification does not entirely rule out plaque, as newer plaque may not be calcified.

Happy Cholesterol

HDL cholesterol helps to take cholesterol out of the arteries and dump it into the liver, where it is processed so that it can be eliminated from the body. (Think of *H* as being "happy.") In general, the higher your HDL cholesterol, the less likely it is that atherosclerosis will develop.

There is really no such thing as an HDL that is "too high." As a rule, HDL should be more than 50 mg/dL for women and more than 45 mg/dL for men.

Just like LDL, HDL subclasses can also be measured. The smaller HDL particles are thought by some experts to be less protective, because they carry less cholesterol out from the arteries. This matter is still under debate.

To confuse the issue further, HDL typically has anti-inflammatory effects on the heart arteries. However, when there is widespread inflammation in the body, the HDL may lose its ability to protect the heart. Many factors affect inflammation: Smoking, obesity, and a diet of fast foods and processed foods are common triggers.

Regular exercise, moderate alcohol use, and avoidance of tobacco smoke are all great ways to boost your HDL cholesterol. Raising your HDL cholesterol naturally via a healthy diet may provide more health benefits than taking a pill to improve them. Conversely, a diet loaded with sugary and starchy foods (often referred to as high-glycemic-index foods) such as white bread, white potatoes, white rice, and pasta will lower your HDL cholesterol (see the "Carbohydrates"section on page 55 to learn more about these foods).

The Liver's Role

Your liver is a central player on the cholesterol team. This multitasking organ manufactures cholesterol from the food you eat, but is also involved in clearing cholesterol and fat from the bloodstream. It is highly efficient at turning saturated fat (from meat, dairy, and tropical oils) and trans fat (from hard margarine and shortening) into cholesterol, but it also makes cholesterol, to a lesser extent, from carbohydrates.

Not all livers are alike, and some people are able to gobble up large amounts of fat without its having a huge impact upon their blood cholesterol levels. Other people are genetically burdened with very high cholesterol levels, no matter what they do.

MY PATIENT FELICIA is a perfect example. A slender, vegetarian runner whose diet is textbook perfect, Felicia had

an LDL cholesterol level, before medication, of 250 mg/dL—
about twice what is considered normal. The only way to
get her level down and protect her from heart disease
and stroke was with medication, which has worked
beautifully.

Your Total Cholesterol Count

What about your total cholesterol level? As a stand-alone number,
it really is not very meaningful. Total cholesterol includes HDL and
LDL cholesterol; it also includes VLDL cholesterol, which is essentially a hybrid of cholesterol and triglycerides (see page 34).

A very high HDL cholesterol could raise your total cholesterol
reading to well over 200 mg/dL (formerly considered the cutoff point
for a desirable cholesterol level), but your LDL might still be low, giving a heart disease risk well below normal. That's why treatment of
cholesterol is no longer focused on the total number; rather, it's important to know your HDL and LDL levels.

Control Your Cholesterol with a Heart-Healthy Diet and Lifestyle

Even when medication is required, improving your diet will limit
the amount of medication you need. Popping a pill is easy, but taking
medication does not relieve you of the responsibility you have to yourself to follow a healthy diet and lifestyle. Heart disease is much more
than a simple set of numbers, and no drug can substitute for healthy
living.

Smoking can be detrimental to both HDL and LDL levels, whereas
exercise and alcohol in moderation promote healthy lipid levels. For
most people, limiting saturated fats, trans fats, and fast foods can
effectively reduce LDL cholesterol levels and, thus, the risk for heart
disease and stroke. Choosing a Mediterranean-style diet rich in monounsaturated fats (see page 115) can help to optimize your LDL particle
size and boost your HDL cholesterol levels at the same time.

CHOLESTEROL INTAKE AND HEART HEALTH

People whose diet is exceptionally high in cholesterol are more likely to suffer heart disease and strokes, it's true; but in general, the connection between cholesterol intake and heart disease is quite modest. On average, the body manufactures three times more cholesterol from scratch than is found in the typical American diet. Cholesterol plays a critical role in the protection of nerve fibers, supports hormone production, and maintains the integrity of cell membranes, but most of us get more than we need. The recommended daily intake of cholesterol is 300 mg for most people, although if you have heart disease, the American Heart Association recommends no more than 200 mg each day.

To give some perspective, a meal that includes a quarter-pound burger with cheese and a large order of french fries will supply more than 50 grams of total fat and about 20 grams of "bad" fats (saturated plus trans), but only 95 mg of cholesterol. One egg, on the other hand, contains 190 mg of cholesterol, but only 4.6 grams of fat.

Unless beef, pork, cheese, and eggs are regulars on your menu, the old-school advice to follow a low-cholesterol diet may be well intentioned but is unlikely to have a major impact on your cholesterol levels by itself.

BEST PRACTICES:
CHOLESTEROL

* If you are at low risk for heart disease, your LDL cholesterol should be less than 130 mg/dL; otherwise, less than 100 mg/dL is optimal.
* If you have heart disease, diabetes, or are at high risk for heart disease, strive for an LDL below 70 mg/dL. This will probably require medication.
* Cut back on saturated fats, trans fats, and dietary cholesterol to lower your LDL cholesterol. And quit smoking!

* Your HDL should be at least 50 mg/dL if you're a woman and 40 mg/dL if you're a man, but the higher the better.
* Exercise regularly, don't smoke, and enjoy alcohol in moderation to raise your HDL levels.
* A low-glycemic diet, reducing your intake of sugars and starches, will increase your HDL. Aim for no more than 300 mg of cholesterol daily, or no more than 200 mg if you have any form of heart disease.

TRIGLYCERIDES

Triglycerides are another important element of the lipid profile. Triglyceride levels greater than 150 mg/dL increase the risk of heart disease, particularly in women (see "Know Your Risk Factors," page 349). An optimal triglyceride level is considered to be 100 mg/dL or less.

Although triglycerides are usually measured in the fasting state, high nonfasting levels may be even more predictive of heart disease risk. High triglycerides often go hand in hand with low HDL cholesterol, a pattern that is common in diabetics. When high triglycerides are combined with low HDL or high LDL, the risk for heart disease is greater than for either one alone. Extremely high triglycerides (usually more than 1,000 mg/dL) can increase the risk for pancreatitis, a dangerous inflammation of the pancreas, which sits near the stomach.

High triglycerides may be the consequence of an inherited genetic disorder, but more commonly, diet and lifestyle are the roots of the problem. Tellingly, as a nation, our triglyceride levels have quadrupled since 1980. Simple carbohydrates, such as white bread, white rice, and white potatoes, along with saturated fat, are the usual suspects. Both of these also contribute to diabetes.

Tackle Your Triglycerides

Not surprisingly, triglycerides levels can often be brought down to normal levels with a combination of a heart-smart diet, regular exercise, and weight loss.

Fish oil, either from the diet or from omega-3 fish oil capsules, can often lower your triglycerides substantially. Your doctor may consider a prescription form of fish oil if you have very high triglycerides (see chapter 13, page 223). Monounsaturated fats such as olive oil can have favorable effects, as well. Small amounts of alcohol (one or two drinks daily) can bring about very healthy changes in your lipid profile, but more than that will tend to raise your triglycerides.

MY PATIENT BRYAN used to go out for a few beers with his buddies after work at least three nights a week. Cheese fries, burgers, and shakes were his lunchtime staples. It was no surprise that his triglycerides hovered around 600 mg/dL and his weight around 250 pounds. When he rolled into the emergency room with a 95 percent blockage in a major coronary artery, Bryan resolved to take his lifestyle seriously. He cut back to no more than one drink per day, chucked the burgers in favor of light tuna sandwiches on whole wheat bread, and started working out at the gym after work instead of going to happy hour. He shed 50 pounds, his triglycerides dropped all the way down to 170 mg/dL, and he felt better than he had in fifteen years.

If you're eating well, exercising, and keeping your weight in a healthy range, but your levels are still too high, take a look in the medicine cabinet. Triglycerides can be affected by a variety of prescription drugs. Estrogen replacement therapy may elevate triglycerides in susceptible women. This effect is seen with the pill forms of estrogen, but usually not with the estrogen patch. Some blood-pressure medications, including diuretics and certain beta-blockers, may adversely affect triglycerides. An underactive thyroid gland is often associated with high triglycerides; this condition can usually be diagnosed with a simple blood test.

LP(a)

Lp(a), referred to by those in the know as "el-pee-little-a," is a tiny relative of LDL cholesterol. High levels are associated with a greater risk for heart disease and stroke for both genders. However, after the age of 65, testing for Lp(a) appears to be more useful for men than for women. This test must be specifically requested by your doctor, as a routine cholesterol test will not detect this dangerous little particle.

Lp(a) is predominantly determined by genetics, and elevated levels (generally considered to be more than 50 mg/dL) are frequently found in people who have heart attacks early in life (i.e., men before the age of 55, women before 65).

Lower Your Lp(a)

Unfortunately, while testing for Lp(a) is easy, treatment is not. Exercise has little bearing on Lp(a). A diet high in trans fats may increase the Lp(a) concentration in the blood by 20 to 70 percent. Paradoxically, a low-fat, high-carbohydrate diet may also raise Lp(a) levels. But there is good news: The healthy fat found in fish oil might reduce Lp(a) levels modestly.

Current research on medical treatment of high Lp(a) still lags far behind that on LDL cholesterol. Most lipid-lowering drugs such as statins have no significant effect on Lp(a). Pharmaceutical-strength niacin is one drug that can be used to treat this condition because, when given in adequate prescription-strength doses, it will lower the level by an average of about 25 percent (read more about this drug in chapter 13, page 220). There is even some evidence that aspirin might help to lower levels in people with very high Lp(a).

BEST PRACTICES:
LP(a)

* To lower your Lp(a) levels, eliminate trans fats, found in hard margarine and many commercial snack foods, and limit simple carbohydrates, such as sweets, white bread, and potatoes.

HOMOCYSTEINE

Homocysteine is not actually related to cholesterol or to lipids, but because it has been associated with a higher cardiovascular risk, a test for it is sometimes ordered along with a lipid profile. Simply put, homocysteine is derived from the breakdown of methionine, one of the essential amino acids found in protein. Its measurement is expressed as a number followed by "µmol/L."

Extremely high levels of homocysteine are generally the result of a genetic abnormality, whereas moderately high levels may be the result of a deficiency in vitamins, specifically folic acid, B_6, and B_{12}. Dietary and lifestyle habits have a sizeable effect on homocysteine. Although levels as high as 15 µmol/L are considered to be in the normal range, readings over 9 µmol/L correlate with a higher risk of atherosclerosis. People with very high levels (more than 15.8 µmol/L) may have triple the risk of a heart attack, when compared to those with a level in the normal range.

Although it was once thought that a high homocysteine level itself caused the problem, it has since been found that (except in those with genetic abnormalities) homocysteine is merely a marker for important lifestyle factors, rather than being the guilty party itself. Essentially, a high level is a red flag that we need to do more to ensure a healthy heart. Lowering homocysteine itself won't do any good, unless we are changing the issues that caused it to be high in the first place.

A diet high in saturated fat tends to raise homocysteine levels. People who drink three or more cups of coffee daily are more apt to have a high level, as are smokers and heavy drinkers.

Hold Down Your Homocysteine

Those who eat fish or take fish oil capsules tend to have lower levels, particularly when B-complex vitamin intake is high. Exercise may lower homocysteine, and so may eating more foods with high folate content, such as green leafy vegetables, peppers, cruciferous vegetables (including broccoli and cauliflower), and fortified cereal products. Wine in moderation, nuts, olive oil, and mushrooms have been linked to lower homocysteine and lower heart disease risk; likewise dairy products, such as milk and yogurt.

Beware of Megadose Hype

For people with elevated levels of homocysteine, some doctors used to advocate megadoses of vitamins, including folic acid, B_6, and B_{12}. We now know, however, that although homocysteine levels can be lowered substantially with such supplements, there is no benefit to heart health.

One important study of nearly four thousand heart attack survivors found that while high-dose vitamins did indeed reduce homocysteine levels substantially, their use was actually associated with a slightly higher risk of heart disease and a trend toward a greater incidence of cancer.

BEST PRACTICES:
HOMOCYSTEINE

* Homocysteine is a marker of an unhealthy lifestyle. Cut out trans and saturated fats, smoking, and excessive coffee to reduce your homocysteine level.

- Alcohol in moderation (1 to 2 drinks daily) is associated with lower homocysteine, but in excess, it will raise levels.
- Exercise, coldwater fish, nuts, green leafy vegetables, dairy, and mushrooms will also lower your homocysteine.

C-REACTIVE PROTEIN

High-sensitivity C-reactive protein (hs-CRP, or simply CRP) is a protein that increases in the body in response to inflammation. Keeping your CRP level down is important, as inflammation of the lining of the heart arteries is often a trigger for heart attacks. A cholesterol-laden plaque in a heart artery may be present for years but not be large enough to cause any symptoms whatsoever, until inflammation within the plaque causes it to become unstable.

The Harvard Women's Health Study found a high CRP level to be even more strongly predictive of a future heart attack than a high level of LDL cholesterol. Studies of people tested just once and then followed for up to twenty years have shown a very strong connection between high CRP and subsequent heart attacks and strokes.

A number of different factors can affect CRP levels. CRP is made in the liver, and fat tissue itself can produce CRP, particularly the visceral, or deep abdominal, fat. Obesity is the factor most strongly associated with high CRP levels.

Because inflammation related to an infection or injury can temporarily raise CRP, a second, confirmatory blood test should be done at least two weeks later if your level is very high. Values greater than 3 mg/L are considered elevated and are associated with a heart attack risk of at least one and a half times normal; values less than 1 mg/L are considered optimal. If your level is greater than 10 mg/L, chances are good that an inflammatory process such as arthritis or infection is going on, so further investigation into those issues should be considered.

Estrogen replacement therapy and oral contraceptives have been found to increase CRP. Smoking will also bump up CRP levels. Severe stress may raise CRP, although generally the elevation is self-limited and will drop back to normal once the problem is gone.

Like homocysteine, CRP appears to be most valuable as a marker of an unhealthy lifestyle. Complicating the picture is the fact that some people have genetically high CRP. However, they do not necessarily have a higher risk for heart disease than do those without the gene. It can be difficult to sort this out without genetic testing, which is not widely available.

Curb Your CRP

What do you do if your CRP is elevated and infection and other inflammatory problems have been ruled out? A healthy diet and weight loss, when needed, are always your first line of defense. Keeping stress under control may help as well.

Statin drugs, which are used to treat high cholesterol, have shown promise in reducing inflammation, even though there is no relationship between cholesterol levels and CRP. For this reason, high CRP levels are sometimes treated with a statin drug. Aspirin, which is well known to reduce the risk of heart attacks by making the blood platelets less prone to clot, may also act on the heart arteries by reducing inflammation, as its preventive effects have been found to be more powerful in those with high CRP.

Alcohol in moderation will lower CRP, whereas heavy alcohol use will raise it. Not surprisingly, a diet high in saturated and trans fats can lead to inflammation of your heart arteries and high levels of CRP. Reducing harmful dietary fats will lower CRP; so will a high-fiber diet.

A German study found that a diet loaded with red meat, margarine, poultry, and sauces was associated with a more than fourfold increase in CRP when compared with those who opted for a vegetarian, Mediterranean-style diet which included plenty of veggies and whole grains, and moderate amounts of wine. (You will learn much more about the Mediterranean diet in chapter 7; see page 115.)

Weight loss will often lower CRP. Exercise, with or without weight loss, can lower CRP by more than 35 percent.

BEST PRACTICES:
CRP

* Hs-CRP (or CRP) is a marker for inflammation. Obesity and smoking are common causes of high levels of CRP.
* Lower your CRP with exercise, moderate alcohol, nuts, high-fiber foods, green leafy vegetables, and fruit.
* Ask your doctor about alternatives to your present regimen of estrogen replacement or oral contraceptives if your CRP level is high.

LP-PLA2

Lp-PLA2 (lipoprotein-associated phospholipase A2) is another inflammation marker that has more recently garnered attention from researchers hoping to predict who might be at risk for cardiovascular disease. A high level of Lp-PLA2 indicates that cholesterol plaques may be inflamed and unstable and is associated with a twofold risk of stroke and heart attacks. Obesity can raise Lp-PLA2, so weight loss and exercise can help. Smokers also tend to have higher Lp-PLA2 readings. A Mediterranean diet, including nuts and lean protein along with moderate alcohol use, has been associated with lower levels. Cholesterol medication can also improve this measurement. The blood test for Lp-PLA2, which is known as the PLAC test, is not recommended for everyone; however, people with intermediate risk of heart disease are good candidates. A normal level is considered to be less than 200 nanograms per milliliter.

BEST PRACTICES:
LP-PLA2

* Lp-PLA2 is a marker for inflammation, and may help predict who is at higher risk for heart attacks or strokes.
* Obesity, smoking, and a high-fat diet can raise Lp-PLA2 levels. A Mediterranean diet and regular exercise may bring Lp-PLA2 down.
* Testing is not necessary for everyone. If your risk for heart disease is intermediate, ask your doctor if you might be a candidate for the PLAC test.

Careful attention to diet, exercise, and lifestyle will make a vital difference to your lipid levels. In the next section, you'll learn which foods should become your core menu for heart health.

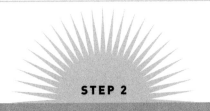

STEP 2

Eat Well to Live Better

EATING WELL SHOULD be a pleasure, but sometimes it all seems so darn complicated. The truth is, it really doesn't have to be that way. Understanding the fundamental building blocks of a heart-healthy diet will pave the way for a lifetime of good health and great food. And once you know the basics, separating the wonder foods from the nutritional evildoers will be a snap. What's more, you'll be able to tune out all those trendy, elaborate, and sometimes downright mystifying diets that seem to sprout up every time swimsuit season rolls around. The ultimate payoff: a healthier heart, increased vitality, and a body that is leaner, fitter, and ready to take you where you want to go.

4

Diet: Why You Really Are What You Eat

FRESH, NUTRIENT-RICH, VIBRANT foods are the foundation for a healthy life and a vigorous heart. Eating well is not complicated and should never make you feel miserable or deprived; nevertheless, making a fresh start may be challenging at first. Yes, changing the way you eat requires some discipline and tenacity, and the strength to say no. But when you nourish the body that works so hard for you, you will begin to notice a profound change in your sense of well-being and vitality. It won't happen overnight, but your cravings will gradually diminish, and you will discover that although you may still enjoy some of the same high-calorie foods that were once your downfall, it will take much less to satisfy your hunger. You will find yourself slowing down at the table, and taking the time to really savor the nuances and flavors of the foods you eat.

Learning how to live a heart-loving lifestyle begins with understanding some important terminology. Such words as *calories*, *fats*, *proteins*, and *carbohydrates* are part of our everyday vocabulary, but what do they really mean to your health?

CALORIES REALLY DO COUNT

A *calorie* (or kcal if we use scientific terminology) is a unit of energy. You take in calories when you eat or drink—be it a carrot stick, potato chip, or cola. Your body burns up calories each time you move, whether you're watching television, gardening, or jogging. If you want to lose weight, you must use up more calories than you consume. It is that simple. You make it hard on yourself if you don't balance out the equation. If you don't burn off what you eat, then your body is forced to store it as fat.

Calories are present in virtually every food, be it carbohydrate, protein, or fat. Most nutritional measures use the metric system. Ten grams equals about ⅓ ounce. However, all grams are not created equal. A gram of fat contains 9 calories. On the other hand, carbohydrates and protein each have 4 calories per gram. So what you eat is just as important as how much you eat. The Institute of Medicine, a nongovernmental advisory group of national health experts, breaks down our calorie requirements this way:

SOURCE	PERCENTAGE OF DAILY CALORIES
fat	20 to 35
carbohydrates	45 to 65
protein	10 to 35

How Many Calories You Need

The average person requires somewhere from 1,600 to 2,200 calories each day to maintain a healthy weight. But, depending on your activity level, degree of physical fitness, age, and gender, your needs may differ. For example, women typically require fewer calories than do men, simply because the average woman is smaller and has less muscle mass than the average man.

To figure your personal caloric needs, you first need to calculate your basal metabolic rate (BMR), more commonly known as your metabolism. This will show you the number of calories your body needs to function properly at rest—that is, before you factor in activity and exercise.

There is more than one way to calculate your BMR. You can easily find an online BMR calculator to plug your stats into, or you can do the math yourself. To roughly estimate your BMR, multiply your current weight in pounds by 10. If you weigh 150 pounds, for instance, your BMR is roughly 150 x 10, or 1,500 calories. A more complicated formula, known as the Harris-Benedict equation (see the equation and the sample calculations that follow), takes into account gender, height, and age. This is more accurate, because younger people have a higher BMR, as do taller individuals and men.

None of these formulas is perfect. Many factors affect your BMR. The leaner you are, the higher your BMR, which is a great incentive to exercise; this also accounts for the higher BMR that most men enjoy, as their body composition tends to skew more toward lean. Conversely, the more fat your body carries, the lower your BMR will be.

Children, especially as they go through rapid growth spurts, have a higher metabolism, as do pregnant women, whose body must work harder to develop the growing fetus and prepare to nourish the new baby. Stress, some illnesses, and constant exposure to extremes of temperature (think the Arizona desert in summer or the Alaskan wilderness in deep winter) raise the BMR. Malnutrition and starvation will lower the BMR, which is one of the many reasons why radical diets fail.

THE HARRIS-BENEDICT EQUATION
FOR BASAL METABOLIC RATE

THE BASAL METABOLIC rate (BMR) defines the number of calories your body needs simply to sustain life in a resting state. Although you can get a very good estimation of your basal metabolic rate simply by multiplying your body weight in pounds by 10, the Harris-Benedict equation provides a more precise, although still imperfect, approximation.

W = weight in pounds
H = height in inches
A = age in years
For women: BMR = 655 + (4.35 x W) + (4.7 x H) – (4.7 x A)
For men: BMR = 66 + (6.23 x W) + (12.7 x H) – (6.8 x A)

For instance, a 45-year-old woman who is 5 foot 4 (or 64 inches) and 150 pounds would calculate her BMR this way:

655 + (4.35 x 150) + (4.7 x 64) – (4.7 x 45) = 1,396.8 calories daily

For a man of the same age, with the same height and weight, the BMR would work out to 1,507.3 calories, a difference equal to about one small chocolate chip cookie.

Once you calculate your BMR, it's easy to establish how many calories your body needs, based on how much energy you burn. This can be worked out fairly precisely. You can obsessively calculate the exact amount of time and energy spent doing everyday activities such as sleeping, standing, sitting, and exercising. Or, you can simply estimate based upon your average activity level.

To figure out the number of calories you need to maintain your current weight, start with your BMR. If you are inactive, spending most of the day sitting at your desk or at home on the couch, multiply your BMR by 20 percent (for example, 1,500 × 0.2 = 300). Then, add the number you get from that calculation to your BMR (1,500 + 300 = 1,800) to get the number of calories you need.

If you engage in light activity, such as walking around at work for several hours over the course of the day, multiply your BMR by 30 percent (1,500 × 0.3 = 450) and make the addition (1,500 + 450 = 1,950).

If your fitness level is moderate—say, you exercise several times a week or have a physically active job—multiply your BMR by 40 percent (0.4).

Finally, if you are extremely active at work or get moving at least four hours every day and rarely sit still, multiply by 50 percent (0.5).

Now that you know how many calories you need, calculate the number of calories you actually eat every day. A number of good references are available for this purpose. Try www.nal.usda.gov/fnic/foodcomp/search for a wide range of foods, or www.myfoodapedia.gov for a more streamlined search. Most chain restaurants and fast-food companies will post detailed calorie and nutrition information on their own Web sites. The important thing is to be honest with yourself about portion sizes and not leave anything out.

HOW MANY CALORIES DO YOU REALLY NEED EACH DAY?

FIRST CALCULATE YOUR BMR (multiply your weight in pounds x 10, or use the Harris-Benedict equation).

Then multiply your BMR by the appropriate percentage below.

If your activity level is:

Sedentary	20%
Mild	30%
Moderate	40%
Heavy	50%

Next, add the two numbers together. The total is how many calories you need each day.

When it comes to food, size really does matter. A 10-ounce steak is not the same thing as a 6-ounce steak. Two cups of even a heart-healthy, flake-type cereal is four times the recommended serving size of ½ cup of flakes. This sounds logical, but study after study shows that most people are not aware of their portion sizes and habitually underestimate the amount that they eat.

HOW FAST CAN CALORIES ADD UP?

IT'S EASY FOR empty calories to "nickel and dime" you into gaining weight. Let's look in on Kate—a self-described couch-potato mom of two teens, who works as an office administrator. Kate, who weighs 150 pounds, usually skips breakfast because her mornings at home are rushed and chaotic. It's a chore just to get the kids dressed and off to school, and she barely has time to be sure her shoes match. To jump-start her morning commute, she stops by her local coffee bar to grab a large latte (270 calories).

At the office, doughnuts magically appear. Feeling the need for a little indulgence, Kate grabs two (420 calories) to eat at her desk. She barely tastes them as she plunges into her inbox.

By lunchtime, Kate is starving, but crunched for time. A quick bite with friends at a nearby fast-food joint includes a cheeseburger (530 calories), small fries (320 calories), and a soft drink (150 calories). At 3:00, a coworker offers to swing by the convenience store, and Kate puts in her order for a candy bar (250 calories) and a soda (150 calories). She is exhausted and hopes the snack break will give her enough energy to make it through the day. That evening, Kate is too sapped to cook, but the family is clamoring for something to eat. A quick call for pizza delivery takes care of dinner.

Kate eats three slices (750 calories) of sausage and mushroom pizza, a glass of whole milk (150 calories), and two chocolate chip cookies (250 calories). Then she takes in a couple hours of television, nibbling absentmindedly on a bag of pretzels (150 calories).

By day's end, Kate's calorie count is 3,390 and she's burned off only 1,800—a net excess of 1,590 calories. At this rate, she could easily gain more than 10 pounds a month. Using our BMR calculations, she is eating enough to maintain a weight of 270 pounds. If she eats this way only twice a week, she will still gain more than 3 pounds per month, or nearly 40 pounds a year.

Worse, her diet is loaded with fat and critically deficient in fruit, vegetables, and whole grains, essential for a healthy heart, mind, and body. Although she blows two hours in front of the TV nightly, Kate makes no time to exercise. It is no wonder she is exhausted.

Kate's story is no exaggeration. Could it be yours?

Keep Track of Calories and Nutrients with a Food Diary

A food diary is a powerful tool that will force you to be honest with yourself about the food you eat. Here are two examples that will help you see just how enlightening a food diary can be: a sample food diary for a heart-smart diet, and Kate's food diary.

BEST PRACTICES HEART-SMART FOOD DIARY

MEAL	FOOD	QUANTITY	CALORIES	TOTAL FAT [G]	SATURATED FAT [G]	CHOLESTEROL [MG]	FIBER [G]	SODIUM [MG]
Breakfast	Oatmeal	1 cup	200	4	0	0	5	0
	Soy milk	6 oz	70	3	0	0	1	90
	Blueberries	⅓ cup	30	0	0	0	1	0
	Black tea	8 oz	0		0	0	0	0
	Honey	2 tsp	45	0	0	0	0	1
Snack	Apple	1	70	0	0	0	3	0
	Almonds	10	55	5	0	0	1	0
Lunch	Greek yogurt (nonfat)	6 oz	100	0	0	1	0	80
	Whole wheat bread	2 slices	140	2	1	0	4	200
	Natural peanut butter	1½ tbsp	150	12	2	0	2	68
	Grapes	1 cup	60	0	0	1	1	1
	Dark chocolate	1 square	65	5	3	0	1	3
Snack	Low-fat string cheese	1 stick	70	4	3	10	0	190
	Whole-grain crackers	4 crackers	70	2	0	0	2	91
Dinner	Mixed greens salad	2 cups	15	1	0	0	1	65
	Balsamic vinaigrette	2 tbsp	60	5	1	0	0	280

MEAL	FOOD	QUANTITY	CALORIES	TOTAL FAT [G]	SATURATED FAT [G]	CHOLESTEROL [MG]	FIBER [G]	SODIUM [MG]
Dinner *(continued)*	Grilled marinated salmon	6 oz	245	14	2	70	0	270
	Baked sweet potato wedges	1 potato	100	0	0	0	4	41
	Red wine	3½ oz	75	0	0	0	0	5
Snack	Soy ice cream	½ cup	140	8	1	0	1	125
	Slivered almonds	1 tbsp	35	3	0	0	1	0
	Strawberries	5 medium	20	0	0	0	1	0
Totals			1815	68	13	81	29	1510

KATE'S FOOD DIARY: COULD IT BE YOURS?

MEAL	FOOD	QUANTITY	CALORIES	TOTAL FAT [G]	SATURATED FAT [G]	CHOLESTEROL [MG]	FIBER [G]	SODIUM [MG]
Breakfast	Large latte	20 oz	270	14	9	61	0	219
	Doughnuts	2	420	26	12	0	2	210
Lunch	Double cheeseburger	1	530	32	6	90	1	1070
	Small fries	1	320	16	3	0	4	350
	Small soda	12 oz	150	0	0	0	0	10
Snack	Candy bar	1	250	17	7	5	2	65
	Canned soda	12 oz	150	0	0	0	0	30
Dinner	Sausage and mushroom pizza	3 slices	750	24	11	60	3	1650
	Whole milk	8 oz	150	8	5	35	0	125
	Chocolate chip cookies	2	250	24	5	10	2	240
Snack	Pretzel crisps	15	150	2	0	0	1	450
Totals			3390	163	58	261	15	4419

The differences between Kate's food diary and the heart-smart food diary are striking. Kate's diet is much less diverse, yet supplies nearly twice the number of calories. While saturated fat should be kept to 20 grams or less, Kate exceeds this limit by nearly threefold. She also consumes three times more sodium than recommended. Most adults do best with 20 to 35 grams of fiber daily, but Kate's diet is seriously lacking. And although Kate comes in just under the 300 mg threshold for cholesterol, the heart-smart diet includes only 80 mg. It's easy to see how poor choices can quickly add up. But it's also clear that heart-smart options do not need to be expensive or time consuming.

Start your own food diary using a simple notebook, a smartphone app, or a Web site service. (I especially like Lance Armstrong's LiveStrong.com/myplate, SparkPeople.com, and MyFitnessPal.com, all of which are free of charge.)

To start, record the nutrition data for all your food, including snacks and nibbles, for a week. (You don't have to record every nutrient, but it's useful to tally fats, cholesterol, fiber, sodium, and, of course, calories.) To correctly track your intake, you may have to get a little compulsive about portion sizes. Invest in a kitchen scale and make use of your measuring cups and spoons to weigh and measure all of your food. Then consult the nutrition data and serving size on the labels to calculate your daily calorie and nutrient intake.

MY PATIENT JONATHAN'S roommate once confided to me that Jonathan's cereal bowl was in reality a mixing bowl that could easily hold half a box of cereal. Jonathan was being honest with me when he said that he only had "one bowl of cereal" each morning, but when proportions are this skewed, it's virtually impossible to lose weight.

For the calorie counts of foods that don't come with a label, consult an online resource such as the USDA Nutrient Database (nal.usda.gov/fnic/foodcomp/search) or the more streamlined

Myfoodapedia.gov. Many chain restaurants also offer nutritional information on their Web sites.

After doing this faithfully for a few days, you will have trained your eye to roughly calculate portion sizes and learned just how many calories you consume, and then you will be able to start finding simple ways to reduce how much you eat.

How to Lose a Pound a Week

If reducing your caloric intake seems daunting, consider this: One pound of body fat equals 3,500 calories, so cutting out *just 500 calories* daily will help you lose 1 pound a week! That's one serving of large fries, a couple of snack bars, or a small milkshake. You'd hardly miss them. Even cutting back by 250 calories each day will earn you a 2-pound weight loss by month's end. Add exercise to the plan and the pounds will peel off faster and more efficiently.

BEST PRACTICES:
YOUR CALORIE COUNT

* Food supplies calories, exercise burns them up. It's that simple.
* Calculate how many calories you need. Most people need 1,600–2,200 calories daily, but most underestimate their caloric intake by 300–500 calories. Snacks and between-meal beverages count.
* Don't just guess how much you're eating. Read package nutrition labels and measure portion sizes to know for sure.
* Fill up on foods that are less dense in calories: Gram for gram, carbohydrates and proteins pack less than 50% of the calories of an equivalent amount of fat, while providing your body with vital nutrients.
* One pound of weight equals 3,500 calories. Cut out 500 calories each day, and in a week you'll have lost a pound!

CARBOHYDRATES

Lettuce, cookies, apples, pasta, whole wheat bread, doughnuts. What do these foods have in common? Although their nutritional values differ tremendously, they are loaded with carbohydrates—nutrients vital to the body and the brain that supply both immediate energy and long-term energy reserves.

Carbohydrates (affectionately known as carbs) are an essential part of a healthy diet, but thanks to a revival of trendy low-carb diets, they took a bad rap in the early 2000s and have never quite recovered their reputation.

The problem is that many people don't understand exactly what constitutes a carbohydrate. Although we've been conditioned to think of them as starchy, sugary junk foods, carbohydrates are also a critical energy source, and many carbohydrate-rich foods are high in important nutrients and fiber.

Carbohydrates can be divided into three major groups: sugars, starches, and fiber.

The Sugars—Simple

Sugar appears in your diet in many more forms than just the old familiar white stuff. Monosaccharides, such as glucose, fructose, and galactose, are found in most foods, including fruit, honey, and milk. Disaccharides, such as sucrose, lactose, and maltose, include the sugar considered "table sugar," as well as sugars found in fruit, vegetables, milk, and even beer.

Apart from being a natural component of such healthy foods as milk or fruit, sugar often turns up in commercially prepared products, such as pasta sauces, in addition to such obvious culprits as sodas and juice-flavored drinks, and many breakfast cereals and baked goods. You can read more about sugar and other sweeteners, including high-fructose corn syrup, in chapter 8 (see page 130).

There is nothing intrinsically bad about sugar. What's important is the amount you consume. There are only 16 calories in a teaspoon of sugar, but up to 25 percent of the total calories of the typical Western diet come from sugars. When we add it all up, the average American eats and drinks nearly half a pound of sugar every day.

The Starches—A Little More Complex

Starches are more complicated. Essentially long strings of glucose, they are bound together in various forms and fashions that require more work for the body to break down. They are commonly found in beans and peas, onions, potatoes, bananas, rice, pasta, and grains, including corn, cereal, and flour.

Fiber

Fiber is more resistant to digestion, so it is able to pass right through your digestive system. Fibrous foods include whole grains, most fruit, and green leafy vegetables. Fiber is critical to heart and digestive health, and will be featured in more detail later in this chapter (see page 64).

The Glycemic Index

The words *simple* and *complex* are often applied to carbohydrates, but more important than the distinction between them is something called the glycemic index. It measures how fast a carbohydrate-based food is likely to raise your blood glucose, or sugar, levels. The higher the number, the more quickly your blood sugar level will rise.

Foods rated high on the index typically contain more sugar or are considered to be more starchy. These include the so-called "white" foods, such as white bread, bakery goodies, rice, pasta, and potatoes. (Carrots, cornflakes, and raisins also rate high on the index, but as I'll explain, that doesn't necessarily mean that these foods are unhealthy.)

Foods loaded with fiber, such as most fruit, nonstarchy vegetables, and whole grains, have low glycemic indices, and therefore will have a more subtle influence on blood sugar.

The more high-glycemic carbs you eat, the faster and steeper your blood sugar level will soar. That is why the often overlooked concept of "glycemic load" is so important. The term *glycemic load* refers to both the glycemic index and the typical amount of food per serving. This is important, because the tables used to determine the glycemic index, which are widely available online, do not compare foods based on the serving size; rather, they relate them carb gram to carb gram. Being that not all foods contain the same amount of carbohydrate grams, such direct comparisons can be tricky.

For example, the glycemic indices of potatoes and carrots are similar, yet the glycemic load of a baked potato is more than four times that of a ½-cup serving of carrots, because the total carbohydrate content of a serving of potatoes is four times higher than that of carrots. The glycemic indices of wild rice and white rice are nearly identical, but because the carbohydrate content of white rice is twice that of wild rice, the glycemic load of white rice is also two times higher. On the other hand, the glycemic load of a glass of orange juice is very similar to that of a can of regular cola.

As a rule, snack foods and "white" foods tend to have a high glycemic load, whereas more complex foods such as whole grains, sweet potatoes, nuts, and seeds have a lower glycemic load.

Although I don't expect you to track your daily glycemic load, understanding this concept will give you a smarter perspective on the foods you choose. You can easily track down detailed tables of the glycemic load of a variety of foods by searching online. You can also look for Dr. Jennie Brand-Miller and Kaye Foster-Powell's book *The Low GI Shopper's Guide to GI Values* for complete information on nearly 1,300 common foods.

■ WHAT YOUR GLYCEMIC LOAD TELLS YOU

Why should you care about the effect your diet may have on your blood sugar levels? To put it simply, what goes up must come down. In general, high sugar levels cause your body to release the hormone insulin. Insulin allows you to process the sugar you eat so that it can be stored in your cells for usable energy. More sugar in the blood means your body must release more insulin.

In diabetics, the body often is not able to make enough insulin to keep up with the dietary sugar load. It is not surprising that people who consume a high-glycemic-load diet are more likely to become type 2 diabetic. For instance, the risk of developing diabetes in women who have the highest glycemic load and the lowest fiber intake is about two and a half times that of women with very healthy eating habits.

It also turns out that the higher the daily dietary glycemic load, the greater the heart disease risk for women, although the same connection has not been proven in men. The Harvard-based Nurses' Health Study found that women who consumed the highest glycemic load were nearly two times more likely to suffer heart attacks and coronary heart disease than were those whose intake of these foods was very low. The heart disease risk was greatest in overweight women.

Other studies have found an association between a high-glycemic-load diet and high blood pressure, high LDL (bad) cholesterol, and reduced levels of HDL (good) cholesterol. Elevated levels of CRP, a substance in the blood linked to inflammation of the heart arteries, are also common.

A high-glycemic diet has even been associated with early age-related macular degeneration, a condition of the retina associated with blindness. Breast cancer, pancreatic cancer, and uterine cancer have all been linked to a high-glycemic diet.

Even if you're not diabetic or prediabetic, a high-glycemic diet will sap your strength. The rapid rise in blood sugar is typically followed by a speedy fall in sugar levels, and this is one reason that high-glycemic foods can leave you feeling groggy, grouchy, and unmotivated. The sugar swings can also lead to sugar cravings, as your body chemistry tries to get you back your sugar buzz.

This unhealthy oscillation of blood sugar creates a vicious cycle of hunger, brief spurts of energy, and rapid fatigue. That, in turn, will goad you into eating more, to recapture that fleeting sense of sugar-induced euphoria. Some people, including children and teens, become virtual carb addicts, craving the highs and dreading the lows. Ultimately, the result will be all too familiar: weight gain, sluggishness, and diminished productivity.

Think back to Kate and her fast-food lunch. When her sugar lows hit, she reaches for her afternoon candy bar and soda, and the dangerous cycle begins again. It is easy to understand why Kate goes home exhausted and too tired to exercise. And it's a safe bet that she is not nearly as satisfied or happy with her life as she could be.

BEST PRACTICES:
CARBOHYDRATES

* Limit high-glycemic foods, particularly starchy "white" foods such as white bread, white rice, white pasta, and white potatoes, as well as sugary products. All raise your blood sugar quickly and substantially.
* Try a low-glycemic diet to reduce your risk for diabetes, heart disease, high cholesterol, and cancer—and avoid sugar surges that can negatively affect your energy level and mood.

FRUITS AND VEGETABLES

Despite the stunning variety of fruits and vegetables cultivated by our nation's farmers, the two most commonly eaten "produce" items in this country are (in order) various forms of potatoes and iceberg lettuce. A full 25 percent of all the so-called vegetables Americans consume are french fries, which are loaded with an enormous amount of fat, plenty of salt, and very few nutrients.

Most Americans have access to a bounty of fresh fruits and vegetables, yet produce remains the underdog of the food world. Although absolutely critical for good health, far too often fruits and vegetables are treated as an afterthought, served on the side or as a sad, wilted garnish. So many of us have grown up in a home in which mass-marketed processed snacks were the norm, and were never taught the pleasures of biting into a juicy, crisp apple; whipping up a vibrant multicolored salad; or brewing a spicy ratatouille. But it's never too late to learn.

How Much Is Enough?

Current U.S. dietary guidelines recommend five to seven servings of fruit or vegetables daily, but most of us eat far less. More recent medical research has suggested that eight to ten servings are probably optimal. A study from the University of Oxford found that people who ate at least eight servings of fruit and veggies each day were substantially less likely to die from heart disease than were those who ate less than three servings daily, even taking into account such variables as smoking, dietary fat, and body weight. A serving is generally considered one piece of fruit, 1 cup of raw leafy vegetables, ¼ cup of dried fruit, or ½ cup of other fruit or vegetables.

Although achieving this goal might sound a little intimidating, it is as easy as tossing a handful of berries onto your breakfast cereal, choosing a big green salad for lunch, scooping up a couple of helpings of veggies at dinnertime, and enjoying a piece of fresh fruit for dessert or a snack. Although ¾ cup of juice is sometimes considered a serving of fruit or vegetable, it does not appear to offer the same protection. This is because the juice is only a fraction of the fruit, and the health benefits come from the full symphony of nutrients and antioxidants working together. Besides, the calorie count of a cup of juice is often substantially higher than a piece of fruit, particularly if the juice has added sweeteners.

Heart-Healthy Produce

Which fruits and vegetables are best? Truthfully, they are all worthy of a place at the table, as long as you keep margarine, butter, cheese, and other unhealthy additives to a bare minimum. However, the more colorful a fruit or vegetable is, the more nutrients it is likely to offer. Aim for a broad variety of fruits and vegetables, to maximize and balance out their heart-healthy qualities. Dark green, leafy vegetables, bright red tomatoes, and rich golden-orange nectarines and peaches are especially good choices. Berries are also wonderfully heart protective.

Although potatoes provide reasonable amounts of vitamin C, potassium, and fiber, they are typically prepared with copious amounts of fat and salt. Consider substituting sweet potatoes, a fabulous source of vitamin C, beta-carotene, and fiber. They have much more flavor than white potatoes, so they don't need to be gussied up to make them taste good. Try them simply baked in foil or roasted in the oven with your favorite spices, a touch of olive oil, and a pinch of salt.

Have fun and experiment with Mother Nature's bounty. Eating well does not have to be expensive. While organic foods might be more environmentally sound, they are often more costly, and the nutritional difference appears to be minimal. Shopping for fruits and vegetables may require a little strategizing, as they do have a limited shelf life. Unless you are freezing or canning, buy only what you will eat in the next several days, so you don't end up with a fridge full of spoiled produce. If it is too time consuming or expensive to buy all the fixings for a salad, check out your grocery store's salad bar. That will allow you to pick and choose just the right amount of fresh ingredients for your meal. Keep your plate colorful, and your heart will be happier.

BEST PRACTICES:
FRUITS AND VEGGIES

* Try to include 8–10 servings daily (french fries don't count). One serving is ½ cup of most fruit or vegetables, or a full cup of raw leafy vegetables.
* Choose a variety of brightly colored fruits and veggies to get the widest variety of vitamins and other nutrients.

WHOLE GRAINS

It's hard to imagine life without bread, cereal, and pasta. We humans have depended on grains for nourishment since the beginning of recorded history. For centuries it was women who threshed the wheat, kneaded the dough, and baked the bread that sustained their family. But over the last fifty or so years, factory-refined flours have far over-taken whole grains in the Western diet. Only about 20 percent of bread now sold in the United States is whole grain; likewise, less than 5 percent of the grains we eat every day are whole.

After millennia of consuming humble, coarse-milled flours, people came to believe lily-white refined flours were purer, more sophisti-cated. Now we know that the milling process actually removes the most nutritious (and delicious) part of the grain, leaving behind only the starchy middle layer, called the endosperm. This part of the grain is rapidly digested and broken down by the body into sugar, which accounts for white bread's notoriously high-glycemic reputation.

The bran (outer layer), and the inner layer known as the germ (or embryo) get lost in the refining process, essentially ending up on the cutting-room floor. These important parts of a grain are rich in fiber, B vitamins, vitamin E, minerals, and often omega-3 fatty acids, as well. Refining removes about 70 percent of the minerals, 80 percent of the fiber, and 25 percent of the protein contained in the grain.

Other vital nutrients lost when the germ is stripped away include phytoestrogens and antioxidants, which may have important protec-tive effects for the heart and other organs. Scientists are still studying these substances, but some of them have been found to lower blood glucose, insulin levels, and cholesterol. Refined flour is found in most of the breads and baked goods sold in grocery stores. Pasta, muffins, pizza, and even most breakfast cereals are also manufactured using refined flour. In many cases, that flour is enriched with niacin, iron, thiamine, riboflavin, and folic acid. This is a major improvement over the bare stuff, but does not go nearly far enough.

Add Whole Grains to Your Diet

Studies show that those who eat about two and a half servings of whole grains daily have as much as a 30 percent lower heart disease risk, when compared to people whose diets include no whole grains at all. A diet that includes whole grains may help lower blood pressure, and is also associated with reduced likelihood of cholesterol plaque buildup in the carotid arteries, which supply blood to the brain. Not surprisingly, whole grains appear to lower the probability of developing type 2 diabetes. People who eat more whole grains are also less prone to colorectal and breast cancer. What's more, whole grains are associated with reduced blood levels of inflammation and may even cut your risk of periodontitis (gum disease).

It's easy to get whole grains into your diet. A serving can be a slice of whole-grain bread or a standard serving size of cereal that contains at least 25 percent whole grain or bran by weight. This is a great example of how simple choices can have a substantial impact on your health and the health of your family.

DECODING LABELS

FOR THE FULL whole-grain experience, whole wheat bread is your best bet. That's not to say that other breads are unhealthy, but they may lack the full kick of nutrients and fiber that whole grains offer. Labels can be confusing. The word *wheat* on a label merely refers to the original source of the flour. The term *wheat flour* or *unbleached flour* is not in of itself an indication that the flour is whole grain. *Unbleached flour* may sound healthier and more natural, but in fact, about 80 percent of its bran has been removed. Wheat bread is whole grain only if one of the first ingredients listed is "whole wheat flour."

Aside from wheat, a world of whole grains is waiting for you to discover. Millet, oats, quinoa, and amaranth are nutritious, tasty, and worth exploring. They are great options for people who are not tolerant of wheat. These grains are often sold in the form of flour or incorporated into breakfast cereals. And don't forget brown rice, a much smarter choice than its plain white cousin.

To be sure, whole grains do require more care than refined flour. To keep them fresh, store flour in the refrigerator or freezer if the package is open for more than a few days.

BEST PRACTICES:
WHOLE GRAINS

* Have 2½ servings of whole grains each day—you'll cut your risk of heart disease by 30%, help prevent type 2 diabetes and protect against colorectal cancer. (One serving is one slice of whole-grain bread or a standard serving of whole-grain cereal.)
* Look for products that contain whole wheat flour, as well as alternative healthy grains such as millet, oats, quinoa, and amaranth.
* Choose whole-grain pastas and brown rice, instead of "white" grain products.

FIBER

Whole grains are a rich source of fiber, but fiber is also abundant in fruits and vegetables. *Fiber* is defined as the indigestible parts of the plants we eat. Your grandmother may have called it roughage. A diet high in fiber is associated with a lower risk of heart disease and high blood pressure and may even play a key role in maintaining a healthy weight.

People who eat more fiber tend to weigh less and to gain less weight over time. The American Heart Association recommends a fiber intake of 25 to 30 grams daily, including 10 to 25 grams of soluble fiber (see the next paragraph for details). Yet the average American consumes only 15 grams of any kind of fiber.

Fiber and Your Cholesterol Levels

There are two types of fiber: soluble and insoluble. Soluble fiber particles attract water and form a sort of gel in the digestive tract, which traps cholesterol-containing bile acids making their way through the intestines and passes them out of the body in the stool. Without soluble fiber, cholesterol is usually absorbed back into the bloodstream.

Fill Up on Fiber

Soluble fiber from sources such as oat bran, apples, oranges, prunes, and legumes (beans) can help lower your cholesterol, mainly by decreasing the absorption of cholesterol through the gastrointestinal tract. The insoluble form of fiber that comes from seeds, whole grains, and brown rice does not have the same cholesterol-lowering effect, but has other benefits.

Both soluble and insoluble fiber allow sugar to release more slowly into the bloodstream, avoiding sudden peaks and valleys in blood glucose. As a result, less insulin is required. People whose daily diet includes the recommended 25 to 30 grams of fiber tend to have lower levels of CRP. And fiber helps maintain good digestive health.

A diet with plenty of fiber will make you feel fuller faster. My patient Jessica credits her before-meal apples for her 20-pound weight loss this year, a claim backed up by research from Brazil and Florida, both well known for their bikini-centricity.

Psyllium is a type of soluble fiber that is usually used as a supplement, rather than a food. Learn more about it in chapter 15 (see page 288).

BEST PRACTICES:
FIBER

* Follow a high-fiber diet to lower your cholesterol, reduce your risk of heart disease and high blood pressure, and boost your digestive health. Fiber will help you feel fuller faster and slow the release of glucose into your bloodstream.
* Strive for 25–30 grams of fiber each day, including 10–25 grams of soluble fiber, which is found in oat bran, apples, oranges, prunes, and legumes.

PROTEIN

Proteins are made up of any number of twenty building blocks known as amino acids. They are involved in all of your body's most important functions. Growth, reproduction, maintenance, and repair of muscle and body organs—you name it, proteins are there. The adult human body is capable of manufacturing all but eight of the amino acids. These eight, dubbed the essential amino acids, must come from the food you eat; without them, your body simply cannot perform normally.

A food that provides all eight of the essential amino acids in proportion to your needs is known as a complete protein. With the exception of soy and some grains, such as quinoa and amaranth, complete proteins are found mainly in foods that come from animals—meats (including poultry, beef, pork, and fish), eggs, and dairy products.

A vegan (a vegetarian who eats nothing of animal origin) can easily obtain all the essential amino acids by including foods from a variety of vegetable, bean, and grain sources. Infants and young children, however, require a ninth amino acid, histidine. (By adulthood, the body is capable of producing this amino acid, so there is no daily requirement). Moderate amounts of histidine are available from soy and nuts, but the nutrient is most abundant in dairy, red meat, poultry, and fish. If you are raising a vegan kid, it's important to keep this in mind and to discuss dietary options with your pediatrician.

Not all protein is the same. For instance, a diet high in vegetable-based protein may help to lower blood pressure, whereas red meat and processed meat (such as lunch meat) are associated with a greater risk of high blood pressure.

We know a lot about carbohydrates and fats, but the role that protein plays in promoting heart health is not as well understood. There is no question that an extremely low-protein diet may severely weaken the heart. This is all too common in impoverished Third-World countries and may also occur with anorexia nervosa.

Protein: How Much Is Enough?

To be precise, most of us require 0.8 mg of protein per kilogram of body weight daily to maintain good health. To find out how much you need, multiply your body weight in pounds by 37 percent (0.37). For example, $150 \times 0.37 = 55.5$ tells us that a 150-pound person will need about 55 grams of protein each day.

The Institute of Medicine has recommended a safe range of protein intake of anywhere between 50 and 175 grams daily. Of course, your protein needs will vary depending on your health and activity level. A highly competitive athlete requires considerably more protein than does a more sedentary individual.

Carnivore or vegetarian, it is easy to get enough protein, and it is usually not necessary to routinely count every gram. The USDA considers 2 to 3 ounces of lean meat, poultry, or fish to be one serving, and our daily requirement to be two to three servings.

Most 3-ounce portions of red meat, fish, and chicken contain 15 to 25 grams of protein. The leaner the cut, the more protein per ounce it will contain. An ounce of cheese or a cup of milk will give you 8 grams of protein, and one egg supplies 6 grams. Tofu is a protein powerhouse, with 20 grams per ¼ cup and 25 percent fewer calories than a 3-ounce piece of steak. You also get small amounts of protein from grains and vegetables, even though these foods are often categorized as carbohydrates.

If your diet skews toward vegetarianism, ½ cup of beans, ½ cup of tofu, one egg, 1 cup of milk or yogurt, a 2½-ounce soy burger, 2 tablespoons of peanut butter, or ⅓ cup of nuts equals the protein equivalent of 1 ounce of meat.

Don't Overdo It

Chances are, the amount of protein in your daily diet is more than sufficient to meet your needs. You can buy a variety of protein supplements, including powdered amino acids, but you really don't need them. Although manufacturers tout their ability to improve strength, muscle mass, and endurance, these claims are not much more than wishful thinking. For a strong, fit, and lean body, you've got to amp up your exercise program. Simply eating large amounts of protein will not boost your muscle mass, although the extra calories may increase your girth. In those whose kidney function is marginal, excessive amounts of protein can even damage the kidneys and the liver.

BEST PRACTICES:
PROTEIN

* Calculate your daily protein requirement in grams by multiplying your body weight in pounds by 0.37 (or your weight in kilograms by 0.8). Between 50 and 175 daily grams of protein is safe for most people.
* Don't overlook the protein "hiding" in healthy food: Although meat, fish, poultry, eggs, and diary are great sources of protein, it can also be found in grains and seeds, legumes, and vegetables.
* Don't bother with protein supplements—there's usually no need to take them, as there's no benefit to excess protein.

THE SKINNY ON FAT

For years, many of us in the medical profession have badgered our patients to follow the "low fat, low cholesterol" mantra. We have blithely promised a lifetime of good health to those who pursue a fanatically low-fat diet, without fully understanding the consequences of our advice.

Thanks to our fat phobia, our grocery stores are now stocked with a mother lode of low-fat snacks. These highly processed goodies, packed with sugar and simple starches, threaten to sabotage our health by tricking consumers into believing that "no fat" equals "healthy."

Simply Put, Fat Is Complicated

Fats are the most concentrated and efficient sources of energy available and are responsible for a great deal of the flavor we associate with good food. Fats will produce a feeling of satiety, or fullness, much more quickly than will protein or carbohydrates, which helps cut food cravings. Most important, fats are involved in virtually all the functions of the body, including those of the brain. Some are even vital for maintaining optimal cardiovascular health.

High-fat diets have been clearly linked to heart disease, stroke, and cancer. Too much of the bad kind of fat can raise your LDL cholesterol and harm your arteries. However, too little good fat can also have a negative impact on your lipid profile. People who choose a diet that is extremely low in fat and high in carbohydrates may find their lipids turned topsy-turvy, with lower levels of HDL and higher levels of triglycerides. Turn to Sherry's story (page 110) to see how the best intentions can go awry.

A prudent diet can include 25 to 30 percent of calories from fat. For someone who requires 2,000 calories a day, a reasonable fat intake should run between 55 and 65 grams—as long as those fats come from the right sources.

All Fats Are Not Alike

Like carbohydrates, not all fats are created equal. There are three major types of fat: saturated, unsaturated, and trans fat. While all fat packs the same number of calories per gram, the type of fat you eat, even more than the amount, is what impacts your cardiovascular risk.

Fat is made up of fatty acids, essentially long chains of carbon atoms. Whether a fatty acid is saturated or unsaturated depends upon its chemical structure. If each one of the carbon atoms has a hydrogen atom attached, we call it saturated. Conversely, if even one carbon atom is missing a hydrogen atom, then it is unsaturated. When unsaturated fats are treated by a process called hydrogenation, their chemical structure is altered in a fundamental way. These modified fats are called trans fats. Retailers like them because they don't go rancid easily, and restaurants like them because they are cheap. They reach our grocery shelves and restaurants as partially hydrogenated oils, most commonly in the form of solid (stick) margarine and vegetable shortening.

Heart-Healthy Unsaturated Fats

Let's start with the good guys. Unsaturated fats are a vital part of good nutrition. The best sources are vegetable oils, olive oil, nuts, grains, and fish. Poultry, beef, and pork also provide modest amounts of unsaturated fats mixed in with a good measure of saturated fats. Unlike saturated and trans fats, unsaturated fats are usually liquid at room temperature.

■ MONOUNSATURATED FATS

Monounsaturated fats (sometimes referred to as omega-9 fatty acids) are found in abundance in olive oil, canola oil, nuts, and avocados. This heart-friendly type of fat has beneficial effects on the cholesterol profile and may also enhance the ability of the heart arteries to respond normally to stress. A number of studies worldwide have established that people who eat more monounsaturated fats significantly lower their risk of developing heart disease and stroke. Monounsaturated fat may even favorably affect your body's response to insulin and help lower your blood pressure.

According to one Spanish study, people who consumed 4 tablespoons of olive oil daily had an 82 percent lower risk of heart disease than did those whose diet included little or no olive oil. This effect can be attributed in large part to a monounsaturated fat called oleic acid, which makes up 55 to 85 percent of olive oil by weight. Olive oil's other components, including antioxidant vitamins, polyphenol antioxidants, and other types of polyunsaturated fats, are probably also heart protective.

Olive oil labeled "extra virgin" or "virgin" contains more of these naturally occurring nutrients and antioxidants than does regular olive oil, and has a more favorable effect on HDL cholesterol, making it a smarter choice.

■ POLYUNSATURATED FATS

Polyunsaturated fats, found in coldwater fish, nuts, grains, and vegetable oils, are essential for good health. This type of fat has a powerful impact on the cholesterol profile. Although we doctors used to counsel our patients to follow a strictly low-fat diet, people who choose a diet high in polyunsaturated fats tend to have lower cholesterol levels and a lower risk of heart disease than do those whose diets are low in fat but high in carbohydrates.

Polyunsaturated fats include two types of essential fatty acids—omega-3 and omega-6. The human body cannot manufacture these from scratch, so you must obtain them from the foods you eat. Both omega-3 and omega-6 fatty acids are vital for the healthy function of all your cells, hormone-producing glands, immune system, cholesterol transport system, and brain. Omega-3 fatty acids have been associated with a lower risk of blood clots, heart attacks, dementia, and strokes, and a decreased likelihood of potentially fatal heart rhythms. They may even help to protect your eyes against macular degeneration. Omega-6 fatty acids may help your body ward off type 2 diabetes when included in a well-balanced diet.

Omega-3 and omega-6 fatty acids compete in your body for enzymes that break them down and allow them to perform their vital functions. It is important to maintain a healthy balance between these two types of fat. For example, excessive levels of omega-6 may contribute to inflammation of your blood vessels, raising your risk of cardiovascular disease and perhaps even diabetes.

■ OPTIMIZING YOUR OMEGAS

Substituting omega-9–rich olive oil for butter or choosing a diet with more nuts and less (or no) meat may reduce your LDL cholesterol by as much as 15 percent and raise your HDL cholesterol by about 4 percent.

Balancing omega-6 and omega-3 fats gets a bit more complicated. The optimal ratio of omega-6 to omega-3 is approximately 5:1 or less. That means you should get no more than five times as much omega-6 as omega-3. Unfortunately, the typical American diet includes somewhere between fourteen and twenty times more omega-6 than omega-3. That means that you are probably seriously lacking in the omega-3 department and need to boost your omega-3 intake. Omega-3 fatty acids are found in walnuts, soybeans, flaxseed oil, and coldwater fish like salmon and tuna. While maximizing your omega-3 fat is good, you also need to reduce your consumption of foods that contain omega-6. Omega-6 can be cut by drastically curtailing your use of most vegetable oils (substitute heart-healthy olive oil instead). Observing these best practices will not only improve your cardiovascular health, but may have other important effects on your health. You'll learn more about omega-3 fats in chapters 5 and 15 (see pages 80 and 283).

Saturated Fat

There is no doubt that saturated fat is a major contributor to heart disease. We get most of our saturated fat from meat, poultry, and dairy products. Coconut and palm kernel oils, commonly used in processed snack foods, are the main plant sources of this type of fat. Saturated fats are usually unappealingly solid and greasy at room temperature, but melt at cooking temperatures, providing the yummy mouthfeel that we crave in high-fat foods.

A study conducted by the Los Angeles Veterans Hospital found that people who substituted unsaturated fat for saturated fat in their everyday diet could reduce their risk for coronary heart disease by more than 30 percent. Similarly, the Nurses' Health Study reported in 1997 that replacing calories from saturated fats with an equal amount of unsaturated fat calories would reduce the risk of heart disease by 42 percent; comparable results were found in a 2005 study from Finland.

Saturated fats raise the LDL cholesterol more than does any other fat except for trans fats. Even a single meal high in saturated fat can be harmful. As they slide though your arteries, saturated fats impede your blood vessels' ability to respond normally to stress, and increase your likelihood of developing potentially fatal blood clots.

Although most studies concerning saturated fat have been done with animal fats, this same effect has also been seen with coconut oil, putting a hole in the popular theory that plant-based saturated fats are healthful. Manufacturers of tropical oils like coconut oil and palm oil are eager to promote their products as "functional foods," but there is not much science to support the hype. It is true that these saturated fats are probably a little less harmful than are those from animal sources, but they are clearly linked to a higher risk for heart attacks, and it's best to avoid them.

A meal high in saturated fat may also trigger an abrupt rise in CRP and other inflammatory substances, and at the same time inhibit HDL cholesterol, making your arteries more vulnerable to injury.

Fats are generally understood to increase our sense of fullness, or satiety, but an intriguing study from the Netherlands reported that when compared to unsaturated fat, saturated fat actually had minimal effect on this sensation. Maybe this explains why so many people can eat a double cheeseburger and still have room for fries.

Unless you're a vegan, it's hard to avoid saturated fat altogether. Try to keep it to less than 7 percent of your total caloric intake, or no more than 20 grams daily; you'll do even better if you strive for a daily limit of only 15 grams of saturated fat. You can get a good sense of the fat content of your food from free online sources such as Nutritiondata.self.com.

■ SAY NO TO SATURATED FAT

To minimize saturated fat, eat less red meat or, better yet, avoid it altogether. Even if you chop off all visible fat and choose leaner cuts, fat is marbled within the muscle fibers and is difficult to remove completely. Poultry supplies less saturated fat if you cut off the skin and remove all visible fat, but is still a significant source.

Although seafood also contains small amounts of saturated fats, many varieties of fish are rich in heart-healthy polyunsaturated omega-3 fats. To keep saturated fats at bay, think of poultry and meat as side dishes, keeping portions small, eat fish more often, and give vegetables and grains the starring role on the plate.

As dairy products are also chock-full of saturated fats, be aware of the amount of cheese and butter you eat, including cheese in pizza, sandwiches, and salads; and butter smeared on steaks and fish. A large slice of cheese pizza serves up as much as 55 grams of saturated fat, or more than twice one day's allotment. That's not to say that dairy products are completely off limits. There is some evidence that whole-fat dairy products can help fight diabetes and may have favorable effects on cholesterol when eaten in moderation.

SATURATED FAT CONTENT OF COMMON FOODS

Food	Serving Size	Saturated Fat
BEEF (70% lean)	3 ounces	6.1 grams
CHICKEN (with skin)	3 ounces	3.3 grams
HAM (regular)	3 ounces	2.7 grams
BEEF (95% lean)	3 ounces	2.5 grams
SALMON (farmed)	3 ounces	2.1 grams
HAM (extra lean)	3 ounces	1.5 grams
SALMON (wild)	3 ounces	1.1 grams
CHICKEN (skinless)	3 ounces	0.9 gram
TOFU (firm)	3 ounces	0.6 gram
BUTTER (stick)	1 tablespoon	7.3 grams
MARGARINE (stick)	1 tablespoon	2.1 grams
CHEESE (cheddar)	1 ounce	6.0 grams
MILK (whole)	8 ounces	4.6 grams
MILK (2%)	8 ounces	3.0 grams
SOY MILK (plain)	8 ounces	0.5 gram
MILK (skim)	8 ounces	0.4 gram

SOURCE: USDA NATIONAL Nutrient Database for Standard Reference, Release 24 (2011)

Low-fat and nonfat dairy foods are a great option if you want a high-quality source of calcium and protein without all the calories and saturated fat. Choose skim milk on your breakfast cereal, or make the switch to soy milk, which is great for your heart and has additional health benefits that you'll read about in chapter 5 (see page 89).

Snack foods and even some protein bars may be land mines of palm and coconut oil, so be sure to glance over the package label before you buy these products. Better yet, avoid processed foods altogether.

Trans Fats

Trans fats lurk just about everywhere mass-produced food is found. Vegetable shortening, solid margarines, crackers, popcorn, candies, baked goods, cookies, chips, fried foods, and salad dressings all are typical hiding places for these bad guys. Trans fats begin life as relatively inoffensive polyunsaturated fats, such as soybean oil or even fish oil. Through a chemical process, more hydrogen atoms are added—this is where we get the term *partially hydrogenated*—to make these oily fats more solid, which lengthens their shelf life.

The process, however, creates a type of fat that is chemically and biologically different from its original source. Trans fats occur in miniscule amounts in nature. But the wide acceptance and commercial success of partial hydrogenation, to the tune of $2.4 billion per year, has created an enormous source of trans fats—overloading your system with far greater amounts than your body is designed to handle.

■ BAD, BAD, BAD

Trans fat hits a triple whammy on your cholesterol levels, raising your LDL, lowering your HDL, and boosting your triglycerides. Overall, the detrimental effect of trans fats on your cholesterol profile is more than double that of saturated fats.

Trans fats have been linked to an increase in belly fat, which is just the kind of fat you want to avoid, because it is more dangerous than body fat stored in other areas.

What's more, trans fats may increase the risk of blood clots in the arteries of your heart and other organs, leading to a higher risk for heart attacks and stroke. They can make your cells more resistant to insulin, leaving you more susceptible to type 2 diabetes and its associated complications. CRP is higher in people whose diets include trans fats. Women who breast-feed pass their trans fats along to their infants, exposing the babies to possible harm during a critical point in development.

Based on an overwhelming body of data showing trans fats to be harmful, manufacturers must now include their data on standard nutrition labels. However, restaurants and fast-food restaurants, some of the worst offenders, are not usually required to provide this information, although many will do so if you ask. Following New York City's trail-blazing example, some cities are considering an all-out ban on trans fats, and many restaurant chains, wary of consumer backlash, are choosing healthier alternatives. (Do your research before dining out: Many chains have a Web site where you can look up the cholesterol and fat content of their standard menu items ahead of time.)

HOW HARMFUL CAN TRANS FATS BE?

AREN'T TRANS FATS better than saturated fats, anyway, and isn't this just another trendy "don't"?

Far from it. Consider these facts:

* The dangerous effects of trans fats have been recognized since 1994, when Harvard researchers estimated that at least 30,000, and perhaps as many as 100,000, deaths per year from heart disease could be directly linked to trans fats.
* A report published in 1997 from the ongoing Nurses' Health Study suggested that if we were to take the 2% of average daily calories that come from trans fats and replace them with polyunsaturated and monounsaturated fats, we could lower the relative risk of heart disease by more than 50%.
* Between 1997 and 2007, Americans' average daily trans fat intake increased more than 25%. The average American in 2003 consumed nearly 6 grams of trans fat every day, much of it from cakes, cookies, crackers, and other baked goods.
* Studies from around the world have shown that people who eat an average of 6 grams of trans fats daily have a 39% higher risk of dying from heart disease as compared with those who eat a single gram daily.

* If fast food is part of your diet, your trans fat load may be higher than you think. A single serving of large fries cooked in partially hydrogenated vegetable oil assaults you with more than 8 grams of trans fats, in addition to nearly the same amount of saturated fat. When deep-fried in trans fat, chicken nuggets and fried fish burgers dish up a good 5 grams or more each.
* A piece of pie can amount to about 4 grams, and doughnuts and Danish pastries pile on 3 grams apiece.
* A typical serving of solid margarine contributes 1 to 2½ grams of trans fats.

The bottom line: There is really no safe amount of trans fats to consume, and your best bet is to avoid them altogether.

■ TURN AWAY TRANS FATS

Become a label reader. It's guaranteed to make you smarter about how much trans fat is really in the products you buy. Although manufacturers of packaged foods are now required to list trans fat content, if a standard serving size contains less than half a gram, it can claim to be "trans fat free." These half-grams can add up quickly, so to be sure, look for "partially hydrogenated oils" in the list of ingredients, and avoid those products that include them.

Stay away from solid margarines and shortening. Softer (tub) margarines are less hydrogenated and are a safer choice, although olive oil is an even better option.

Curb your sweet tooth for all the reasons already discussed, but also because so many packaged and bakery goodies contain margarine or vegetable shortening, and so are likely to be loaded with these deadly fats. I have found partially hydrogenated soybean oil in a wide variety of seemingly innocent products, including baby crackers, breakfast cereal, whole-grain bread, and "nutrition bars."

Do not be fooled by labeling that proclaims a product is "cholesterol free" or "cooked in vegetable oil." Although these statements are truthful, they can be misleading and don't mean that the product is healthy.

You've got to stay alert to be heart smart. Now that trans fats have reached our national consciousness, some companies have made an ironic about-face, substituting lard, a saturated fat, for trans fats, which allows them to promote their products as trans fat free.

Perhaps even more insidiously, palm oil is increasingly replacing trans fats in a wide range of snack foods, despite the fact that it is dangerously high in saturated fat. And it's no better for the environment than it is for us: Although it's promoted as a more natural alternative, the industrial production of palm oil endangers a wide range of indigenous Southeast Asian rain forest vegetation and wildlife, including the Sumatran tiger, orangutans, and native elephants.

BEST PRACTICES:
FATS

* Your daily fat intake should be 25–30% of calories consumed, as long as you choose the healthier forms of fat.
* Switch to olive oil and canola oil. They contain monounsaturated fats (omega-9s), which reduce the risk for heart disease and stroke and improve the lipid profile.
* Don't neglect omega-6s: In moderate amounts, these fatty acids are important for good health, but too much can lead to inflammation. A good proportion to maintain of omega-6 to omega-3 is 5:1. Omega-6s come from most vegetable oils.
* Boost your omega-3s by consuming fish, flaxseed oil, and walnuts. Omega-3s reduce the risk for heart attacks, dementia, stroke, and heart rhythm abnormalities.
* Saturated fat, found in animal products and coconut and palm kernel oils, raises the risk for heart disease, stroke, and dementia. It is associated with higher LDL, lower HDL, higher CRP, and an increased risk for blood clots.

Limit your saturated fats to less than 20 grams daily.

* Even more importantly, stay away from the trans fats found in solid margarine, vegetable shortening, and many snack foods. These are the worst forms of fat for heart health; they're even worse than saturated fats.

* Read labels carefully. The FDA allows a label to state "no trans fats" if the amount per serving is less than ½ gram. If the phrase "partially hydrogenated oil" appears on the ingredient list, trans fats are there.

The food we choose can grant us power or take it away. The effect on your pants size notwithstanding, these very simple changes in your diet will have deep, powerful, and lasting effects on your quality of life, and the lives of those around you.

5

The Truth About
the Wonder Foods

NOT ONLY DOES the food we eat nourish and sustain us, but some foods can actually help us to heal, safeguarding our health and vitality. Medical science is only beginning to unlock their secrets, but these "wonder foods" have all been studied with a scientifically objective and open-minded approach.

THE FATTIER THE FISH, THE BETTER

A delicious and versatile fish rich in heart-protecting omega-3 fatty acids, salmon is a nutritional multitasker. When you add to your plate fish that are high in omega-3 fatty acids, not only do your taste buds celebrate, but you also provide your heart with hard-core protection, and probably your skin and nervous systems, too. Eating fatty fish such as salmon just once or twice a week appears to cut the risk of death from cardiac disease by about a third and *to reduce mortality from any cause* by more than 15 percent.

Although salmon usually takes the spotlight, other coldwater fish, including bluefin tuna, mackerel, herring, and sardines, are also excellent sources of omega-3 fatty acids. And while not considered to be omega-3 powerhouses, oysters, mussels, rainbow trout, and swordfish do supply moderate amounts of the good stuff.

Most of the leaner and warmer-water fish are fairly meager sources of omega-3s. That doesn't mean you should overlook them, as they are still excellent choices for healthy protein that is low in saturated fat.

Just in case you're wondering: Nope, fried fish won't cut it. Once the fish is fried in its toxic greasy bath and slathered with mayonnaise, it loses all of its heart-smart power. In fact, a typical fast-food fried fish burger packs more calories and fat than a double cheeseburger.

Fish and Your Heart

Marine omega-3 fatty acids provide several kinds of heart protection. The theory is that when the heart is under severe stress, such as during a heart attack, the fatty acid is released and helps to stabilize its cells, thereby protecting that organ from a potentially deadly rhythm disturbance.

This is important when you consider that more than half of sudden deaths from heart disease (what we doctors call sudden cardiac death) occur in people who have no prior history of heart problems. Fully 300,000 sudden cardiac deaths in this country occur every year due to a catastrophic heart rhythm abnormality that affects the ventricles, the lower pumping chambers of the heart. This can be the result of a heart attack, a weakened heart muscle, or from an electrical malfunction of the heart. Many survivors of cardiac arrest suffer irreversible brain damage and damage to other vital organs. Rather than deal with the aftermath, it is best to prevent such a tragic event, and that's where omega-3s may help.

Omega-3 fatty acids provide other benefits to the heart, including decreased susceptibility to blood clots, lower triglycerides, lower blood pressure, improved blood flow, and reduced inflammation.

Numerous studies conducted worldwide attest to a protective effect of salmon and other omega-3–rich fish. For instance, a study of American women found that those who ate fish two to four times per week had a 31 percent lower risk of heart disease than did those who ate fish less than once a month, as well as a lower risk of sudden cardiac death and stroke. The more fish the women ate, the greater the reduction in risk. However, eating fish as infrequently as one to three times a month reduced cardiovascular risk by an impressive 21 percent.

Japanese men are typically voracious fish eaters, and on average have twice the blood levels of omega-3 fats as white Americans or even Japanese-Americans, who tend to eat less seafood. A joint study from the University of Pittsburg and Shiga University in Japan found about one third the amount of cholesterol buildup in the heart arteries of Japanese men when compared to either white or Japanese-American men in the United States.

Besides the clear cardiac advantages, there is some evidence that eating fish regularly may reduce the risk of prostate cancer, breast cancer, macular degeneration, hearing loss, and depression. Older folks who eat more fish do better on tests of cognitive skills. And omega-3 fats from fish may help you look and feel younger by keeping your skin supple and healthy.

Omega-3s are of critical importance to brain development of the fetus and growing child. They are associated with higher levels of fine motor development, verbal intelligence, and social behavior. Sadly, many pregnant and nursing women simply don't get enough of this vital nutrient, but correcting the problem is not that simple.

Mercury: The Dark Side of Seafood

As with so many good things, there is often a downside. The mercury in our environment comes primarily from coal-burning power plants. In the United States alone, 48 tons of the toxin are released into the environment each year. This and other pollutants found throughout the waters of the world work their way up the food chain, beginning with the tiniest of organisms, and end up concentrated in the fish we eat. When the mercury enters our bloodstream through the digestive tract, it easily slips into our brain and may become trapped there. High levels of mercury can result in neurological symptoms such as tremor, numbness, tingling, and nervousness. When mercury poisoning is suspected, a blood test can readily detect high levels; tests of hair and nails tend to be less accurate.

Fortunately, the adult body is very good at ridding itself of excess mercury, and usually simple avoidance of high-mercury foods will bring levels down over a period of months, without the need to resort to specific treatment.

For infants, children, and the developing fetus, the risk of mercury poisoning is far greater, because high levels of mercury can interfere with normal brain development. Mercury is excreted in the breast milk, making it particularly harmful for nursing infants. The Institute of Medicine recommends that pregnant women, those considering pregnancy, and children eat only 6 to 12 ounces of seafood each week and avoid fish that tend to be especially high in mercury.

The FDA has specifically advised that pregnant women, breast-feeding women, and young children completely avoid these four high-mercury species: tilefish (also known as golden bass or golden snapper), swordfish, king mackerel, and shark. Tilefish have one of the highest mean concentrations of mercury (1.45 parts per million, or ppm, as reported by the Food and Drug Administration), and the other three species also carry very high concentrations (0.96–1.00 ppm).

Although not as toxic as those four fish, ahi tuna (often used for sushi), white albacore tuna, grouper, and Chilean sea bass are also considered high in mercury (0.30–0.49 ppm). The National Resources Defense Council recommends that you limit yourself to three servings or less of these fish per month. Even fish with moderate levels of mercury, such as canned chunk light tuna, mahimahi, and crab (0.09–0.29 ppm), should not be eaten more than twice a week. Salmon, shrimp, scallops, oysters, freshwater trout, and flounder typically have the lowest levels of mercury (0.09 ppm).

■ MERCURY AND YOUR HEART

Although fish is considered a heart-healthy food, mercury can actually cause harm to your heart. One way it does this is by inactivating important heart-protective antioxidants. Mercury may also increase the risk of blood clots. A study from Finland found that men with the highest mercury intake had almost twice the risk of cardiovascular disease as did those whose diet included very little mercury.

That is not to say that fish came out looking bad. The people in that study who consumed the greatest amount of omega-3 fatty acids had a 44 percent lower risk of heart events, compared with those who consumed the least. But when they looked at people with the very lowest levels of mercury plus the highest omega-3 consumption, the researchers found that the risk of heart disease was cut by two thirds. Similar findings were reported in a study involving men in eight European countries and Israel, although a study of 30,000 men in the United States found no definite correlation between mercury and heart disease.

Wild or Farm Raised?

Fish in the wild acquire omega-3 fatty acids from their diet of plankton and algae, natural delicacies that are not available to farmed fish. This is one important reason that wild salmon is usually more flavorful, rich, and colorful. Farm-raised fish may be deficient in omega-3 fatty acids, because they are often fed fish chow that includes less-expensive omega-6 fatty acids. Farm-raised salmon may also be comparatively deficient in vitamin D. Don't be fooled by the brilliant orange-red color. To give it that healthy omega-3 glow, farm-raised salmon is typically cosmetically enhanced with food coloring.

Farm-raised salmon is more likely to have high levels of man-made toxins such as dioxin and PCBs (polychlorinated biphenyls), industrial pollutants that were banned in the 1970s but are still present in our environment. European-raised salmon tends to have higher levels of contaminants than does salmon from North and South America. Salmon farming also contributes to the pollution of the world's oceans, due to the widespread use of pesticides and antibiotics, as well as the waste products that are released into the surrounding waters.

Since the 1980s, shrimp, catfish, tuna, and other fish farmed in Asia have landed on American plates in record numbers. It is estimated that over 90 percent of the shrimp we eat comes from either Asia or

Latin America. Environmental and health regulations are far laxer in these countries than in the United States, and there is little oversight of the industry. As a result, fragile ecosystems and marine animals are threatened or destroyed, and we are exposed to a toxic slew of chemicals, antibiotics, and pesticides.

Although it may sound fresher, your Aunt Betty's catch of the day may not be such a good bet, either. That's because many of our local waterways are contaminated with PCBs. Overall, experts believe that the health risk from toxins such as these is probably fairly low when this type of fish is not part of your usual diet, but high levels have been linked to cancer in animal studies. Neurological problems such as impaired memory have been reported in adults who regularly eat sport fish from polluted waters.

Developmental delays, learning disabilities, and poor immunity are known to occur in children of women exposed to high levels of PCBs during pregnancy. PCBs are generally found in the fattiest part of the fish, including the skin. To determine your level of exposure, blood testing for PCBs is available, but it costs well over $1,000. Limit your exposure to these toxins by avoiding farm-raised salmon and fish caught in polluted local lakes and waterways. Unlike mercury, once PCBs have taken up residence in your body, it may take years to clear them.

What Are the Alternatives?

Omega-3 fats are an important part of a heart-smart diet, but if fish just doesn't float your boat, read on in this chapter to learn about plant-based omega-3 sources, or turn to chapter 15 (see page 283), where you'll learn about omega-3 fatty acid supplements.

Although as yet there are no specific guidelines on fish oil supplements during pregnancy, many obstetricians recommend them as a safer source than fish flesh for omega-3 fatty acids, because the mercury and other toxins are usually filtered out. Of course, if you are pregnant or nursing, be sure to ask your doctor's advice before taking supplements of any kind.

BEST PRACTICES:
FISH

* Eat fish often. Consuming fish 2–4 times weekly is associated with a 30–50% reduction in heart disease risk.
* Your number one choice should be wild salmon, which is a powerhouse source of omega-3 fatty acids. Many other coldwater fish also supply omega-3 fatty acids.
* Avoid tilefish, swordfish, king mackerel, and shark; these fish have been found to be excessively high in mercury, which may increase the risk of heart disease.
* Pregnant women, nursing women, and children should eat no more than 12 ounces of even low-mercury seafood per week, to limit exposure to other toxins such as PCBs.

NUTS—MORE THAN JUST A FUNNY WORD

For years, an earnest low-fat brigade has vigorously preached the evils of nuts, vexed by the high fat content of these crunchy little goodies. The irony is that nuts are a true wonder food, and a tremendous source of healthy fats and plant protein. Nuts not only protect against heart disease, stroke, and diabetes, and possibly lower LDL and Lp(a), but they are also a terrific and satisfying snack.

One of the first studies to look at the heart-protecting effects of nuts found that people who ate nuts more than four times a week had half the risk of fatal coronary heart disease as those who ate nuts less than once a week. The benefits were similar among males and females, elderly and young people, smokers, nonsmokers, and vegetarians. Comparable findings were reported in the Physicians Health Study of more than twenty-one thousand men, followed for seventeen years. Men who ate an ounce of nuts at least twice per week had half the risk of sudden cardiac death as did those who rarely ate nuts.

Other research has found that women who regularly eat nuts at least five times per week may reduce their chances of developing diabetes by more than 25 percent, compared to those who eat no nuts at all. Even eating nuts just one to four times weekly may cut the risk of diabetes by more than 15 percent.

Go Nuts

Although nuts are undeniably high in fat, it is primarily the heart-healthy monounsaturated variety. Per ounce, they supply 160 to 200 calories, 50 to 75 percent of which are fat calories. It's easy to go overboard with nuts, so a good rule of thumb is that 1 ounce amounts to about twenty almonds, pecan halves, or cashews; fourteen walnut halves; or 2 tablespoons of natural (not processed) peanut butter.

Pecans, walnuts, hazelnuts, and almonds are low in naturally occurring saturated fats, and are the best choices. Brazil nuts, with more than 25 percent saturated fat and a high overall fat content, are less heart friendly. Cashews are somewhere in the middle. Macadamia nuts, which are more than 70 percent fat by weight, are very caloric, but in small amounts can be a good source of monounsaturated fatty acids.

Walnuts are particularly dear to our heart, because they supply both omega-6 and omega-3 fatty acids (in a heart-healthy ratio of 5:1), as well as monounsaturated fatty acids. Walnuts provide ten to fifteen times more omega-3 fatty acids than do other nuts, and are high in antioxidants and low in saturated fat.

Nuts are full of a variety of other important nutrients, including vitamin E, magnesium, and folic acid. They are a good source of fiber, including heart-healthy soluble fiber, which is yet another reason why a diet containing liberal amounts of nuts and nut products can improve the cholesterol profile significantly.

The All-American Peanut

Peanuts, an American tradition, are technically not really nuts at all. In fact, they belong to the family of legumes, which also includes beans and peas. Legumes, including soybeans, are outrageously good for you. A large national study reported in 2001 that when legumes were eaten

BEST PRACTICES:
NUTS

* Eat 1 ounce of nuts each day: It may lower your risk of fatal heart disease by 50% and lower your risk for type 2 diabetes by more than 20%.
* Keep walnuts in the mix: They're a good source of omega-3 fatty acids.
* Don't overdo it: One ounce of nuts provides 160–200 calories. Peanut butter serves up 100 calories per tablespoon.
* Avoid peanut butter or nut butters that have been manufactured with partially hydrogenated oils or tropical oils.

four or more times per week, the risk of coronary heart disease was reduced by 22 percent. In 2002, the Nurses' Health Study reported that eating peanut butter five or more times per week was associated with a 21 percent reduction in the risk of developing type 2 diabetes, as compared to that of people who rarely, if ever, touch the stuff.

Peanuts provide considerably more protein than most nuts—about 25 percent by weight—and they are also higher in fiber. They are a valuable source of monounsaturated fatty acids and offer a reasonably good amount of polyunsaturated fatty acids, with only a modest helping of saturated fat.

I personally eat natural-style peanut butter on whole-grain bread or crackers almost every day for lunch. It's super easy, cheap, and delicious. As healthy as peanuts can be, however, peanut butter is not all goodness and light.

Manufacturers typically add partially hydrogenated oils (the dreaded trans fats) or palm kernel oil (saturated fat) to peanut butter to help prolong shelf life. You're much better off choosing the all-natural form of peanut butter. Although it usually has to be stirred before eating, due to separation of the peanut oil, refrigerating after you stir it up will help prevent this separation. If peanuts are not your thing, try experimenting with almond butter, cashew butter, or even sunflower seed butter, which is higher in protein and lower in fat than the nut-based products.

SOY

In 1999, after reviewing twenty-seven important clinical research studies, the FDA allowed manufacturers of soy-based foods to market health claims for soy protein and its role in lowering the risk of coronary heart disease. Soy protein in the range of 25 to 50 grams daily has been associated in some studies with modest reductions in LDL cholesterol and triglycerides, especially in people who have high baseline cholesterol levels.

Soy might even help to lower blood pressure. A Chinese study of people with hypertension found marked reductions in blood pressure in people who ate 40 grams of soy protein every day. In a Boston study of hypertensive postmenopausal women, when just 1 ounce (or 28 grams) of daily protein intake from animal sources was replaced with 1 ounce of soy protein, there was a significant drop in blood pressure (about 10 mm Hg systolic and 7 mm Hg diastolic), which is in line with the results we usually see with a mild antihypertensive drug.

There is a whole host of other ways in which soy can help keep your body healthy and strong. In a study of nearly sixty-five thousand Chinese women, the more soybeans (and other legumes) a woman ate, the less likely she was to develop diabetes. Soy foods appear to be protective against ovarian, uterine, and breast cancers. And good news for both genders: Soy protein may help improve the tone of blood vessel walls and reduce the risk of blood clots.

Soybean oil does not offer the same health benefits. While nearly 80 percent of edible fat consumed in the United States comes from soy oil, this is often in the form of partially hydrogenated oil (that is, the evil trans fat you read about in chapter 4; see page 75). Natural soy oil is better, but it provides none of the heart-protective nutrition of the soybean, such as high-quality protein, fiber, and other plant-based nutrients.

Do Isoflavones Matter?

Isoflavones are chemicals that occur naturally in plants and bear certain similarities to our own estrogen. Plants produce isoflavones to protect themselves from harmful microorganisms and stress. They are nutritionally available to us in important amounts in the form of soy. Chickpeas, also known as garbanzo beans, and a major ingredient in hummus (a Middle Eastern specialty) are another good source.

What can isoflavones do for us? A study from 1997 sheds some light on the subject. Monkeys fed a soy-based diet either with or without isoflavones were found to have major differences in the amount of atherosclerosis they developed. Although the arteries of both groups looked better than those of monkeys on a regular diet, the isoflavone group came out far ahead, with much less cholesterol buildup.

One theory is that isoflavones may act as antioxidants, preventing damage to the artery walls that may lead to plaque buildup and heart attacks. What's more, isoflavones may block the growth of cells in the arterial walls that are involved in the development of atherosclerosis, improve the elastic tone of the arteries, and reduce the likelihood of blood clots.

Where Isoflavones Come From

Soy oil and soy sauce do not contain isoflavones, but soy protein does. However, if the soy protein has been processed with ethanol at the time of manufacturing, the isoflavones are washed away. The closer soy is to its natural state, the more isoflavones it will have. For example, hulled or defatted soybeans have less isoflavones than do virgin soybeans.

The isoflavone content of soy is dependent on the crop and the conditions under which it was grown. The average isoflavone content of soybeans is 1 mg per gram, but the range can be anywhere from 0.4 to 2.4 mg per gram. Therefore, it is difficult for manufacturers to be specific about the isoflavone content of their products, as any given product may include soy from several different sources.

Isoflavones in fermented soy products such as tempeh appear to be easier for the body to utilize than are those in other soy products. Regardless of the source, your body's ability to put isoflavones to work may be inconsistent. Wheat fiber reduces your body's capacity to absorb isoflavones, due to the fiber's binding effect. Moreover, your unique gut microflora (resident beneficial bacteria) may affect your ability to absorb soy isoflavones.

The Safety of Isoflavones

Isoflavones are phytoestrogens, plant-based substances that are structurally similar to estrogen. This is why, for years, breast cancer survivors and women at risk for the disease were warned to avoid soy foods altogether.

Women can now enjoy their soy burgers with a clear conscience, thanks to a large Chinese study of over five thousand breast cancer survivors, run jointly by scientists from Vanderbilt University and the Shanghai Institute of Preventive Medicine. In this study, the more soy foods a woman ate, the less likely she was to have recurrence of her cancer. The benefit was there whether or not the cancer was estrogen receptor positive. Another study of Chinese women without breast cancer also found a protective effect.

Soy foods have been linked to decreased male fertility in animal studies, and in at least one study in humans. Men who were seen at the Massachusetts General Hospital Fertility Center filled out questionnaires about their use of soy products. When the results were analyzed, those who ate the most soy were more likely to have lower sperm concentration. There was no effect on the health of the sperm cells, however. On the other hand, soy does not appear to lower testosterone levels, although the research is fairly limited.

Soy may have a modest effect on thyroid hormones, but as long as you are not iodine deficient, this is unlikely to be a major issue. However, if you eat a lot of soy, let your doctor know, so that routine blood work can be done if needed.

How Much Soy Is Enough?

The American Heart Association (AHA) has specifically advised against isoflavone supplements and other soy-based pills and potions (see chapter 15, page 287), but continues to advocate soy in the diet as an excellent source of protein, fiber, and other nutrients. The AHA points out that perhaps the most important role soy can play is as a heart-friendly alternative to saturated-fat-laden animal protein.

While the FDA suggests a goal of 25 grams per day of soy protein to improve heart health, no definite recommendations have been made regarding isoflavone intake. A typical serving of a soy-based food provides 20 to 35 mg of isoflavones. The Japanese diet includes, on average, about 50 mg of soy isoflavones per day, whereas the average soy-deficient American diet contains about one tenth that amount. Japanese people following a traditional soy-based diet have about half the heart disease risk of Americans. Coincidentally they also have lower risks of breast, prostate, and endometrial cancer—risks that rise in people who move to the United States and take up our typical high- saturated-fat, low-soy Western diet. A traditional Japanese diet contains a number of other heart-smart elements that we'll cover in chapter 7 (see page 120).

Enjoy Soy

So how do you go about adding more soy to your diet? A simple first step is to substitute soy milk for your usual cow's milk in your breakfast cereal and coffee. Don't cringe—soy milk doesn't have to be the watery, grainy liquid you may remember from years ago. There are several terrific brands (Silk, 8th Continent, and Whole Foods house brand, to name a few) that are readily available at the supermarket, in or near the dairy section. These milks can often be used for cooking, and as they tend to be creamier than skim milk (but often just as low in calories), they work well in cream-style soups and other recipes, and even in some baked goods. For variety, you can also buy soy milk in flavors such as vanilla, coffee, chai tea, and chocolate. A typical brand of soy milk provides 6.25 grams of soy protein and roughly 40 mg of isoflavones per 8-ounce serving.

If you like yogurt, it's worth giving soy yogurt a try. It has all the same beneficial bacteria as the traditional dairy yogurt, is a super source of protein, and is naturally low in fat. It's a great option for those who are lactose-intolerant, and, like dairy yogurt, can be used in recipes in place of butter or sour cream.

Edamame, steamed bright green soybeans often served warm in Japanese restaurants, are great all by themselves or in a salad; so are crunchy roasted soy nuts, which come in a variety of flavors. Don't overlook the wonderful (and super easy to prepare) soy sausages and soy burgers, which you can usually find in the freezer case at the grocery store, and which can fool even a committed carnivore, including my dog.

Tofu is another way to add some healthy protein to your diet. Because tofu takes on the flavors of the foods it is cooked with, it is a natural in stir-fries and casseroles, and soft tofu can also be used in desserts because of its creamy texture.

Texturized vegetable protein (TVP) is a great meat alternative. It often comes in a dry form, but increasingly can be found in the frozen foods aisle. When reconstituted and cooked with spaghetti sauce, barbecue sauce, or chili, for example, it is a remarkably good substitute for ground beef. Tempeh is another potent source of isoflavones, although frankly an acquired taste.

BEST PRACTICES:
SOY

* Aim for 25 grams of soy protein per day; 30–50 grams may be even better.
* Try soy protein as a heart-smart replacement for animal products such as red meat. You'll find it in soy milk and yogurt, edamame, roasted soy nuts, soy burgers, tofu, tempeh, and textured vegetable protein.

BERRIES AND OTHER BRIGHT TREASURES—
THE ANTIOXIDANTS

Blueberries, strawberries, raspberries, and cranberries are easy to love. They're gorgeous, they taste great, and they are bursting with heart-protective antioxidants.

Antioxidants block the action of free radicals, which are highly reactive substances we get from food or our environment. Antioxidants have at least one unpaired electron, which makes them unstable, because that electron will do everything it can to pair up. (In the more stable state, negatively charged electrons are paired with positively charged protons, keeping the electrical charge neutral.) Free radicals are not all bad, as, when present in healthy quantities, they help to produce energy and to kill harmful bacteria. Free radicals also protect against cancer by preventing chemical reactions that stimulate the growth of abnormal cells.

But when there is an overabundance, free radicals can cause harmful reactions that lead to serious damage of our cells and arteries. Oxidation of LDL cholesterol by free radicals, for example, is one thing that makes the LDL so dangerous to our arteries. If it never gets oxidized, it is much less likely to cause harm.

While most fruits and vegetables are naturally high in antioxidants, berries, in particular, are superb health boosters. Blueberries have substantially greater antioxidant activity than do most other fruits and vegetables. Truthfully, most blueberry research to date has been done on rodents; nevertheless, blueberries appear to have some very important brain-sustaining properties, enhancing learning ability, and slowing down age-related decline. Along with other brightly colored fruits and veggies, blueberries may help to lower blood pressure in people who enjoy them regularly.

Strawberries and raspberries are also antioxidant powerhouses. Studies of raspberries have shown that the darker the berry, the greater the antioxidant activity. And don't wait for Thanksgiving to enjoy cranberries. Preliminary research suggests that they may contain substances that aid in relaxation of the arteries and perhaps even help to reduce the chance of blood clots.

Pomegranate juice has impressive antioxidant properties as well. A research trial of people with heart disease, funded by the pomegranate industry, reported significant improvement in stress test results in pomegranate juice drinkers. The most active component of pomegranate juice appears to be ellagic acid, an antioxidant that is also found in red raspberries, strawberries, cranberries, blueberries, and walnuts.

Lycopene is another notable antioxidant. It provides the red pigment to tomatoes, watermelon, and grapefruit, and has been associated with heart protection and reduced cancer risk.

Oddly enough, lycopene is better absorbed from processed tomato products like spaghetti sauce and tomato paste than from fresh tomatoes, so you don't have to feel guilty about getting your tomatoes from a can. A Finnish study found that people who drank about 14 ounces of tomato juice daily, and also added a little ketchup to their food, had lower cholesterol levels than did those who had no tomatoes in their diet at all. Tomatoes are also a great source of vitamin A and provide a number of other antioxidant nutrients, fiber, and potassium.

Your Antioxidant Palette

Nature is blooming with antioxidants. Berries and tomatoes may give you the greatest bang for the buck, but essentially any highly pigmented plant is likely to supply you with these very important plant chemicals (also known as phytochemicals). To get the most out of your antioxidants, choose a wide variety of pigmented fruits and vegetables. Experiment with color and your life is sure to be richer for it.

BEST PRACTICES:
ANTIOXIDANT FRUIT

* Add blueberries to your breakfast cereal and perk up your morning.
* Ask for mixed berries for dessert when eating out—but remember to hold the whipped cream.

* Create a riotous salad with a variety of green leafy vegetables, colored peppers, and tomatoes, and forgo pale iceberg lettuce, which is a relatively meager source of antioxidants.

* Order a reduced-cheese veggie pizza with tomato sauce on a thin whole wheat crust, and you're good to go.

* Eat an orange, rather than drinking it, as many of the phytochemicals are contained in the fruit pulp itself.

* Don't be afraid of spinach, kale, and other gorgeous dark greens. Remember to add some of the lighter colors, too. Besides adding flavor, onions and garlic also contain important antioxidants.

Food can indeed be powerful medicine, but be skeptical of self-styled experts who attribute fantastical properties to a new and exotic food or juice—particularly if they are selling it. If it sounds too good to be true, it probably is. My goal is to help you achieve a healthy heart without the hype and to make it fun and tasty at the same time. While virtually all foods from nature will promote good health, the "wonder foods" covered in this chapter have the power to enrich, and maybe even to save, your life.

6

The Evildoers:
Fact or Fiction?

DANGER IS LURKING on your dinner plate. The news is streaming from your TV, jumping off the newspaper headlines, and popping up everywhere you look online. The soccer mom down the street, your mailman, even the guy behind the counter at the convenience store know all about it. Sometimes it seems like everyone has the scoop on "good" food and "bad" food.

You know there are healthy fats, unhealthy fats, and downright dangerous fats, yet many people still insist that all fat is bad. Eggs, salt, and chocolate are other dietary taboos, but do they really deserve their evil reputation?

BUTTER OR MARGARINE: JUST LET IT SLIDE?

For years, doctors and dieticians urged us to dump the butter in favor of what was thought to be the obvious healthier choice: margarine. Although this butter-impersonator has no cholesterol and little to no saturated fat, solid margarine, with its abundance of trans fats, may be even more harmful to the arteries than real butter. While the labels proclaiming margarine to be "all vegetable oil," "high in polyunsaturated fat," and "cholesterol free" are true, these claims ignore trans fat, a truly bad actor.

Vegetable shortening, commonly used as a butter substitute in baking, is often loaded with trans fats, although, in the wake of bad trans fat publicity, many manufacturers have come up with alternatives. Ironically, some of these "new and improved" products contain lard, the greasy animal fat that old-style shortening was designed to replace.

Butter is virtually trans fat free and provides a calorie and total fat content similar to margarine, albeit with three to six times the saturated fat. Ounce for ounce, trans fat is more harmful to your heart than saturated fat is, but both are best avoided. That's where soft margarine comes in. Per serving, tub margarine contains one fourth to half the amount of trans fats of stick margarine; liquid margarine in a squeeze bottle is even better, with minimal amounts of trans fats per portion.

In an effort to boost the nutritional value of margarine and other spreads, some companies have incorporated plant sterols and their derivatives, plant stanols. These products include Benecol and Smart Balance soft margarines. They work by decreasing the amount of cholesterol the intestinal tract can absorb. When used regularly, LDL cholesterol may be lowered by as much as 10 to 20 percent.

The hitch is that this sort of effect is achieved only when substantial amounts, typically 2 grams or more, of the stanols and sterols are consumed on a daily basis. To get that much, you would need about 4 tablespoons of the margarine product each day, for a total of about 300 calories. There are other ways to get these natural cholesterol reducers (see chapter 15, page 290).

Of course, you really don't need butter or margarine. Olive oil is a much healthier alternative, chock-full of antioxidants and healthy monounsaturated fat. Although olive oil cannot be used as an across-the-board substitute, it works beautifully with bread and vegetables and is a perfect complement to salads. Like all fats, butter and margarine included, the calorie count ranges between 100 and 120 calories per tablespoon, so it's important to work this into your daily calorie equation.

What if you, like me, find the taste of fresh butter irresistible, and don't want to give it up entirely? If you choose to indulge in this little luxury, make sure you do it in moderation. One teaspoon contains 35 calories and has 2.5 grams of saturated fat, or about 15 percent of your daily allotment. That doesn't sound too bad, but if you bump it up to a tablespoon, suddenly you've reached half of your recommended daily saturated fat intake, and 100 calories.

EGGS: IS THERE A SUNNY SIDE?

Years ago, our grandparents, following the wisdom of the day, took it for granted that eggs were part of a healthy and hearty breakfast, second in importance only to bacon and nearly as integral to the morning meal as fried toast. Eggs are still part of many people's mornings, but now that we know about the dangers of cholesterol, they are, often as not, served up with a heaping helping of guilt. Do they deserve this villainous reputation, or have eggs been the victim of a nutritional smear campaign?

We know that cholesterol is linked to heart disease, but in truth, the cholesterol in your diet has a fairly modest impact on your blood levels. That is because your body manufactures about three times as much cholesterol from other types of food you eat, including saturated and trans fats. While it's smart to shy away from high-cholesterol foods, all told, eggs account for only about 30 percent of the cholesterol in the average American's diet. The rest comes mainly from meat and dairy products. One egg provides about 5 grams of total fat, only 1.5 grams of saturated fat, and 200 mg of cholesterol. The total recommended daily intake of cholesterol for most of us is 300 mg; people with heart disease should stick to 200 mg or less.

Although the landmark Framingham heart study, which enrolled thousands of everyday residents of a small Massachusetts town, found no clear association between eggs and blood cholesterol level, another large study found that people who ate six or more eggs per week had nearly three times the risk of heart disease as did those who ate less than one egg per week, all other factors being equal. For reasons that are not entirely clear, diabetics may be especially vulnerable to the harmful effects of eggs.

Eggs are big business, so marketing geniuses have been hard at work trying to turn them into health food. For instance, eggs that are higher in omega-3 fatty acids are now widely available. You may also find "free-range" eggs at your grocery store; the chickens that lay these do not necessarily produce better eggs, unless they are genuinely free-wandering, free-feeding birds like the ones you might find on a small family farm.

Eggs do promote a sense of fullness much more effectively than carbs, so having an egg for breakfast instead of a bagel or muffin may help to cut your cravings for a midmorning snack. They may even give your healthy HDL cholesterol a boost.

My take on eggs is this: It appears that eating one or two eggs once or twice a week is not especially harmful, unless you are diabetic. However, if you choose to eat eggs, it's important to cut back on your other sources of cholesterol.

If you like eggs, you may want to opt for an egg-white omelet, instead of using whole eggs, because the cholesterol is concentrated in the yolk. Eggs are a good source of protein (about 6 grams per egg), a little over half of which is found in the white. If you really enjoy the yolks, use one whole egg together with two or three egg whites, and be sure to cook in olive oil or canola oil, rather than in bacon grease. Egg Beaters and other similar products made from egg whites are a simple way to avoid egg yolks without the mess. Add vegetables, including peppers, tomatoes, onions, and mushrooms, for flavor and texture, and you'll be surprised by how little you miss the yolks.

For baking, egg substitutes are easy to find, and often work remarkably well; tofu and bananas may also be substituted as binders in some recipes.

SODIUM: SHAKING THE HABIT

High blood pressure, or hypertension, is a problem of epic proportions in the United States, afflicting over 70 million Americans, or one in three adults over age 20. High blood pressure is a major contributor to nearly 900,000 heart attacks per year and is also the most important and preventable cause of stroke (see " Know Your Risk Factors," page

349). Each year, up to 2 million more people will develop hypertension, yet only two thirds of those who have high blood pressure even know that they have it. It has been estimated that fewer than half of those treated have an adequately controlled blood pressure of less than 140/90.

There are many factors that contribute to high blood pressure (this will be covered in more detail in chapter 13; see page 203), but for many people, sodium in the diet is a major troublemaker. The chief source of sodium in your diet is salt, although monosodium glutamate (MSG) may also be an important player, particularly in Asian diets. If you have hypertension, especially in the early stages, you may avoid the need for medication simply by cutting back on salt.

The daily minimum requirement of sodium is a mere 500 mg, or about ⅕ teaspoon of salt. Yet the average American consumes on the order of 4,000 mg of sodium a day, or nearly 2 teaspoons of salt. The recommended maximum daily intake of sodium is 2,300 mg for people under 45 and 1,500 mg for people 45 and older and for those with high blood pressure. Fewer than one in ten of us actually meet that goal.

Stanford University researchers estimate that if American adults age 40 and up were able to scale back salt intake by as little as 10 percent, we would prevent more than half a million strokes and nearly as many heart attacks over the course of our lifetime, and save over $32 billion in health-care costs. Other studies suggest that cutting our average sodium by half could save 150,000 lives each year. That's one reason why the government is working with industry to try to make important voluntary changes in the way processed and restaurant foods are prepared.

Who really needs to worry about sodium? People with borderline to high blood pressure stand to benefit most from reducing sodium intake. African Americans, who tend to be more salt sensitive, should be especially vigilant about salt. It behooves anyone with heart disease to cut back. Decreasing salt intake by about half can often drop blood pressure substantially, reducing the risk for stroke, heart attack, kidney failure, and congestive heart failure. A high-salt diet has also been linked to stomach cancer.

Salt and Congestive Heart Failure

Congestive heart failure is an increasingly common condition that occurs when the heart's ability to pump is not sufficient to meet the body's demands. It is characterized by fluid buildup, most notably in the lungs, but also in the soft tissues, especially the legs. (Don't panic. Not everyone with swollen legs has heart failure, although many people do experience swelling in the hands and feet after a salty meal.)

Congestive heart failure may be caused by weakness of the heart muscle, stiffness of the heart muscle, or both. Many factors may play a part in the development of heart failure, but a major player is high blood pressure. People who are afflicted with congestive heart failure are often exquisitely sensitive to salt. For some of these folks, a pepperoni pizza can mean a trip to the emergency room.

Salt may affect overweight people more seriously than those of normal weight. If you are overweight and you eat more than the recommended amount of salt, your risk of congestive heart failure will be 40 percent higher than that of someone whose salt intake falls within the recommended levels.

Who Hid the Salt?

Most of the salt in your diet doesn't come from the salt shaker, but from the salt that has been added to your food before it ever makes it onto your plate. At least 75 percent of the salt you eat is hidden in fast or processed foods. Lunch meats, ham, hot dogs, soups, pizza, pasta sauces, pickles, crackers, chips, and cheeses are all major sodium offenders.

Fast food is a sodium land mine. When you combine a quarter-pound cheeseburger with large fries, you have not only a day's supply of fat, but also nearly 1,500 mg of sodium, or a whole day's worth of sodium if you are over 45. Four slices of sausage pizza or a typical fast-food chicken dinner supplies about 2,300 mg.

Breakfast foods are not necessarily any better. Choose a salted bagel, and you've bought yourself over 4,500 mg of the bad stuff. Even scones have been known to hide upward of 1,750 mg of sodium in their sweet little bodies.

Whether your meal out is a quickie or a fancy sit-down dinner, most chefs play fast and loose with the salt shaker. Pasta dishes and sauces are especially treacherous. Asian food, which is often laced with liberal amounts of soy sauce and MSG, can easily rack up as much as 15 grams of sodium, a staggering ten times the recommended daily limit.

Home cooking doesn't guarantee salt safety if you use premade sauces, packaged products, or canned ingredients. To the uninitiated, product labels can be truly mystifying, so it's important to know how to crack the code before you buy. For instance, "reduced sodium" does not necessarily mean low in sodium. For a product, such as soy sauce or soup, to be labeled this way, it merely needs to contain at least 25 percent less sodium than the regular product. "Light in sodium" is better; that product must contain no more than half of the sodium found in the regular equivalent. "Low sodium" means 140 mg sodium or less per serving, and "very low" means 35 mg sodium or less. The sodium content is included on the standard nutrition labels on all prepared foods, so be sure to check it out before buying.

Getting used to a reduced-salt diet may take a little time, but studies have shown that after two to four months on a low-salt diet, your taste buds will adjust. Cut back gradually and you're more likely to be successful.

KENT, A 50-YEAR-OLD accountant with high blood pressure, was accustomed to meeting with clients at lunchtime, usually at chain restaurants known for their quick lunch service. He never frequented fast-food joints, and assumed that by avoiding burgers and fries, he was being smart about salt. When he came in with a high blood pressure of 150/90 despite taking two blood pressure medications, we took a closer look at his diet and lifestyle. Nutritional information from the restaurant chains was readily available on the Web, and Kent was shocked to find that his meat-and-three-sides meals were loaded with sodium. By making simple changes in his meal choices, asking for sauces on the side, and choosing fresh steamed vegetables, he was able to drop his blood pressure a good 12 points, lose 10 pounds, and avoid a third prescription.

DIVINE CHOCOLATE

In chocolate's scientific name, *Theobroma cacao*, "*theobroma*" translates to "food of the gods," and who can argue with that? A taste of the divine—could it really be so bad?

To the great delight of chocolate lovers everywhere, chocolate turns out to be a very good source of antioxidants known as flavonoids. These antioxidants can prevent LDL cholesterol from inflicting damage on the heart arteries and may reduce inflammation, as measured by CRP. Cocoa also appears to inhibit blood platelet function slightly, meaning that it may have the power to lower the risk of dangerous blood clots. It may even help to bring down blood pressure. All these beneficial properties may account for the happy discovery in 2010 by German scientists that chocolate lovers have about 25 percent fewer heart attacks and nearly 50 percent fewer strokes than those who hardly ever touch the stuff. The catch? Apparently Germans are a bit more restrained than we here in the States. The amount of chocolate eaten each day by the high consumers was on average only about ¼ ounce.

Dark chocolate is much more heart friendly than milk chocolate. When chocolate is combined with milk, its antioxidant properties drop off dramatically. White chocolate, which contains cocoa butter but not cocoa solids, seems to have no antioxidant effect at all.

Complicating matters further, much of the popular dark chocolate that is widely available in this country is actually low in flavonoids. It is the flavonoids that give dark chocolate its bitter taste. Because many Americans have yet to develop a liking for this bitterness, manufacturers often remove the flavonoids from their products. To get your full quotient of antioxidants, look for extra-dark chocolate with high cacao levels of 70 percent or greater.

Despite its potential health benefits, chocolate often travels with some bad-guy ingredients, including sugar, butter, and cream. For instance, a typical 1.6-ounce milk chocolate bar contains 225 calories, 26 grams of carbohydrates, and about 13 grams of fat, 8 of which are saturated fat. Definitely not a heart-smart choice, no matter how loudly it may call your name.

These negative aspects may account for the results of a study conducted by Harvard researchers in conjunction with scientists at Sweden's Karolinska Institute. They found that women who enjoyed anywhere from 1 ounce of chocolate per month to 3 ounces per week had a substantially lower risk of heart failure compared to those who ate no chocolate at all. However, women who ate more than that were statistically more likely to suffer from congestive heart failure, most likely due to the extra calories and saturated fat.

Healthier ways for you to enjoy chocolate include cocoa nibs, which are nuggets of coarsely ground cocoa beans, usually with a little sweetener. Also, you can substitute 3 tablespoons of cocoa powder plus 1 tablespoon of oil for an ounce of baking chocolate in recipes, and while this will not save any calories, it will allow you to substitute a polyunsaturated fat for one that is saturated. Personally, I like to splurge on a really high-quality chocolate bar and savor a small square or two every day. However you choose to enjoy it, it's good to know that this little taste of heaven is no longer entirely taboo.

BEST PRACTICES:
THE EVILDOERS

* If you choose butter, use it in moderation. One teaspoon of butter has 35 calories, 11 grams cholesterol, 4 grams total fat, and 2.5 grams of saturated fat, or about 15% of your daily saturated fat allotment, and virtually no trans fats.

* Avoid stick margarine; it's a potent source of harmful trans fats. Tub or squeeze forms of margarine are safer, since softer margarine has less trans fat.
* Limit whole eggs to 4 or fewer per week. One egg has 5 grams total fat, 1.5 grams saturated fat, and 200 mg of cholesterol. (The total recommended daily intake of cholesterol is 300 mg; 200 mg if you have heart disease.)
* Keep sodium to 2,300 mg daily if you're under 45; cut back to 1,500 mg if you're 45 or older, or have high blood pressure or heart disease.
* Join the dark side: Unlike milk chocolate, dark chocolate is a very good source of antioxidants and might improve lipids, reduce inflammation, lower blood pressure, and reduce the risk of blood clots.
* One quarter of an ounce of dark chocolate daily is all it takes to reduce heart attack risk. More than that and the risk goes up, thanks to excess calories and saturated fat. So do indulge . . . in a square or two per day.

7

The Battle of the Diets

IT'S ONE THING to understand the basic building blocks of a healthy diet. But putting those pieces together can be downright puzzling, especially if you want to lose weight and get healthier at the same time. It's easy to get lured into the newest fad, but fashionable diets tend to run in cycles, just like hemlines and lapels. What's trendy today may not always be what's best for you.

Among the most intriguing and enduring of the popular diets are the high-carbohydrate, low-fat diet; the high-protein, low-carb diet; the Mediterranean diet; the Japanese diet; and the vegetarian diet. Each has its own unique appeal.

Only the high-carb, low-fat and Mediterranean diets have been rigorously studied with respect to their effects on heart health. Both diets came out way ahead when compared to a traditional Western diet.

The high-protein, low-carb diets have been studied in people without heart disease for up to a year, but their long-term effects on heart health and overall health are not known. We do know, however, that a diet high in saturated fat can have harmful effects on the heart and blood vessels, so there is good reason to be suspicious of a regimen that allows unlimited quantities of bacon, beef, and cheese. Remember what your parents and your financial advisor told you: If it sounds too good to be true, it probably is.

THE HIGH-CARBOHYDRATE, LOW-FAT DIET

Given what we know about the importance of fruit, vegetables, and whole grains, it is no wonder that many cardiovascular specialists have recommended choosing a diet chock-full of these healthy high-carb foods. In the 1980s, Dr. Dean Ornish, a cardiologist and research scientist who is a prominent advocate of a high-carbohydrate, low-fat diet, proposed a radical shift in the way Americans eat and live. He advised that no more than 10 percent of our daily calories should come from fats and that complex carbohydrates should account for the majority of calories (about 70 percent). This recommendation is in stark contrast to the typical American diet, which breaks down to about 35 percent fat, 50 percent carbohydrate (primarily simple carbs), and 15 percent protein. Dr. Ornish's plan also bans cholesterol entirely, whereas the standard-issue American diet includes up to 500 mg of cholesterol daily.

The complex carbs in Dr. Ornish's diet specifically include whole grains, fruit, vegetables, and legumes. Highly processed, high-glycemic carbs such as cookies, white breads, and white pasta are not permitted. Limiting these "white" foods is crucial, as a diet with a high glycemic load is linked to a greater likelihood of heart attacks, stroke, and diabetes.

In a study of forty-eight highly motivated people with heart disease (thirty-five of whom actually stuck it out and completed the study), Dr. Ornish and his colleagues at California Pacific Medical Center were able to show a modest reversal of cholesterol plaques in the heart arteries after just one year by introducing a whole-foods vegetarian diet, combined with an intensive lifestyle modification, blending aerobic exercise, yoga, stress management, group therapy, and smoking cessation. In contrast, those people enrolled in the study who turned down the opportunity to take part in Dr. Ornish's admittedly rigorous therapy showed measurably more cholesterol buildup.

After five years, the results were even stronger for the low-fat vegetarian group, whereas people who did not participate had further growth of their cholesterol plaques. What's worse, their blockages were more unstable, putting them at higher risk for a heart attack. In fact, the risk of a heart attack or other cardiovascular problems was nearly two and a half times greater in those who did not follow Dr. Ornish's regimen. People who stuck to the program also lost weight (about 24 pounds on average) and kept about half of that weight off over five years.

Was it the low-fat vegetarian diet, was it the dramatic lifestyle changes, or were both equally important? There is no way to know for sure. One blow to the theory that it was the low-fat diet alone that made the difference was the Women's Health Initiative Dietary Modification study of nearly sixty thousand women, which found no reduction in cardiovascular or cancer risk in postmenopausal women who followed a diet that limited fat to just 20 percent of daily calories for eight years. Nevertheless, Dr. Ornish has convincing, long-term data, a claim that devotees of most other diets cannot make.

Why Doesn't Everyone Eat This Way?

What could be wrong with the high-carb, extremely low-fat approach? It goes without saying that it is tough for most people to stay the course with this type of diet. Furthermore, several decades ago, when the high-carbohydrate diet was originally developed, research regarding the importance of healthy fats was just emerging. A diet this restrictive essentially excludes nuts, seeds, and fish, all of which are now known to be associated with a lower risk of heart disease, stroke, and, in the case of nuts, diabetes.

Only small amounts of omega-3 fatty acids are allowed on a very low-fat diet. That's a serious omission, because these good fats, along with monounsaturated fats such as olive oil, benefit cholesterol and other lipid levels.

As it turns out, a diet very high in carbohydrates and very low in fat will lower not only LDL cholesterol, but also HDL cholesterol. Excessively low levels of HDL are associated with a higher risk of heart disease. Proponents of this diet counter that the reduction in HDL produced by this regimen may not bring on the same repercussions as low HDL due to other dietary and lifestyle conditions, but the issue remains controversial.

Triglycerides may also increase with a high-carb diet, although this is more of an issue with simple "white" carbs, which are not sanctioned by Dr. Ornish. Finally, in a very low-fat diet, vitamin D levels may be inadequate, particularly if the diet includes few or no animal products.

LET ME SHARE one example with you of how following a high-carb diet can go awry. My patient Sherry, a diabetic, was 58 years old and determined to get back into shape after her office visit revealed high blood pressure and a weight gain of 15 pounds over the past year. She and her husband joined a gym, signed up with a personal trainer, and began working out religiously. When Sherry came back to see me a few months later, her blood pressure was nearly normal, and her weight had dropped a full 10 pounds.

At first, I couldn't explain why, with these stellar improvements, her HDL cholesterol had dropped by more than 30 percent, her triglycerides had doubled, and her blood sugar was elevated, while her LDL had not budged. When I quizzed her about her diet, the puzzle was solved.

Sherry's trainer, an enthusiastic guy in his early 20s, had explained that because she was working out harder, she needed to eat more simple carbs such as pasta and rice, and Sherry had followed this recommendation with gusto. Unfortunately, this was absolutely terrible advice. Even worse, Sherry was diabetic, so she was extremely sensitive to the sugar-raising effects of these simple carbohydrates. Many trainers are simply not qualified to give nutritional guidance, no matter how sincere their intentions may be. Fortunately, we caught the problem early, and Sherry is now back on track.

THE HIGH-CARBOHYDRATE, LOW-FAT DIET

BENEFITS

* Seventy percent of calories come from carbohydrates, 20% from protein, and 10% from fats, with no cholesterol.
* Highly refined, high-glycemic carbohydrates such as "white" foods are not part of this plan. Better choices include whole grains, fruits, vegetables, and legumes.
* Combining this diet with intensive lifestyle changes helps reverse heart disease.

DRAWBACKS

* This regimen can be difficult to stick to because you may not feel full.
* The original diet lacks nuts, seeds, and fatty fish, which means that you will not get enough omega-3 fats for optimal heart health. Your HDL (good) cholesterol may drop and triglycerides may increase.
* Your vitamin D level may drop.

THE HIGH-PROTEIN, LOW-CARBOHYDRATE DIET

It is hard to imagine that a diet that is, in essence, the opposite of Dr. Ornish's program, could inspire similar weight loss and health claims—but that is exactly what devotees of the high-protein, low-carb, high-fat diets contend.

This regimen, sometimes referred to as a ketogenic diet, takes many forms. Versions of it have been around since the 1860s. Contemporary adaptations include the Atkins and Stillman diets, the South Beach Diet™, and the Zone Diet™.

In general, a high-protein, low-carbohydrate diet provides 30 to 60 percent of its calories from protein, 5 to 15 percent from carbohydrates, and up to 55 percent from fat. Because free access to protein-rich, high-fat foods, such as steak, eggs, and bacon, is a cornerstone of many of these diets, they have been wholeheartedly adopted by millions of people who have found the low-fat approach too difficult or unpalatable. Many people have indeed lost weight using these programs. Whether they've kept it off is another story. Most have not.

Just how does a high-protein diet work? Like other diets, it restricts the number of calories consumed. A diet like this also holds a few tricks up its sleeve. Although the pounds may seem to melt off very quickly in the beginning, most of this early weight loss turns out to be water loss, or what we medical types call diuresis. Because high-carb foods often hold water within people's intestines, doing away with these foods means there is less water in the body, and hence a lower number on the bathroom scale.

After one to two weeks on the diet, ketosis begins. In ketosis, fat is broken down for use as fuel by the body. This fat breakdown produces substances called ketone bodies. You can even test your urine with special dipsticks to see if this process is taking place. (This type of ketosis should not be confused with diabetic ketoacidosis, a life-threatening condition that may occur in uncontrolled diabetics, but has only been reported on rare occasion in people following an extreme low-carb diet.) Although advocates of low-carb diets may claim otherwise, ketosis is not necessary for weight loss, nor is it desirable.

Ketosis in animals has been well observed, particularly in dairy cattle following calving. I found this description of ketosis in cattle, published in the Pennsylvania State Extension circular #372: "The animals usually have a gaunt appearance and milk production is decreased. Cows may appear depressed, restricted in their movements, their hair coat may appear rough, and their eyes may be glazed. Their breath may have a characteristic odor of ketones." Happily, "death from ketosis rarely occurs." Still, not very attractive, is it? In fact, ketosis is well known to cause halitosis (bad breath—or should we call it cow breath?) and constipation in humans. Ketosis breath has even been mistaken for the presence of alcohol, as one hapless airline pilot on this diet discovered when he was detained by airport police.

Does a Low-Carb Diet Work?

On the surface, the low-carb, high-protein, high-fat diet appears to be counterintuitive and perhaps even harmful. Indeed, it may well be, but some interesting research studies do validate some of the many claims made.

Without a doubt, such diets may help to improve the lipid profile, facilitate weight loss, and reduce body fat when combined with exercise and a good dose of motivation.

In fact, the high-protein, low-carb diet comes out a little ahead of the low-fat diet in terms of weight loss and lipids. However, the fix is not that simple. Overall, it appears that the weight loss achieved on a low-carb diet is not due to any magic formula, but simply to a reduced caloric intake. Although it is true that both high-fat and low-fat diets may improve blood pressure, this benefit appears to be directly related to weight loss. High-fat diets in which weight loss does not occur are well known to elevate blood pressure, and we have known for centuries that a richer diet raises the risk for gout.

It may just be that these diets are easier to stick with than those of the low-fat variety. This was the conclusion of a group from Stanford that painstakingly evaluated 107 articles in the medical literature that reported data on a combined total of 3,268 participants. And there are some potentially harmful side effects of this diet that its proponents do not publicize.

The Perils of the High-Protein, Low-Carb Diet

The high-protein, low-carb diet poses significant dangers for anyone at risk for heart disease, and may lead to osteoporosis, kidney disease, or cancer.

After a meal high in saturated fat (for instance, steak, pork, or cheese), a load of these nasty fats is dumped into the bloodstream and circulates through the arteries, reaching every organ in your body. The immediate result is that the arteries become stiffer and less flexible. This effect lasts at least six hours, increasing your vulnerability to heart attacks.

Higher-fat diets also are associated with higher levels of fibrinogen, a clotting factor, in the bloodstream, raising the susceptibility to blood clots, strokes, and heart attacks. Saturated fats may also increase blood levels of LDL, homocysteine, CRP, and Lp(a) (see chapter 3, page 26).

A study from Oxford University in England evaluated the effects of a high-fat diet on mental function in healthy men in their 20s. After five days on a 75-percent fat diet (probably typical dorm room fare), the guys had a harder time concentrating, showed slower thought processes, and were more likely to be moody and negative. Despite their youth and good health, most participants' hearts also became measurably stiffer.

A high-protein diet can deplete calcium levels, which may lead to osteoporosis, or weakening of the bones. In fact, bone fractures are more common in women who eat excessive amounts of protein. Because calcium loss occurs through the urine, kidney stones are another unintended side effect of a high-protein diet.

In people who have chronic kidney disease, high-protein diets may stress the kidneys beyond what is safe and contribute to the progression of kidney failure. The American Kidney Foundation has advised against extremely high-protein diets and has suggested that the maximum safe level of protein intake in healthy people without kidney problems should be considered 2 grams per kilogram of body weight. For a 150-pound person, this would equal about 140 grams of protein, which is still substantial.

Finally, by avoiding healthy carbohydrates such as fruit, vegetables, and whole grains, and by increasing red meat, the probability of developing colon and rectal cancers rises. Women who eat more red meat also appear to be more prone to breast cancer, particularly the hormone receptor positive form of the disease.

If a high-protein diet still intrigues you, consider going vegetarian. Tofu and other high-protein soy foods are cheap, versatile, and heart friendly. Harvard researchers who evaluated up to twenty-six years of diet diaries from over eighty-five thousand women and forty-four thousand men reported that those who followed a meat-based low-carb diet had a 23 percent greater risk of death compared to those who chose a high-carb diet. In contrast, a vegetarian low-carb diet meant a 20 percent lower risk of dying over the study period.

THE HIGH-PROTEIN, LOW-CARBOHYDRATE DIET

BENEFITS

* Weight loss in the first 2 weeks is mainly water. After that, the diet works by simply reducing calories consumed.
* The diet may improve lipids and blood sugar, but this is mainly due to weight loss.

DRAWBACKS

* Stiffening of arteries
* Increased risk of blood clots
* Increased levels of LDL, homocysteine, CRP, and Lp(a)
* Decreased mental clarity and mood
* Osteoporosis
* Increased risk of breast cancer and colorectal cancer
* Kidney stones, and worsening of kidney function in diabetics and others who have kidney disease

THE MEDITERRANEAN DIET

As a nation, we are unrivaled in our innovation, leadership, and individualism. But when it comes to diet, we still have a lot to learn.

In 1970, the landmark Seven Countries Study began to explore heart disease risk factors in seven countries, including five European nations, Japan, and the United States.

Overall, the investigators tracked more than twelve thousand men aged 40 to 59, in sixteen different centers. In 1995, twenty-five years later, researchers reported follow-up data on these men, who had by then reached the age range of 65 to 85.

Across the years, clear-cut differences in health and prevalence of disease emerged, fundamentally transforming our understanding of nutrition and culture. The divergence in mortality rates was stunning. After statistical adjustment to account for the variations in the ages of the men who were studied, the Japanese mortality rate from heart disease was only 3.2 percent at the twenty-five-year point; in Mediterranean Europe, 4.7 percent. The highest mortality from heart disease was found in Northern Europe, weighing in at 20.3 percent, followed by the United States at 16 percent.

Even more intriguing was the observation that at similar cholesterol levels, the Japanese and Mediterraneans had only half to one third the number of heart disease deaths as did citizens of the United States and Northern Europe.

For example, at a total cholesterol level of 210 mg/dL, the twenty-five-year mortality rate from heart disease in Japan and Mediterranean Europe was 4 to 5 percent, as compared to 10 percent in inland Southern Europe, 12 percent in the United States, and 15 percent in Northern Europe. It was obvious that there was something that the Mediterranean and Japanese people were doing right which people in the other countries were doing wrong. That vital factor turned out to be the traditional diets of these regions.

Although it may sound exotic, the Mediterranean diet is based on whole grains, green vegetables, fruit, olive oil, and fish—foods that are readily available, easy to prepare, and, for the most part, reasonably familiar to our taste buds. Tomatoes, onions, garlic, and herbs are also integral to this cuisine. Wine is part of the culture and typically enjoyed with the evening meal.

The Seven Countries Study focused on the diet of the inhabitants of the Greek island of Crete, an ecosystem that provides an exceptionally rich variety of heart-protecting foods. Citizens of Crete consumed up to thirty times more fish than did a typical North American in the 1970s. And although beef is eaten on occasion, the cattle in Crete are traditionally grazing animals, resulting in higher levels of omega-3 fatty acids in Mediterranean beef than in typical factory farm–raised American animals.

Likewise, the chickens in Crete are free-roaming, with a substantial portion of their diet coming from local plants, including purslane, which is rich in omega-3 fatty acids. Consequently, the omega-6 to omega-3 ratio in Cretan eggs is estimated to be 1:3, as compared to the U.S. ratio of 19:4 (see page 71 for more about this ratio).

Countering the conventional low-fat wisdom, the fat content of the Mediterranean diet works out to about 30 to 35 percent of daily calories. The critical difference is that its artery-clogging saturated fat content is no more than 8 percent, and there are no trans fats whatsoever.

On this diet, the daily intake of protein is around 15 percent, and of cholesterol, approximately 200 mg (about the equivalent of one egg). Not only do people on the Mediterranean diet have lower cholesterol levels than inhabitants of the United States and Northern Europe (averaging 200 mg/dL as compared to 240–255 mg/dL), but also, even when we compare people with the same cholesterol levels, we find a lower risk of heart disease among Mediterranean diners. This finding is thought to be due to the effect of dietary antioxidants on LDL cholesterol in the bloodstream, which prevents LDL cholesterol from becoming oxidized and thus more damaging to the blood vessel walls.

It doesn't hurt that people who follow a Mediterranean diet are 40 percent less likely to be obese than are those whose diet more closely resembles our standard Western diet.

Adding Years to a Healthy Life

Although this healthy way of eating makes sense, some would debate that perhaps it is not the diet at all but something else the Mediterraneans are doing right. Without a doubt, they do have a more active lifestyle and perhaps a lower level of stress as well.

To help shed some light on the matter, in the late 1980s to early 1990s, researchers in Lyons, France, decided to put the diet to the test in heart attack survivors. About six hundred patients under the age of 70 who had suffered a heart attack within the past six months were randomly assigned to a Mediterranean diet plan or usual care. The experimental subjects were told to increase green vegetables, root vegetables, breads, and fish and to reduce the amount of red meat in their diet by replacing it with poultry. They also ate fruit every day and replaced their butter with a special canola oil–based margarine and olive oil. Wine with meals was encouraged.

A little more than two years later, sixteen people had died of heart disease in the usual care group, as compared to only three in the Mediterranean diet group. When adjusted for other variables, the overall risk reduction for cardiovascular death in the Mediterranean group was a stunning 76 percent, despite the fact that there was no major difference in cholesterol profiles between the two groups.

Four years later, this way of eating provided sustained protection, with a 47 percent reduction in the combined incidence of heart attack, unstable heart disease, stroke, heart failure, pulmonary emboli (blood clots in the lungs), and blood clots in the legs. Even more surprising, there were no major differences in weight, blood pressure, or cholesterol profiles between groups, although those with lower cholesterol levels fared even better.

Those whose blood work indicated a high level of dietary omega-3s (meaning that they ate more fish) were at a greater advantage, because their risk of heart disease was lower still. Remarkably, the Mediterranean group also benefited from a 61 percent reduction in the risk of cancer, including breast cancer. Other studies report a lower likelihood of colorectal cancer.

More recently, researchers in Greece followed more than twenty-two thousand apparently healthy adults for nearly four years and reported their findings in 2003. Those who adhered to a more traditional Mediterranean diet had one third fewer deaths from heart disease and 24 percent fewer cancer deaths than did those whose diet skewed more Western. The benefit held true irrespective of gender, smoking status, or physical activity. When the elements of the diet were broken down, there was no one food or component of the diet that appeared to be more important than the others.

In other studies, the Mediterranean-style diet consistently comes out ahead. Blood glucose levels, insulin levels, and blood pressure are lower, and the cholesterol profile improves. People with the metabolic syndrome (see chapter 13, page 235), who are at high risk for diabetes and heart disease, have been able to slow down or even reverse this process by following a Mediterranean-style diet. The immune system improves, and blood levels of inflammation drop.

Mental health also improves with a Mediterranean diet. Depression is less prevalent, and, in the elderly, brain function seems to be more stable and less prone to decline.

Remember, this diet is based on the heart-healthy diet of the Greek isle of Crete, not the menu at your favorite Italian restaurant! Foods of the Mediterranean are easily found at your grocery store and, depending on your taste, can be prepared very simply or with great complexity. The effects can be profound. A 50 to 70 percent reduction in heart attacks and strokes is far greater than can be achieved with almost any single drug. These nourishing foods have the potential to add years of good health to your life.

Your shopping list is simple: fresh vegetables and fruit, nuts, legumes, unrefined cereals, fish, and monounsaturated fats such as olive oil and canola oil. If wine is appropriate for you, enjoy it in moderation. This diet is easily adaptable to a vegetarian or vegan regimen.

For recipes and meal plans to get you started, check out Dr. Angelo Acquista and Laurie Ann Vandermolen's *The Mediterranean Prescription: Meal Plans and Recipes to Help You Stay Slim and Healthy for the Rest of Your Life* (Ballantine Books, 2006).

THE MEDITERRANEAN DIET

BENEFITS

* Thirty to 35% of calories come from fat (but only 7–8% from saturated fat), 15% from protein, and 50% from carbs.
* The Mediterranean diet may lower heart disease risk by 33–70%, and cut cancer risk by 25–60%.
* Blood glucose levels, insulin levels, and blood pressure are lower, and the cholesterol profile improves.

DRAWBACKS

* None

THE JAPANESE DIET

While the Mediterranean diet is easy for our Western palate to love, the Seven Countries study also highlighted the diet and way of life in Okinawa, a dazzling string of 161 islands located between Japan and Taiwan. Traditional Okinawans enjoy excellent health and remarkable longevity.

Until 1985, when fast food began oozing its way across Japan, the age-adjusted death rate from cardiovascular disease in Okinawa was less than one fifth that of the United States and 30 to 40 percent lower than Japan's national average.

The traditional Okinawan diet is really very humble. The Japanese sweet potato (*Ipomoea batatas*) takes the place of rice and provides a major source of energy. Austrian researchers have found that an extract from this sweet potato may help to improve diabetes control and possibly even lower cholesterol.

Seaweed, soy, herbaceous plants, fish, and jasmine green tea are also important elements. Protein accounts for just 10 to 20 percent of daily calories. Fish and soy are the chief sources of protein, with negligible amounts coming from meat, poultry, and eggs. At least 80 percent of the diet is plant based, and the fat content, at about 30 percent, is mainly polyunsaturated.

One fascinating aspect of the traditional Okinawan diet is its low caloric content. The people of this culture follow a charming custom of eating until just about 80 percent full. Not only does this restriction help to keep them lean (the average BMI in Okinawan elders is 18 to 22), it also may help to explain why they live longer.

There seems to be a key difference between maintaining weight by burning off more energy than we eat, and simply eating fewer calories. The major theory that explains this important effect of calorie restriction upon life span is that of reduced oxidative stress. What this means is that free radicals, which are generally damaging to the cells of the body and are considered to be responsible in large part for the aging process, are limited when we eat less. Less food means fewer of the harmful chemicals that are part and parcel of the food we eat. For traditional Okinawans, daily caloric intake is estimated to be 17 percent lower in adults and 36 percent lower in children than the Japanese national average.

Back home in the United States, the Harvard Alumni Health Study and the Nurses' Health Study have both found overall lower mortality in people with a BMI 15 to 20 percent below average. Whether these slimmer folks ate less or exercised more is not established, but most likely both healthy habits contributed to the lower body weight.

Perhaps as important as diet is the Okinawan lifestyle. Members of this culture tend to be physically and mentally active throughout their entire lives. Moderation is viewed as a virtue, smoking is uncommon, and optimism is rampant. Spirituality is an important part of traditional daily life. Not surprisingly, the incidence of dementia is low.

Because of the global reach of Western diet and lifestyle, many younger Okinawans have fallen prey to fast food. In fact, Okinawa can now boast the greatest concentration of fast-food restaurants per capita in all of Japan, and Okinawans on average are currently the heaviest people in the country. Longevity has plummeted, especially for men, who seem to be more easily influenced by the abundance of fast food.

THE JAPANESE DIET

BENEFITS
* In this diet, 20% of calories come from protein, 30% from fat (mostly polyunsaturated), and about 50% from carbs.
* The principal protein sources are fish and soy. The diet also includes sweet potato, seaweed, herbaceous plants, and green tea.
* Okinawans stop eating when they are 80% full. Studies show restricted calories lead to a longer life.
* Okinawan elders have one fifth the risk of heart disease as Americans, and live healthier and longer lives.

DRAWBACKS
* To Westerners, the optimal foods of this diet may not be as appealing as other healthy diet choices.

THE VEGETARIAN DIET

The term *vegetarian* is rather vague, and encompasses a diverse group of vegans and variously lacto-ovo vegetarians. A vegan eats absolutely no animal-derived products and therefore avoids dairy foods and eggs. Lacto-ovo vegetarians include dairy (lacto) and eggs (ovo) in their diet; some vegetarians are strictly lacto or ovo. These distinctions are important, because dairy products and eggs are important sources of protein, but they also supply saturated fats and cholesterol. Vegans by and large consume extremely low amounts of saturated fats and no cholesterol.

The Oxford Vegetarian Study, based in England, included six thousand vegetarians and five thousand nonvegetarians. The meat eaters included in this study were friends and relatives of the vegetarians who were recruited for the study. Detailed information on diet and lifestyle was obtained, and the participants were followed for about twelve years.

Taken as a whole, everyone, vegetarian or not, had a lower death rate than the national average. The investigators speculated that this was because the vegetarians tended to be healthier people in general, and so their nonvegetarian friends and relatives were also more likely to lead a healthy lifestyle.

Despite the overall good health in this study, some very important differences emerged. For instance, after twelve years, the vegetarians had a 20 percent lower risk of death from all causes and a 27 percent lower risk of death from heart disease. Among the meat eaters, the risk of heart disease death progressively climbed as their animal fat intake rose, such that the top third of animal fat consumers were more than three times as likely to die from heart disease, when compared to their veggie friends.

A National Institutes of Health study of about half a million Americans aged 50 and up confirmed the potential harm of a meat-based diet. Those who ate just 4 ounces of beef or pork every day had a 30 percent higher mortality, including heart disease and cancer, compared to those who ate no red meat at all.

Finding Balance

Is a vegetarian diet all good? Not necessarily. Vegans, and some vegetarians, are more likely to be deficient in vitamin B_{12}, a condition that can usually be rectified with supplements. We all need B_{12}, but the issue becomes critically important during pregnancy. (Read more about B vitamins in chapter 14; see page 259.)

As with any sort of diet, balance is essential. Lacto- and/or ovo-vegetarians have it a little easier than vegans, as the former eat complete proteins, which supply all the essential amino acids, in the form of dairy products and/or eggs. (Essential amino acids are those that the body cannot manufacture itself, making the diet the only source of these nutrients.) For vegans, obtaining a sufficient amount of protein may get tricky but is usually not a major problem. For example, soy, unlike most plant products, is a complete and versatile protein. Other vegan protein sources include grains, seeds, nuts, and legumes.

Although it is not crucial to incorporate all of the essential amino acids at every meal, it is important to get an adequate amount of essential amino acids over the course of the day. This requirement is not complicated. Broadly speaking, a complete protein meal can be accomplished by combining legumes with grains. That can be as simple as beans with brown rice or peanut butter on whole wheat bread.

AFTER HER SECOND heart attack, my patient Lila decided that enough was enough. Due to side effects, she was only able to tolerate a low dose of cholesterol medication, and her LDL remained much higher than was optimal. Although she came from a family of meat eaters, she decided that it was time for a change and made the switch to a vegetarian diet. Three months later, her LDL had dropped 40 points, her mind felt clearer, and her energy level soared.

Getting Enough Omega-3s

Although it's easy to get plenty of protein with a vegetarian diet, it can be difficult for vegetarians to include enough of the omega-3 fatty acids that are vital to cardiovascular health.

Flaxseeds and walnuts are two good vegetarian sources of omega-3 fatty acids. However, although walnuts supply more omega-3s than other nuts, the percentage of these fatty acids in walnut oil is fairly low, weighing in at less than 10 percent. Flaxseed oil is a great supplemental choice for vegetarians, as it contains 57 percent omega-3 and 17 percent omega-6 fatty acids. Flaxseed oil must be refrigerated, or it quickly goes rancid. And because it breaks down when exposed to direct heat, this oil cannot be used in cooking, although it is a heart-smart complement to salads, pasta, and vegetables. Some people even drizzle it on their morning oatmeal.

Flaxseed oil capsules, which you'll read more about in chapter 15 (see page 283), are a reasonable alternative. Whole flaxseeds are not useful because they just pass through the body undigested; flaxseeds need to be ground or crushed to be digestible. Ground flaxseeds (look for these in the specialty flours aisle) can be sprinkled on salads and cereal, and, when beaten with water, can even serve as a vegan substitute for eggs in baked goods.

One caveat: Excessive amounts of flaxseed oil can interfere with normal functioning of the thyroid gland by affecting iodine uptake. For this reason, limit flaxseed oil to no more than 4 tablespoons per day.

Although it is the best vegetarian alternative, flaxseed oil cannot hold a candle to fish oil. Whereas your body can put fish oil to work right away, the omega-3 fatty acid that comes from plant sources (known as ALA, or alpha-linolenic acid) must be converted by special enzymes before it can be used effectively. This chemical process is slow and not very efficient, and it can be hindered by saturated fat, trans fat, cholesterol, and alcohol. An extremely low-protein diet can also impede this process.

Because omega-3 and omega-6 fatty acids compete for the same enzymes, foods high in omega-6 fats, including corn oil, sunflower oil, and safflower oil, can interfere with the body's ability to make use of the omega-3 fatty acids. A smarter choice is olive oil, a monounsaturated fat that minds its own business and does not influence this conversion process.

THE VEGETARIAN DIET

BENEFITS

- Vegetarians tend to live longer and have less heart disease than nonvegetarians do.
- Protein sources for vegans include soy (a complete protein), grains, seeds, and nuts. Lacto-ovo vegetarians also get protein from dairy products and eggs.

DRAWBACKS

- Vegetarians may lack omega-3 fatty acids. However, flaxseed oil and walnuts are reasonably good sources.
- Strict vegans need vitamin B_{12} supplements to maintain good health.

BATTLE OF THE DIETS: WHO WINS?

When it comes down to it, what you really need to know is: What is the "right way" to eat?

■ LOW-FAT: THE ORNISH WAY

The results achieved by Dr. Ornish and others who espouse the low-fat approach are impressive, but diet was only part of the program. Lifestyle modification was tremendously important in the studies reported, and the drop-out rate was high.

■ HIGH-PROTEIN: THE ATKINS ROUTE

If you take the other extreme, by following an Atkins-style high-protein, low-carbohydrate diet, you will lose weight more quickly, but much of that will be an illusion, as the initial weight loss is substantially water weight. Longer term, the weight loss may be a little more significant than with the low-fat approach, but that is due to reduced calorie consumption, not to any magical effect of ketosis.

Fruit, vegetables, and whole grains are critical for a healthy heart, brain, and digestive system, but are in short supply in most diets of this type. People who choose these diets run the risk of being deficient in the many phytochemicals (vitamins, minerals, and more) present in produce.

Because we do know that saturated fats, abundant in meat and dairy products, have both immediate and long-term harmful effects on the heart arteries, I can't recommend this type of diet to you, especially if animal fats are the principal fat source. If you'd like to try a modified and more heart-smart version, cardiologist Dr. Arthur Agatson's *The South Beach Diet* (St. Martin's Griffin, 2005) is a sensible option.

The Three Most Heart-Healthy Diets

■ DINING ON THE MEDITERRANEAN

The Mediterranean style of eating makes a great deal of sense and is my diet of choice. Fruit, vegetables, monounsaturated fats, omega-3 fatty acids, and moderate amounts of alcohol are the backbone of this regimen. All of these elements are easy to find, taste great, and require as much or as little effort as you are willing to spare. There is enough healthy fat so that you won't feel deprived, and the variety of foods and flavors is broad. This nutritional approach has been studied in non-Mediterranean cultures and even in vegetarians with highly favorable outcomes. Who can find fault with a simple and delicious diet that has the potential to reduce heart disease by 50 percent or more?

■ HOW THE OKINAWANS DO IT

Likewise, the diet of the Okinawans gives us plenty of food for thought. We have gotten ourselves into a world of trouble by believing that we must continue to eat until our ever-expanding belly tells us to stop. The importance of finishing a meal before feeling completely full is profound and may be the most important lesson the Okinawans can teach us. (Whatever diet you choose to follow, stopping before you feel full is a healthy practice to begin.) While the joys of Japanese cuisine may elude you, the key components of the Okinawan diet—fish, soy, brightly colored vegetables, and green tea—are known for their heart protective effects and are readily available at virtually any grocery store. Give at least some of these elements a try.

■ LIFE AMONG THE VEGGIES

A vegetarian lifestyle makes a great deal of sense on many levels. The only important drawback from the standpoint of heart health is the absence of coldwater fish, with their rich supply of omega-3 fatty acids. Flaxseed oil is a reasonable alternative, but vegetarians will need to pay close attention to get enough omega-3 fatty acids to achieve heart protection on par with fish eaters. Vegans need to be sure to supplement with vitamin B_{12}.

BEST PRACTICES:
YOUR DIET

* In my view, your best bet is the Mediterranean diet, which offers the broadest menu and heart-health benefits of fresh produce, whole grains, fish, legumes, and healthy oils.
* If the Japanese diet as a whole is too stringent to appeal, at least incorporate its philosophy—stop before you feel full—and some of its foods into your lifestyle.
* Likewise, if going the vegetarian route feels difficult for you, just scheduling a meatless day once or twice per week will be beneficial to your health. Vegetarian and vegan cuisine has come a long way since the earnest yet inedible fare you may remember from the 1960s and '70s!

You might not be ready or inclined to go whole-hog vegetarian, so to speak, but planning a meat-free day or two each week is a smart way to begin making simple and life-affirming changes that may have far-reaching effects on your health and well-being. Integrate elements of the Mediterranean and Okinawan diets, and the food you eat could truly save your life.

8

The Big Fake-Out: The Skinny on Sweeteners and Other Food Fakes

A RE SUGAR AND FAT substitutes better for you? Are they even safe?

SUGAR: THE REAL THING

When it comes to sugar, our brain tends to go a little gooey. Sugar is the original sweetener, and the average American shovels in more than 135 pounds of it per year, much of it from sugar-saturated soft drinks; children may put away even more. Our addiction to sugar has fueled the burgeoning rates of diabetes and obesity in adults and kids alike. Pancreatic cancer has also been linked to high levels of sugar consumption. How can something so sweet be so destructive?

Most table sugar, or sucrose, starts out as sugar cane and sugar beets. That sounds simple enough. Your body breaks the sugar molecule down into glucose and fructose, two simpler sugars that are easily absorbed. Fructose, which is also the sugar found in fruit, is taken up by your bloodstream a little slower than glucose is, because it has to be converted into glucose by your liver before it can be used.

Despite its bad rep, sugar delivers only 16 calories per teaspoon. So a teaspoon or even two in your tea is really no big deal, unless you're a diabetic. But a soft drink is not such innocent fun. Chug a single can of soda pop, and you've bought yourself the equivalent of a whopping

10 teaspoons of table sugar. Just for kicks, measure out 10 teaspoons of sugar and see what that looks like. Shocking, isn't it? And when taken in quantities that large, sugar, the ultimate simple carbohydrate, provokes wild swings in blood glucose levels, setting you up for the cycle of sugar highs followed by those awful sugar cravings that will inevitably sneak in, fooling you into thinking you're hungry for more.

High-Fructose Corn Syrup

Corn syrup is the base for most commercial sugar sweeteners. In its natural state, corn syrup is mainly glucose, but it is chemically processed in such a way that it becomes higher in fructose, making it more stable. This form of sugar, known as high-fructose corn syrup (HFCS), is typically found in soft drinks and snack foods such as cookies, cakes, and crackers. Manufacturers prefer HFCS because it is less expensive than sugar, mixes well with other ingredients, and helps to retain product freshness. Thanks to HFCS, commercially baked goods, such as breads and cookies, stay soft and chewy.

Fructose occurs naturally in fruits and vegetables, honey, and molasses, but we eat relatively modest servings of these foods. Thanks to the pervasiveness of HFCS-loaded commercial products, Americans glug and gobble on average about 63 pounds of HFCS each year, about half of our entire sugar consumption and up to 10 percent of our total caloric intake.

Our industrial reliance on HFCS has spawned a number of myths as well as legitimate concerns about its use. One myth, that HFCS affects our ability to sense fullness, or satiety, was disproven in two studies reported in 2007, one conducted by research scientists at the University of Toronto, and the other by Dutch researchers. So far there is no convincing evidence that HFCS, in and of itself, leads to overeating any more than do other forms of sugar. But, like other refined sugars, HFCS clearly contributes to high triglycerides and low HDL cholesterol.

A legitimate concern is the possible connection between excessive fructose and pancreatic cancer. At the University of California, Los

Angeles, research lab, pancreatic cancer cells were fired up by fructose, using it to rapidly create new cancer cells, whereas sucrose had a much less powerful effect.

The Sugar Trap

Sugary soft drinks are an unmitigated health hazard, concealing 150 calories in one 12-ounce can. They are the greatest single source of sugar, typically in the form of HFCS, in the American diet and one of the easiest ways there is to pack on the weight. Drink twenty-three sodas in a month, less than one per day, and you've just bought yourself a pound. Voilà! In a year, you've gained 12 pounds, without even trying. Women who drink at least one soda a day are nearly twice as likely to become diabetic as are those who rarely drink these beverages.

▪ SACCHARIN

Saccharin is three hundred to seven hundred times sweeter than sugar. Although high doses of saccharin have been linked to the development of bladder tumors in rats, a human cancer connection has never been proven. The FDA considers saccharin safe for human consumption. (Nevertheless, you might want to avoid feeding it to your pet rat.) The sweetener Sweet'n Low contains saccharin.

▪ ASPARTAME

Aspartame, a chemical blend of two amino acids, phenylalanine and aspartic acid, is about 200 times sweeter than sugar. It is used in many commercial foods, including cereals, yogurt, ice cream, and, of course, soft drinks and other beverages. NutraSweet and Equal are well-known brands containing aspartame. The maximal accepted daily dose is 40 mg per kilogram of body weight, or about 2,800 mg for a 150-pound person. A can of diet soda contains less than 100 mg of aspartame.

A HEALTH WARNING:
IF YOU HAVE PHENYLKETONURIA, AVOID ASPARTAME

BECAUSE PEOPLE WITH phenylketonuria cannot break down phenyl-alanine, those with this rare genetic abnormality must steer clear of aspartame. This condition is typically diagnosed at birth with a routine blood test. A phenylketonuric person exposed to phenylalanine may suffer severe brain damage. This is why standard label warnings are required for packaged products made with the sweetener.

Is Aspartame Safe?

Since aspartame's approval by the FDA, many anecdotal reports have suggested neurological dangers, including brain tumors, seizures, and headaches. The aspartame brain cancer scare, which arose in 1996, was quickly debunked when it was shown that aspartame could not have contributed to a reported rise in brain cancer, as the cases of brain cancer cited had already begun developing prior to the introduction of aspartame.

A study published in the *New England Journal of Medicine* in 1995 reported on eighteen people with seizure disorders who claimed that aspartame provoked their seizures. When these people were studied continuously for five days with brain-wave monitors and given high doses of aspartame or a placebo (unaware of which option they were receiving), there were no seizures observed, effectively disproving the connection.

In other studies, researchers found no effect of aspartame on brain-wave activity, mood, psychological function, headaches, or any other measures of neurologic or psychologic function. A 1994 Vanderbilt study reported no effect on cognitive performance or behavior in children, even at high doses. In people with Parkinson's disease, research has likewise shown no evidence of ill effects.

Some People Could Have Problems

Other smaller reports have been less favorable, although far from definitive. Some people probably do have an increased susceptibility to headaches with aspartame. Children with certain types of seizures may be more prone to seizure activity if they consume aspartame. And a small study in 1993 suggested that individuals with bipolar depression may become more depressed if they use aspartame.

Aspartame appears to be safe for most people, but some are sensitive to it, and these individuals should avoid using this sweetener. As long as you do not suffer from phenylketonuria, there is no convincing evidence that aspartame use will cause you permanent harm.

▪ ACESULFAME-K

Also known as acesulfame potassium, this artificial sweetener is 200 times sweeter than sugar. It is used in thousands of products around the world, and marketed under the brand names Sunett and Sweet One. Unlike with aspartame, prominent package labeling is not required, as this chemical is not known to adversely affect people with specific health problems. In the United States, it is found in soft drinks, chewing gum, dessert and beverage mixes, dairy products, and candy, among other things. Acesulfame-K is sometimes used in conjunction with aspartame. There is no proof that this sweetener is harmful, although concerns regarding a possible cancer risk, at least in animal studies, continue to surface.

▪ SUCRALOSE

Sucralose (commonly marketed as Splenda), derived from sugar, is free of calories but 600 times sweeter than sugar. Sucralose has been studied for about twenty years, and there are no confirmed adverse effects on human health. Animal studies have shown that the majority of sucralose that is consumed is simply excreted by the body and not absorbed.

▪ NEOTAME

Neotame, marketed by the same company that makes NutraSweet, is 7,000 to 13,000 times sweeter than sugar. Like the other artificial sweeteners, it is used in soft drinks, chewing gum, yogurt, candy, and desserts. Extensive research reviewed by the FDA prior to neotame's approval found no compelling evidence of detrimental health effects.

■ STEVIA

Stevioside is an extract from the leaves of a shrub native to Paraguay and Brazil known as stevia. It is noncaloric and said to be 250 to 300 times sweeter than sugar. The FDA considers stevia to be a supplement, rather than a food additive, and so has limited regulatory power over its use. Thus, stevia has not been subject to the intensive scientific scrutiny required for other sweeteners (see chapter 14, page 274, for more about the FDA and supplements). There is very little human research available on stevia, although it has been studied in rodents and appears to be safe. To date, some studies have shown that stevia may have a beneficial effect upon blood pressure and blood sugar, but it might also reduce male fertility by lowering levels of testosterone.

■ SUGAR ALCOHOLS

The sugar alcohols are a class of sweeteners that can occur in nature, so they are not considered artificial. Examples of sugar alcohols include sorbitol, xylitol, mannitol, hydrogenated starch hydrolysates, and maltitol. The sugar alcohols provide 1.5 to 3 calories per gram as compared with sugar, which weighs in at 4 calories per gram. Despite the name, sugar alcohols do not contain ethanol, and they are not exactly sugars. Because they are absorbed very slowly from the gut and require very little insulin to metabolize, sugar alcohols are commonly used by diabetics seeking a sweet treat without the risk of high blood sugar. Dentists like the sugar alcohols because they do not cause tooth decay, another important advantage over regular sugar.

Sugar alcohols are found naturally in many foods, including plums, pineapples, carrots, asparagus, apples, mushrooms, berries, and lettuce. In moderate to large amounts, they may cause intestinal bloating, gas, and diarrhea, because they are not completely absorbed from the intestine and may act somewhat like a laxative. Prunes are a great example of a food with high sugar alcohol content and a potent laxative effect.

FAKE FATS

You have probably eaten fake fats without even realizing it. Products labeled "light," "reduced fat," "low-fat," or "fat-free" are likely to be manufactured with fat substitutes, particularly if they are modified versions of higher-fat foods. You will find them in low-fat salad dressings, low-fat dairy products, low-fat spreads, and some bakery products.

Most fat substitutes are derived in some way from carbohydrates or from egg or milk protein. They help processed foods retain moisture, increase thickness and texture, and provide what is known as a mouthfeel reminiscent of the real thing. Although these fat substitutes may not completely fool your senses, they are safe and have not been shown to affect overall nutritional status or digestion. The same can probably be said about some unique types of fat known as caprenin and salatrim, which are chemically modified fats that provide 5 calories per gram, as compared to real fat's 9 calories per gram. A more controversial fake fat is a substance known as olestra.

Is Olestra Diet Magic?

Olestra is a chemical melding of sucrose and fatty acids that is indigestible by the body. Simply put, it passes right through the gastrointestinal tract and is excreted unchanged. It is used in a few brands of low-fat potato chips.

Because it is not really a food but merely a traveler, many concerns have been raised about olestra's effects on the intestinal system itself. There is no evidence that olestra affects the mucosa, or lining, of the digestive tract, but it may interfere with the absorption of vitamins and other nutrients. Increased flatulence and softer stools are unfortunate side effects of olestra. That's probably why it has all but disappeared from the market.

BEST PRACTICES:
FAKE-OUT FACTS

* Don't be fooled: Raw and brown sugars, honey and syrups, and other natural sweeteners such as agave nectar or brown rice syrup are still sugar.
* Don't rely on artificial sweeteners alone to help you lose weight; they may cause you to compensate with other high-calorie foods.
* When it comes to sugar alcohols such as sorbitol and mannitol, "sugar-free" does not mean noncaloric. These lower-calorie sugar substitutes are safe, but may cause gassiness and diarrhea.
* "Fake fats" are probably safe, but don't necessarily help in weight loss.

Learn How to Take a Break (Without Checking Out)

LIVING HEART SMART doesn't mean you can't have a little good, clean fun. A mug of joe or a bracingly strong cup of tea not only gets the morning off to a good start, but also delivers a stream of healthy antioxidants that may help to fight the effects of aging and support the health of the heart and nervous system. A few times a week, a leisurely glass of wine with dinner may feel just right, and it might even help keep your blood vessels clean and healthy.

But it's important to know when to say when. One, and occasionally two, cups or glasses of your brew of choice is fine, but more is just too much. If caffeine or alcohol push the wrong buttons, keep your distance. After all, there's more than one way to keep a smart heart ticking.

And when it comes to tobacco and illicit drugs, the best answer is no. You have too much life to live to waste it on smoky weeds and toxic chemicals.

9

Rituals, Vices, and Addictions, Oh My! The Truth About Caffeine, Alcohol, Tobacco, and Recreational Drugs

CROWDED IN BY our daily responsibilities and obligations, we may find ourselves looking for a way to open a little space in the day, to take time to pause and reflect, and to reenergize. Many of the small rituals we create and embrace over time are harmless and unobtrusive; some may even offer unexpected blessings of good health.

Yet our rituals can also be terribly destructive. As a smoker lights her first cigarette of the day, she does so knowing full well that this habit is dangerous and addictive. Alcohol in excess contributes to a world of misery for the drinker, for the ones who care about him, and for those who may be harmed by his booze-tainted lapses of judgment. Even caffeine, when taken to extremes, can be detrimental. And while every small child knows to say no to illicit drugs, many drug users do not realize the damage they may inflict on their heart and body.

CAFFEINE: PICK YOUR POTION

Anyone who has ever pulled an all-nighter knows that too much caffeine can cause the heart to race, the hands to shake, and the eyes to twitch. As a cardiologist, I frequently meet with patients referred to me for palpitations (pounding heartbeats). After a complete consultation, evaluation, and round of testing, the culprit often turns out to be none other than an oversized java habit. To put the issue into perspective, check out the caffeine chart:

BEVERAGE	CAFFEINE CONTENT
Energy drinks (size varies)	80–1,800 mg
Coffee (8 oz)	100–250 mg
Black tea (8 oz)	40–60 mg
Cola (12 oz)	35–50 mg
Green tea (8 oz)	15–20 mg
Decaffeinated coffee	2–5 mg

Daily doses of more than 300 mg of caffeine are considered potentially harmful. Some people are supersensitive to caffeine and should avoid it completely. And while you may enjoy your morning coffee buzz, caffeine is active in the bloodstream for up to nine hours, so it is best to switch to unleaded after noon.

Coffee

Unfiltered coffee, including French press, espresso, and old-fashioned boiled coffee, contains an active ingredient known as cafestol, which is well known to raise cholesterol levels. This chemical is easily removed by using a simple paper filter. In countries where most coffee is filtered (as it is, for the most part, in the United States), studies have found no significant effect upon the lipid profile, unless you are a smoker. In smokers who drink coffee, LDL appears to increase disproportionately. People who drink more than three cups of coffee daily may also have higher levels of homocysteine, considered a marker for risk of heart disease.

Although we associate the energizing power of coffee with caffeine, there are probably other elements of the magic bean that also contribute to the coffee buzz. A Swiss study evaluated this effect by measuring blood pressure, heart rate, and nervous activity of muscles before and after giving test subjects a triple espresso, a decaffeinated triple espresso, intravenous caffeine in an amount corresponding to the triple espresso, or intravenous salt water. Half of the study subjects were habitual coffee drinkers and half were not.

The study found that in those who did not usually drink coffee, decaffeinated coffee actually raised muscle nervous system activity in a manner similar to pure caffeine, suggesting that something other than caffeine was at work. So when you go home with a case of the coffee jitters after ordering a decaf, don't be too quick to blame the waiter for bringing you the wrong brew.

■ COULD COFFEE BE GOOD FOR YOU?

Although it's possible to overdo it, our beloved bean has received an undeservedly bad reputation. It's starting to look like coffee really is hot stuff, thanks in large part to its rich blend of polyphenols, or plant-based antioxidants. Coffee drinkers appear to be substantially less likely to develop Parkinson's disease than are abstainers, and may even have a lower risk of diabetes and strokes. One study reported that women who drank between one and three 8-ounce cups of coffee daily had a lower risk of death from cardiovascular and inflammatory disease (including infections, diabetes, and rheumatoid disease) when compared to abstainers; there was no effect on cancer deaths. But before you make another lunge for the coffee pot, know that drinking more than three cups of coffee actually diminished the cardiovascular benefit. And four or more cups a day may tend to increase feelings of stress and anxiety.

When tested with CT scans, coffee drinkers appear to have lower levels of calcification in the heart arteries. Arteries become calcified when cholesterol builds up and hardens, so less calcification means a lower likelihood of blocked arteries and heart attacks.

We think of coffee as a trigger for heart palpitations, but when the issue was actually studied by researchers with Kaiser Permanente, the opposite appeared to be true. The medical records and coffee habits of over 130,000 patients were reviewed, and remarkably, those who drank the most coffee were the least likely to be hospitalized for heart rhythm problems. The decaf drinkers showed no such benefit. Of course, we are all different, and some people are extremely sensitive to the effects of caffeine, so it's important to listen to your own body.

Although coffee may transiently increase the blood pressure, the rise is usually small, short-lived, and unlikely to pose a significant risk to most people who drink three cups or less. In fact, one- to two-cup-a-day coffee drinkers appear to have more flexible arteries, which may be beneficial in hypertension.

Decaffeinated coffee does not appear to affect blood pressure, although it may cause more gastric upset, and it may even have undesirable effects on blood lipids. However, like regular coffee, it does appear to grant some protection against diabetes.

Keep in mind that one cup is 8 ounces—not a super-duper mega-mug. Too much of a good thing is usually too much. And side effects are not limited to the heart. People with gastrointestinal problems such as esophageal reflux and irritable bowel may find that coffee intensifies these conditions as well.

Tea

Devotees of tea tend to have slightly lower blood pressure, and may even enjoy a greater sense of serenity than the average java head. A study from the University College, London, found that drinking black tea was associated with lower levels of the stress hormone cortisol and a greater sense of relaxation, when compared to a tea-free drink that was spiked with a comparable amount of caffeine. Blood platelets were also less active in the tea drinkers, indicating a reduced susceptibility to blood clots.

Some 78 percent of the tea consumed in the world is black, 20 percent is green (including white tea), and less than 2 percent is oolong. The classifications depend on the stage at which the leaves were harvested and how they were processed. ("Tea" is made from *Camellia sinensis* only. Herbal "teas" do not count as tea; they are more correctly termed "tisanes").

Green, white, and oolong tea provide powerful flavonoid antioxidants known as catechins, whereas the antioxidants in black tea are somewhat less potent. But let's face it. Green tea is an acquired taste, and not everyone fancies it. Many studies have lumped all tea drinkers together, and most have shown remarkable benefits of tea drinking, regardless of the choice of brew.

■ A HEARTWARMING STORY

In 1999, Harvard researchers reported a 44 percent reduction in the risk of heart attacks in American tea drinkers who enjoyed at least one cup of tea daily. A later study, also from Harvard, found that in the years following a heart attack, tea drinkers were 30 to 40 percent less likely to have died than were the non-tea drinkers. The benefit appeared stronger in those who enjoyed at least a couple of cups each day. Research from the Netherlands looks even better, with a 70 percent reduction in fatal heart attacks for those drinking at least one cup of tea daily.

Also from the Netherlands comes research that suggests that tea may reduce cholesterol deposits, or plaque, in the aorta. Although a single daily cup of tea was protective, the greatest benefit was found in people drinking more than four cups of tea each day.

There is some evidence that green tea may modestly lower cholesterol levels. A collaborative study between scientists from Vanderbilt University and China reported a hefty 16 percent drop in LDL cholesterol when healthy people were given a capsule of green tea extract enriched with theaflavins, which are the antioxidants found in tea. There was no real improvement in HDL or triglycerides.

This sounds great, but before you rush off to brew a pot of tea, I should point out that the capsules, marketed as TeaFlavin, contain the antioxidant equivalent of about thirty-five cups of green tea, without the caffeine.

Studies from the United Kingdom have been less stirring, but it turns out that when it comes to the heart, certain British idiosyncrasies may be counterproductive. First, most Brits add milk to their tea, which appears to neutralize the heart-protective effects. And whereas American tea drinkers tend to be more health conscious, the heavy tea drinkers in the British studies were more likely to be smokers and eat a high-fat diet, skewing the results.

Some scientists have speculated that the antioxidants in green tea may not only prevent damage to arterial walls but also hinder the formation of cancer cells. Small studies support the theory that green tea may lower the risk of developing gastrointestinal, ovarian, and bladder cancer, although at least one study found a possible connection between tea and colon cancer, when at least 32 ounces (1 quart) of tea was consumed every day.

Other potential benefits of tea include stronger bones and a lower likelihood of kidney stones and diabetes. Both coffee and tea have been linked to a lower risk for glioma, an invasive type of brain tumor.

Sodas, Energy Drinks, and Cocoa

What about sodas and energy drinks? These caffeinated products are no substitute for tea or coffee. They are loaded with artificial colorings and flavorings, and provide none of the beneficial antioxidants. Cocoa is another energy booster that may taste good but is unlikely to be of much use to the heart. Although we know that dark chocolate is a great source of antioxidants, adding milk to the mix appears to neutralize the potential benefits (see chapter 6, page 104, for more about chocolate).

BEST PRACTICES:
CAFFEINE

COFFEE

* Go ahead and enjoy caffeinated or decaffeinated coffee in moderation: It may reduce your risk for heart disease, Parkinson's disease, diabetes, and rheumatoid disease.

* Learn your limit: One to three 8-ounce cups per day should be fine for you, but some people experience irregular heartbeats and anxiety with any amount of caffeine.

* Don't let coffee ruin your sleep: Caffeinated coffee is most likely to keep you up at night, but even decaf can trigger nervous system activity in your muscle tissue.

TEA

* Drinking at least 1 cup of tea every day appears to reduce the likelihood of cardiovascular disease by 40% or more. Tea may also help boost bone strength, reduce cancer risk, and protect against kidney stones.

* Green tea may boost your metabolism very slightly, by less than 5%.

* Black, white, green, and oolong tea all supply antioxidants, although they are most abundant in green and white tea. Decaffeinated tea is a little weaker in antioxidants, but still a good source. Herbal "teas" don't count.

* Don't add milk. Adding milk to tea may neutralize its antioxidants.

ALCOHOL: HERE'S TO IT

For centuries, humans have celebrated the secrets of fermentation, and reveled in the pleasures of wine, beer, and spirits. We have also suffered the consequences, great and small, of addiction and overindulgence. Although the enjoyment of wine has long been a part of many cultures, its effects on the heart were not scientifically validated until the 1970s. To date more than sixty studies have affirmed the heart-healthy benefits of moderate drinking, and the list continues to grow.

Although no one will ever do the type of double-blind, controlled clinical trials of alcohol use that we scientific types prefer, the overwhelming consensus is that any type of alcohol, enjoyed in moderation, can help to protect against heart disease. A report published in 2010 followed more than 245,000 Americans who participated in the U.S. National Health Interview Survey for twelve years. Compared with nondrinkers, light to moderate drinkers (seven drinks or less per week for women, and fourteen drinks or less per week for men) had a heart attack risk that was one third lower than that of their teetotaling counterparts, even when other risk factors for heart disease were taken into account. Heavy alcohol use (more than seven drinks per week for women or fourteen drinks per week for men) showed no such benefit. A number of studies around the world have led to similar conclusions.

HEY, BARTENDER!

ONE DRINK IS:
    5 ounces of wine
    12 ounces of beer
    1 ounce of hard liquor

While it's never too late in life to raise a glass, there's no point in trying to make up for lost time, as binge drinking does not offer any benefit. In fact, there is a higher risk of heart attacks and high blood pressure in binge drinkers.

On the other hand, light to moderate alcohol use of any variety may raise HDL cholesterol by 10 percent or more. Alcohol also reduces the stickiness of blood platelets, which are involved in the clotting process, meaning a lower risk for blood clots. Because of its rich array of antioxidants, red wine probably has a more powerful blood-thinning effect than do other types of alcohol.

The risk of congestive heart failure is lower in light to moderate drinkers, even among the elderly. What's more, people who have already suffered a heart attack may reduce their risk of future mortality from heart disease by 20 to 30 percent. Moderate drinkers (one to two drinks per day) fare a little better than light drinkers (less than one drink daily), regardless of the type of alcohol consumed.

Alcohol even improves the body's sensitivity to insulin, resulting in a lower risk of diabetes. The metabolic syndrome (see chapter 13, page 235) is also reduced in mild to moderate drinkers. Even full-fledged diabetics may benefit substantially. There is evidence that diabetic women who drink less than half a drink a day may be able to cut their chances of heart disease by nearly 30 percent compared to abstainers; those who drink one or two drinks daily appear to lower their risk by as much as 55 percent.

A Tonic for the Brain?

The heart isn't the only organ that appreciates a little tipple. The brain, a highly vascular structure, usually benefits from anything that helps the heart. This appears to be true in the case of alcohol in general, but perhaps even more so with wine.

A study from Copenhagen found that drinking alcoholic beverages as infrequently as once a month was associated with a greater than 15 percent reduction in stroke risk. Weekly and daily drinkers' risks were about 40 and 30 percent lower, respectively. Other researchers have reported similar findings. Compared to those who abstain, people who drink one to six drinks per week are about half as likely to suffer from dementia later in life. Women who drink moderately may benefit even more than men do.

But more is not always better. When it comes to alcohol, those who drink more than fourteen drinks a week have a 20 percent higher probability of dementia.

Red Wine: The Cardiologist's Choice

We cardiologists hold a special place in our hearts for red wine. Red wine is rich in chemicals known as phenols, which give it its characteristic body and taste. Phenols are powerful antioxidants and include flavonoids known as catechins, which are also abundant in tea, chocolate, beans, apples, and berries, as well as resveratrol, which is found only in grapes. These antioxidants are not found in beer or spirits and occur at much lower concentrations in white wine.

A Danish study of more than twenty-seven thousand people reported that light drinkers who did not drink wine had about a 24 percent reduction in heart disease risk compared to nondrinkers. Although this sounds impressive, when wine drinkers were singled out, their risk appeared to decline by a striking 42 percent. Red wine has had the edge in a number of other European studies, although research done here in the United States has not shown the same effect. One key difference may be in the way that wine is enjoyed. In European countries it is customary to drink wine with meals, whereas Americans tend to sip wine at social functions. This difference is important, especially with fatty meals, because it appears that wine, via its antioxidant properties, actually tempers the LDL cholesterol that is released into the bloodstream after a meal, rendering it less harmful to the arteries.

Some wines are higher in natural antioxidants, with wines from a specific province in Sardinia, Italy, and those from southwestern France having the most potent effect on blood vessel function. Not surprisingly, people who live in these regions have greater longevity than the average citizen.

It seems that wine can even help keep your tummy trim. At least two studies have found that light to moderate drinkers tend to have a smaller waist and a lower likelihood of obesity than do nondrinkers. The pattern of alcohol use is important, as binge drinkers tended to have the biggest beer bellies.

The Dark Side

It would be foolish to discuss all the wonderful properties of alcohol without acknowledging its dark side. Heavy drinkers who regularly drink more than three drinks a day are at risk for severe weakening of the heart muscle, which can lead to congestive heart failure, disability, and death. High blood pressure and high triglycerides are common among those who drink more than two drinks daily. Heavy drinkers are also more likely to have strokes due to bleeding into the brain. Binge drinking can provoke an erratic and rapid heart rhythm called atrial fibrillation, a common scenario we cardiologists term "holiday heart," and which may lead to strokes.

Many women are unaware that drinking alcohol may raise their risk of breast cancer substantially. Women who regularly drink more than one drink daily have a 28 percent higher risk of breast cancer than do those who drink less or no alcohol. Women who drink this much and take hormone replacement therapy double their risk of breast cancer. That's why women should limit their alcohol to an average of less than one drink per day.

Smokers should be cautious, as smoking combined with moderate to heavy alcohol use is associated with a higher risk of cancers involving the throat and gastrointestinal tract.

A tendency toward alcoholism may be inherited, so if a parent or sibling is an alcoholic, you should be especially judicious. For these reasons and others, alcohol is not for everyone.

Who, then, stands to gain the most from drinking alcohol? Men over 40 and women over 50 are the prime candidates, as this is when the risk of heart disease begins to rise. Those with important risk factors for heart disease, such as diabetes, high blood pressure, and high cholesterol, might benefit from adding alcoholic beverages to the diet at a younger age.

Given all the dangers involved, there is no doubt that if it were invented today, alcohol is a "drug" that would never make it through the FDA's stringent approval process.

What If You Don't Drink?

Because alcohol can be associated with such dire consequences, researchers have turned to grape juice, to see if it might share some of the same properties as wine. Overall the results are encouraging. Red wine that has been de-alcoholized increases blood levels of the antioxidant catechin at least as much as red wine itself. Purple grape juice also appears to help improve the ability of the arteries to dilate and has been found to have antioxidant effects on LDL cholesterol. Cranberry and blueberry juices seem to have similarly positive effects on the arteries.

However, red wine contains far more flavonoid antioxidants than does juice. This is because the wine-making process extracts these substances from the seeds and skin of the grape, where they are concentrated. Nevertheless, 4 to 8 ounces per day of purple grape juice or cranberry juice is a practical substitute for wine or alcohol for those who prefer not to imbibe.

Resveratrol comes from the skin of the grape, and is one of red wine's active antioxidant ingredients. It is often marketed as a supplement for heart health and cancer prevention, but not enough is known about the effects of high doses of this antioxidant. In fact, there is evidence that while low doses, such as what we might get from wine or juice, can protect our heart and other organs, even helping to guard against cancer, very high doses may actually be harmful, leading to cell death. Until we understand more about this important antioxidant, it's best to enjoy it in its natural state, and leave the pills for the laboratory rats.

BEST PRACTICES:
ALCOHOL

* Enjoy alcohol in moderation: It raises your HDL; lowers your triglycerides, C-reactive protein, and Lp(a); and reduces the likelihood of dementia. Three to 7 drinks per week for women and 1 to 2 drinks per

day for men may cut heart attack and stroke risk by 25–40%.

* Don't overdo it: More than 3 drinks per day will increase your chances of heart failure, high blood pressure, high triglycerides, and abnormal heart rhythms. Exceed 14 drinks weekly, and your risk of dementia will begin to rise.

* Choose wisely: Red wines from the southwest region of France and from Sardinia, Italy, have the most potent antioxidants, but any kind of alcohol is protective. Grape juice, cranberry juice, and blueberry juices are good alternatives to alcohol, although they won't supply you with the full balance of antioxidants found in red wine.

TOBACCO: THE EVIL WEED

WHEN I FIRST met Krystal in the ER several years ago, the pack-a-day smoker was pale, clammy, and clutching her chest in pain. The EKG confirmed that this 58-year-old architect was suffering a heart attack. She was rushed to the cardiac catheterization laboratory, and her blocked artery was opened up beautifully.

Krystal thought she was home free, until a routine chest X-ray disclosed a mass in the right lung. Fortunately, we had caught the cancer very early—she had experienced absolutely no symptoms, and the cancer had not spread. In short order, Krystal was seen by the cancer specialist, chest surgeon, and lung doctor, and plans were made to treat the tumor aggressively. I thought for certain that two life-threatening illnesses diagnosed in the span of one week would convince her to lay off the smokes.

To my surprise, Krystal insisted she was not ready to stop yet. "I'm way too stressed out," she told me. "I'll stop when I feel better." Despite surgery to remove half a lung and intensive exercise therapy in cardiac rehabilitation, Krystal continued to smoke for more than a year. Whether it was my nagging that finally wore her down, or that she woke up one day and realized how fortunate she was to still be among the living, I'll never know, but she finally did quit.

The irrational struggles with tobacco addiction faced by this rational and educated woman opened my eyes to the immense hold that this killer can have on a person's life.

ANOTHER PATIENT, CRAIG, is a happy-go-lucky bricklayer who suffered a heart attack at the ripe old age of 39. A two-pack-a-day smoker with a stale haze of smoke that seems to hang over him like a bad aura, Craig sees me every six months and takes his medications like clockwork. I do my best to convince him to stop smoking, but to no avail. I was dismayed, but not surprised, when he showed up in the emergency room with a second heart attack just days before his forty-second birthday.

So much misery in the world is caused by tobacco. In this country alone, more than 430,000 lives are lost each year as a direct result of smoking and other forms of tobacco use. That means that tobacco contributes to about one out of every five deaths. Worldwide, nearly 5 million deaths per year are due to tobacco.

Half of all smokers die prematurely, cutting their lives short by an average of fourteen years because of a senseless but powerful addiction to tobacco. A quarter of smokers die before the age of 70.

About 80 percent of people who currently smoke want to quit, but most are unable to break the addiction. A pack-a-day habit costs over $1,600 per year; in some states, it may reach $2,500 or more. Despite these grim statistics, it is estimated that over 1 million people, mostly teens, join the ranks of smokers each year, and as many as 50 million Americans use tobacco regularly.

Tobacco kills in many ways. Cigarette tobacco contains more than four thousand naturally occurring compounds and scores of additives, many of which cause cancer. Not surprisingly, smoking is responsible for most cases of lung cancer in this country. Chronic lung disease, such as emphysema, is endemic in smokers, often chaining its victims to lifelines of oxygen tubing. Fully one in four smokers will eventually develop chronic lung disease.

Don't Smoke Out Your Heart

While smoking's effects on the lungs are well known, many people are unaware that smoking is a major contributor to heart disease. Smoking even one cigarette per day increases the risk of a heart attack at least 50 percent. Smoking more than forty-five cigarettes per day may raise the likelihood of heart disease to six times normal, and smokers who keep smoking after a heart attack are nearly twice as likely to die suddenly from a fatal heart rhythm disturbance. One hundred thousand deaths from heart disease each year can be blamed on tobacco alone (see "Know Your Risk Factors," page 349).

Smoking affects heart health on many fronts. It increases dangerous LDL cholesterol and triglycerides and lowers the heart-healthy HDL cholesterol. C-reactive protein levels and homocysteine are higher in smokers. Tobacco smoke contains dangerous oxidants that may generate free radicals in the bloodstream, causing widespread damage to the lining of the blood vessels. It saps the body of a host of vitamins, including B vitamins, vitamin C, beta-carotene, and vitamin E.

Smoking also enhances our susceptibility to blood clots and, at the same time, reduces the effectiveness of aspirin as a clot preventer. It is probably this vulnerability to blood clots that causes women smokers who use the birth control pill to have an astounding heart attack risk of forty times normal—a risk that few realize they are taking. Smokers on the pill are also more likely to have a stroke, and the risk increases dramatically after the age of 35.

Smoking is responsible for many disabling and fatal strokes and is a major cause of peripheral vascular disease, or blockage of the arteries of the legs and arms. Diabetics are especially susceptible, and the condition may eventually lead to amputation due to poor healing of infections of the skin and bones. Indeed, smokers are more likely to become diabetic, as they are more prone to insulin resistance.

Smoking will bring on menopause about two years earlier, depriving women of valuable years of natural estrogen. Smokers are 50 percent more likely to develop osteoporosis, a disabling weakening of the bone structure that increases vulnerability to bone fractures. And while lung cancer kills three times as many women as breast cancer does, smoking also increases the likelihood of breast cancer by up to five times the usual rate. Smokers' risk of ovarian cancer is more than doubled, and cervical cancer is more prevalent as well.

Smoking Hurts You and Those You Love

Secondhand smoke increases the risk for heart disease and stroke, and can even harm the reproductive organs. A study from Johns Hopkins University found that nonsmoking women who live with smokers are more than twice as likely to have precancerous cells in the cervix, when compared with women who are not exposed to smoke at home. Women chronically exposed to secondhand smoke are more than 30 percent more likely to develop breast cancer. Smokers' kids are more apt to develop cancer and heart disease as adults, even if they never smoke.

Smokers and people who use other forms of tobacco also dramatically increase their risk for a variety of nasty and disfiguring cancers of the head and neck. Cancers of the stomach, esophagus, pancreas, kidneys, and bladder are all legacies of tobacco use.

Periodontal disease (inflammation of the gum tissue) and bad breath are common side effects of smoking. And for men, smoking at least doubles the chances of developing erectile dysfunction.

Although many smokers feel that tobacco gives them mental clarity and energy, a Dutch study found that tobacco use over time actually speeds up mental decline. Middle-aged and older smokers followed over five years earned lower scores for memory, mental flexibility, and overall cognitive function than nonsmokers, foretelling a higher likelihood of dementia later in life. A British study found that people exposed to secondhand smoke may show similar deterioration in mental function over time.

SMOKING AFFECTS EVERYONE. One patient I will never forget was Patty, a 38-year-old stay-at-home mom with three beautiful children. Patty took low-dose birth control pills. She was not a smoker, but her husband was, and he chose to smoke in their home. Patty came into the ER early one morning in the throes of a heart attack, her frantic husband and children at her side. Fortunately, she survived with no long-term damage, and after exhaustive evaluation, the only risk factor we could find was her birth control pills. Combined with exposure to her husband's tobacco smoke, this was a near lethal mix.

Pipes and Cigars

Once the choice of stodgy old men, cigars suddenly became fashionable in the mid-1990s, even among women, and are still considered cool in some circles. Because cigars are decidedly not cigarettes, many believe that the risks are negligible. Unfortunately, they are mistaken.

Regular cigar smokers and pipe smokers are 30 to 70 percent more likely than nonsmokers to develop heart disease. Nevertheless, cigarette smokers who switch to cigars or pipes do reduce their risk of heart disease by about half, which is probably because they are less likely to fully inhale the tobacco smoke.

How to Quit

On average, people who quit using tobacco cut their risk of dying early by more than 30 percent. Quitting before the age of 30 will eventually bring your risk down to that of a never-smoker, but even quitting by the time you hit 50 buys you several more precious years, an enhanced quality of life, and the gratitude of your friends and loved ones.

Quitting is not easy. Nearly half of all smokers will try to quit each year; most are not successful. I wish I could tell you a foolproof way to kick the habit. Unfortunately, there isn't one. Tobacco is highly addictive in all of its forms. Nicotine, the addictive part of tobacco, affects a complicated array of brain chemicals. It acts as both a stimulant and a depressant, and may suppress the appetite, which is one reason that modest weight gain often follows smoking cessation.

Simply throwing the cigarettes away and resolving never to smoke again works for some people, but not for most. Nicotine replacement products are a reasonably safe option for the short term, even for people with heart problems. These include nicotine gum, lozenges, and patches, all of which can be bought over the counter, and prescription nicotine inhalers and nasal spray. When used according to the directions, they are undoubtedly safer than tobacco, which we know to be highly toxic, and all are about equally effective. Typically, these products should be used for several months. The important thing is to give it time, which many people fail to do. Even when used properly, the success rate with nicotine replacement is modest, with about only 20 to 25 percent of tobacco users quitting by about three months.

Buproprion (marketed as Wellbutrin-SR and Zyban) is a prescription drug that has been approved by the FDA to help smokers quit. Usually buproprion is prescribed for several months. When combined with a healthy dose of motivation and determination, the quit rates in the first few months are on the order of 50 percent. Unfortunately, at least half of the quitters will backslide by a year, so a strong commitment to your health and well-being is essential. Combining buproprion with a nicotine replacement product may boost your chances of quitting.

Some people just feel horrible on this drug, in which case they should discontinue use. Because there is a very small (less than one tenth of 1 percent) risk of seizures with buproprion, people with a seizure disorder or a history of anorexia nervosa or bulimia should avoid this drug, as they are more likely to suffer this side effect.

Varenicline (marketed as Chantix) was developed by pharmaceutical giant Pfizer, and first appeared on the U.S. market in 2006. A prescription drug, it helps to block the receptor in the brain that is associated with tobacco cravings and with symptoms of tobacco withdrawal. Because it can also cause slight nausea, it is not usually associated with weight gain. In a clinical trial, nearly half of those who used the drug quit smoking in the first month (compared to 33 percent with buproprion and 17 percent with a placebo in the same three-month time frame). Treatment with the drug continued for three months.

That sounds great, but at the one-year mark, only 14 percent remained abstinent. Although the stats are dismal, in this particular study Chantix still fared far better than buproprion (6 percent) and the placebo (5 percent). Patients who have taken this medication successfully have told me that they simply "forgot to smoke." Chantix is a reasonably safe drug, but there is some evidence that it might provoke heart problems in a small number of people. Uncommon side effects include depression or other more severe psychological problems, so it's important to follow up with your doctor while on the drug. Chantix should not be used during pregnancy or breast feeding.

Electronic cigarettes have been marketed aggressively online, and have helped some people to quit. However, not much is known about their safety or overall effectiveness. Unlike nicotine replacement products and prescription drugs, they are not approved by the FDA. In 2009, the FDA released a warning that these products contain carcinogens and other toxic chemicals, including diethylene glycol, found commonly in antifreeze.

Don't rule out hypnosis. Although there is really not much in the way of good medical research to back up the use of hypnosis for smoking cessation, when administered by a credentialed practitioner, it may be effective for as many as 20 percent of smokers.

Have You Smoked a Cadillac?

Please don't tell me that it is too expensive to quit. Add up what you spend on your cigarettes, and you will see that the investment is well worth it. A day's worth of nicotine patches or Chantix costs about as much as a pack of smokes. As a lovely and genteel Southern lady once told me, "Honey, I have smoked an entire Cadillac." Another patient put it even more bluntly when she told me that quitting is cheaper than chemotherapy.

If your spouse or roommate smokes, you are much more likely to quit if you do it together. Being around other smokers is a powerful trigger and a quick way to sabotage your best-laid plans.

When you do quit, it's true that you may gain weight. The average person who quits gains about 5 to 10 pounds, mostly because the oral fix that comes from smoking is transferred to food. The younger you are when you quit, the less likely it is that you'll gain weight. And if you do put on a few pounds, believe in yourself and know that you can lose it. Add more fruits and vegetables to boost your antioxidants, increase your exercise, and enjoy the fresh air that you are now free to breathe.

BEST PRACTICES:
TOBACCO

* No form of tobacco is safe.
* Don't be fooled by "low-tar" or "light" smokes: There is no such thing as a low-risk cigarette. They do nothing to reduce the risk of smoking-related illnesses. Not surprisingly, trendy unfiltered cigarettes are even more dangerous than conventional filtered brands.
* If you already smoke, switching to a pipe or cigars may reduce your risk of heart disease, but it is far healthier to stop smoking entirely.
* You can quit, but you will probably need help doing so. Ask your doctor about your medical options. Hypnosis is

also worth a try. Cold turkey usually doesn't work.

* If you share living quarters with a smoker, try to quit together so you won't be tempted to backslide when your partner lights up.

* Transfer your cravings to heart-healthy foods such as fruits and vegetables, which contain antioxidants.

ILLEGAL DRUGS: YOUR HEART SAYS NO

More than 80 million Americans have used marijuana at least once, over 25 million have tried cocaine, and at least 5 million have experimented with amphetamines. Exactly how many people use drugs on a regular basis is a matter of some debate. Understandably, many people will not 'fess up to their drug use, but regular marijuana users probably number around 5 million and cocaine users about 1.5 million or more.

Many of these folks, especially pot smokers, are everyday working people. They may be your neighbors, your grocer, your lawyer, or even you. Everyone knows that heroin and other narcotics are dangerous, but most people don't realize that marijuana, cocaine, and amphetamines can be damaging to the heart.

While research on marijuana and the heart is pretty sketchy, we do know that in the first hour after smoking pot, the risk of a heart attack increases to five times normal. That means that high-risk people like cigarette smokers, diabetics, and people with high blood pressure are especially vulnerable.

Some individuals enjoy the sensation of being "mellowed out," but the heart is far from relaxed when exposed to marijuana. Heart rate and blood pressure rise, but standing up will often cause the blood pressure to fall precipitously, resulting in severe lightheadedness and sometimes even fainting.

My patient Gretchen, a corporate recruiter and self-described former hippie who had smoked more than her share of pot in her younger days, visited Amsterdam on vacation to enjoy the legal marijuana available there. Minutes after smoking what she described to me as "a big fat doobie," she stood up and fainted dead away. She was rushed to a hospital where she endured a number of expensive medical tests before being pronounced safe to travel back home to the States. Gretchen's husband was not amused.

Cocaine poses special dangers to the heart. It causes constriction of the heart arteries, often leading to prolonged spasm that may result in a heart attack. In the first hour after using cocaine, the heart attack risk rises to a staggering rate of twenty-four times greater than normal. Up to 25 percent of heart attacks that happen before the age of 45 are due to cocaine use. Life-threatening heart rhythm disturbances and congestive heart failure are also well-known side effects of cocaine. Repeated use of the drug can lead to permanent damage to the heart arteries, causing widespread cholesterol plaques and aneurysms.

MY PATIENTS Jack and Jane, two well-respected and highly sociable business people, regularly indulged in cocaine, sometimes using it to help them through grueling workdays and even longer evenings spent entertaining clients. They thought it made them look hip and young. Both required bypass surgery before the age of 50 for life-threatening blockages in the coronary arteries. Neither had any other risk factors to explain such extensive disease.

Amphetamines are similarly risky. They raise both blood pressure and heart rate, increasing the risk of heart attacks and heart failure. Amphetamine use can also cause bleeding into the brain, which can have the disastrous outcome of a disabling stroke or even death.

BEST PRACTICES:
CONTROLLED SUBSTANCES

* Don't use recreational drugs: They are not safe for your heart in any amount. In the first hour after smoking marijuana, the risk of heart attack jumps to 5 times normal; in the first hour after using cocaine, it soars to 24 times normal.

A steaming mug of coffee or a bracing cup of tea may help ease you into the morning or revive your dwindling energy in the afternoon. A glass of wine with friends or family may add dimension and structure to a wonderful meal or an evening of stimulating conversation. And your heart will thank you for it. But it's heart smart to say, "No, thanks" to indulging in other recreational stimulants, or even too much of the good stuff.

STEP 4

Get a Move On

EXERCISE MAKES YOU look good and feel great. It keeps your heart beating and your mind clear. Your time on this Earth is a gift that should not be wasted sitting idly in front of the TV or computer. When you get up and move, you are tapping into a force for health that is more powerful than any drug the pharmaceutical industry could dream up. And it can be virtually free of charge, making for a brilliant return on a very small investment.

Find something that motivates you and keeps you going back for more. Run for your life, walk like you mean it, swim like a fish, lift dumbbells for the sheer thrill of feeling your own strength, immerse yourself in yoga, or dance to your own music. Whatever you choose, make it yours.

10

Exercise and the
Active Lifestyle

TO ACHIEVE A healthy heart, mind, and body, exercise is not an option. It's a must. Your exercise capacity, or the amount of exercise that you can do before reaching the point of exhaustion, is a more powerful predictor of your life span than is high blood pressure, diabetes, smoking, or even preexisting heart disease. If you exercise, chances are you will live longer, healthier, and happier.

It is so much easier to make fitness a way of life when you find an activity that inspires you. You may already know what sparks your passion. If not, perhaps now is the time to explore your options and create opportunities that motivate you to move with joy and strength. Whether it is gardening, hiking, tennis, golf, yoga, walking, or any other activity that gets you up and moving, the choice is all yours.

THE GOOD NEWS ABOUT EXERCISE

If you commit to exercise, you are half as likely to become obese as are your couch-bound neighbors. People who exercise regularly have lower levels of triglycerides and higher levels of beneficial HDL cholesterol. Although total LDL cholesterol levels don't usually change with exercise alone, LDL subclasses do improve, so that the LDL that you have is less likely to harm your arteries. And if you lose weight, your LDL will probably fall as well. Inflammation in the body, represented by CRP levels, may be reduced by up to 40 percent with exercise.

Aerobic fitness improves the body's sensitivity to insulin so that diabetes is much less likely to develop. This is due in part to the fact that aerobic exercise is one of the best ways to get rid of that harmful deep abdominal fat, or "belly blubber." Women who exercise are less inclined to develop breast cancer. For men, regular workouts mean a 30 percent lower likelihood of erectile dysfunction compared to those who are inactive—good motivation to get to the gym. And researchers at the University of Washington found that exercise might even help prevent the common cold.

If that is not incentive enough, consider this: People who exercise can actually increase the size of the hippocampus (the memory center of the brain) and reduce the likelihood of dementia and age-related mental decline. A 2011 study from researchers at the University of Pittsburg looking at people over the age of 60 showed that simply walking for forty minutes three days every week was all it took to grow new brain tissue. The results were seen as soon as one year after the walking program began.

Regular workouts will make you smarter and happier, and over time you'll be less likely to suffer from depression and insomnia. People who exercise age more slowly and handle stress better, both physically and mentally. For menopausal women, exercise may be one of the best ways to deal with the capricious effects of fluctuating hormones.

What's more, exercise is nearly free of charge, with a great return on your investment. Most people can put on a pair of walking shoes and head outside or to a nearby mall for a brisk walk. The Centers for Disease Control and Prevention has estimated that if the 88 million or so sedentary Americans would get up off their cabooses and exercise, health-care costs could be slashed by more than $75 billion.

Even folks well into their 80s, including those with physical disabilities, will reap benefits from regular physical training. However, the earlier you start exercising, the greater the rewards will be.

It's a common misconception that exercise will increase appetite and make it harder to lose weight. This isn't necessarily true for most people. Scientists have found that exercise actually has a fairly weak effect on appetite as long as you are getting enough calories for your body's needs. Research shows that after moderate-intensity exercise, such as brisk walking, people generally eat about 35 percent of calories burned, when allowed open access to food. If you're a hard-core athlete, your body may demand more calories. For instance, if given free rein, runners will often consume 90 percent of the calories they worked so hard to sweat off. This just means that if you're athletic and trying to lose weight, you need to be more vigilant about your calories after a hard workout.

EASY NUMBERS

To optimize your health and well-being, commit to 150 minutes of exercise each week. Ideally, this will be at least 30 minutes of aerobic exercise five days a week, because sustained exercise is best for heart health. Incorporating brief bursts of physical activity into your daily life will burn some extra calories and modestly improve fitness, but for true cardiovascular impact, the heart must work for a minimum of 20 minutes straight.

If you haven't been very active for a while, consider using a pedometer to track your steps, and aim for at least ten thousand steps per day. Take a long walk across the parking lot at work instead of circling to find the closest spot. Climb the stairs instead of taking the elevator, and choose a walk break instead of a smoke or coffee break. Although they don't take the place of regular exercise, these mini-workouts are well worth the effort, and will help keep you in an active frame of mind.

If you are working on weight loss, you will need to exercise more and eat less. Don't expect to lose a lot of weight through exercise alone. Every day patients come to me frustrated because they have not lost weight despite regular exercise. It's a simple mathematical equation. Each pound of body weight costs us 3,500 calories, so it's very hard to burn enough calories to lose even 1 pound. For instance, if you weigh 160 pounds, walking for sixty minutes at a brisk pace burns about 360 calories. At that rate, you'd have to walk ten hours to lose just 1 pound.

Although 150 minutes—two and a half hours—every week is ideal, any regular exercise will put you ahead of the curve. The more you exercise, the better off you will be. For people in their 40s through 60s, exercising for at least two hours every week will lower the likelihood of developing heart disease by 60 percent compared to those who do not exercise at all. Just one to two hours each week reduces the risk a respectable 40 percent, and even just a little regular exercise promotes a 15 percent reduction in heart disease risk compared to doing nothing at all.

AEROBIC EXERCISE

Aerobic exercise gets you breathing more deeply and your heart pumping faster and stronger. If you are exercising aerobically, you are working the large muscle groups of your body, typically your arms and legs, and you're probably breaking a sweat.

Brisk walking, jogging, biking, skating, and swimming all get you moving and pull more oxygen into your body. Aerobic exercise classes also fit the bill, as do dancing, mowing the lawn, and playing tennis. Whatever you choose, the ideal aerobic activity is one that you can keep up for at least thirty minutes without stopping.

The goal of aerobic exercise is to increase your heart rate, to strengthen the heart muscle, and to improve your circulation, allowing oxygenated blood to flow throughout your body. "Aerobic" literally means "with oxygen." To learn what your heart rate is at any time, you can check your pulse either at your wrist (the radial artery) or at your neck (the carotid artery). Count how many beats occur in fifteen seconds, then multiply by 4. For example, at rest, you may count twenty beats in fifteen seconds, which gives 20 x 4 = 80, or eighty beats per minute. (If you have an irregular heart rhythm, this method is not likely to be accurate, and you will probably need to count your heartbeats for a full minute.)

You can also buy a monitor to wear on your chest or wrist to check your heart rate, but be aware that these can sometimes misread the heart rate due to interference from muscle movements and contractions.

To be aerobic, exercise must raise your heart rate to 60 to 85 percent of your age-adjusted maximal heart rate. How do you know what your target heart rate is? It's simple: First, subtract your age from 220; this will give you your age-adjusted maximal heart rate. To get 60 and 85 percent of that number, multiply it by 0.6 and by 0.85. This will give you your range. For example:

If your age is 40, then $220 - 40 = 180$

$180 \times 0.6 = 108$ (60% of your maximum predicted heart rate)

$180 \times 0.85 = 153$ (85% of your maximum predicted heart rate)

Your target heart rate range is 108 to 153 beats per minute.

YOUR HEART RATE—DO THE MATH

WHAT'S YOUR HEART RATE RIGHT NOW?

Check your pulse at the wrist or neck: Count how many beats you feel in fifteen seconds, and then multiply by four. A normal resting heart rate may vary considerably from one person to the next. More athletic individuals tend to run heart rates in the 50s and 60s, while others may range between 70 and 90. Some medications (including beta blockers and calcium channel blockers) may lower the resting heart rate. If your heart rate is consistently over 100 or below 50, check in with your doctor.

As long as you have normal blood pressure, it is not usually necessary to monitor your blood pressure with exercise on a regular basis. However, if you have high blood pressure, check with your doctor before you launch into an exercise program. It makes sense for everyone to warm up and cool down for five to ten minutes when doing vigorous exercise, to avoid abrupt changes in heart rate and blood pressure. Stopping suddenly can sometimes cause your blood pressure to fall too quickly, which can lead to dizziness or even fainting.

In general, more energetic exercise is better, as long as you can keep it up without stopping. If you're a walker, pump up your pace to three miles per hour or more, for an optimal cardiovascular workout. If that's too fast, don't despair. Even slow walkers are far better off than those who do nothing.

If you are just starting to work out, begin slowly and work your way up. Don't expect to be able to run an eight-minute mile or to bike for two hours straight if you hung up your tennies right after high school graduation. Overdoing it is often counterproductive, as you are apt to get sore and discouraged and just give up. And don't wait for a sunny day to strut your stuff. Blaming the weather is a tired old excuse for not exercising that will get you nowhere.

Find something that you can do despite the weather or the time of year. An exercise bike or treadmill is a great investment in your future, especially if you are not able to get to a gym regularly. If you have physical limitations, learn to work around them, perhaps with the help of a good physical therapist. Arthritis sufferers or those with back trouble can search out a local pool to swim laps or do water aerobics. Some of the fittest patients in my practice are paraplegics and amputees who don't let their disabilities get in the way of good health.

It's fine to start out at just fifteen minutes per day, if you need to, and increase the time week by week. And despite what the hard-core gym rats might say, it's also okay to read a book or watch TV while you're exercising on a stationary bike or treadmill, as long as that doesn't slow you down. Many people find that exercising to music helps them to stay motivated and keep a steady pace.

If you are over 40 and have not exercised for years, see your doctor and get a thorough checkup before launching into an aerobic exercise program (see "Heart Health Checklist: What Your Doctor Needs to Know," page 347). Not everyone will need a stress test, but if you have high blood pressure, diabetes, or preexisting heart conditions, your doctor may advise that you get this done first. Knowing your aerobic capacity and the response of your blood pressure and heart rate to exercise will give you a good idea of your baseline level of fitness. This information will also help your doctor uncover and treat important risk factors or signs of significant heart disease and ensure your safety as you embark on your new lifestyle.

ANAEROBIC EXERCISE

Aerobic exercise is, by definition, exercise that uses oxygen. Anaerobic exercise, such as weight lifting, uses glycogen, a type of sugar stored in the muscle tissues. A by-product of glycogen breakdown is lactic acid. Contrary to popular belief, lactic acid is not responsible for the "burn" we feel after heavy exercise. We now know that lactic acid is what helps keep the muscle working past the point of fatigue.

Weight lifting, sometimes referred to as resistance training, is a great complement to aerobic exercise, because it works the body and the muscles in a completely different way.

Weight training benefits are seen in men and women of all ages, ranging from teens to the elderly. It's never too late to start. One study showed striking improvements in muscle strength and ability to perform activities of daily living in a group of one hundred frail nursing-home patients whose average age was 87, most of whom required a cane, walker, or wheelchair to get around.

Besides strengthening the muscles, regular weight training actually increases your basal metabolic rate and will burn more calories even when you are doing nothing at all. That's because muscle tissue requires more energy to maintain itself than does fat tissue. Diabetics who combine weight training with aerobic exercise will often see incremental declines in blood sugar levels.

Some women fear that weight training will bulk them up, and so they avoid this type of exercise. That's not a worry as long as you follow my recommendation of twenty to thirty minutes of weight training twice per week. I've been working out with weights for more than twenty-five years and have yet to find a muscle that I don't want to keep. On the other hand, weight lifting shouldn't be counted on as a stand-alone exercise.

Weight lifting uses less than half the number of calories as aerobic exercise in a given amount of time. However, adding weight lifting to aerobic exercise may protect your heart even more than does aerobic exercise alone.

If you're planning to embark on a weight-lifting program, check in with your doctor first. People with hypertension are at greater risk for a stroke if their blood pressure is not controlled, because the strain of weight lifting will briefly raise the blood pressure. With regular workouts, the rise in blood pressure will usually become less substantial, as long as your resting blood pressure is normal. Of course, people with untreated heart problems, such as unstable blockages and congestive heart failure, should not exercise until their problems are under good control. A few heart conditions, such as serious heart valve disease and severely thickened heart muscle walls, make weight lifting unacceptably risky.

DON'T GET HURT AT THE HEALTH CLUB

MOST GYMS WILL provide new members with basic training, including safety precautions, for their machines and equipment. If your health club doesn't offer this service, investing in a few sessions with a well-qualified trainer is usually money well spent. Proper technique is vital if you want to achieve optimal results and avoid injuries and muscle strain. Be sure any workout you choose begins with a warm-up and ends with a cool-down.

A good trainer recognizes that there is no such thing as a typical client, and will work with you to develop a plan that takes into consideration your personal goals and available time, as well as your baseline strength and fitness. Be up front with your trainer about any medical conditions and medications that may affect your particular regimen.

YOGA AND PILATES: MIND AND BODY

Yoga and Pilates are physical exercises that incorporate an awareness of the body and mind through the use of the breath. They are often referred to as "mind-body" disciplines. Through both forms, the body is stretched and made supple, lengthening the muscles and allowing greater flexibility. Tendons and joints become more flexible, the core becomes stronger, the mind becomes calmer, and stamina increases. It is no wonder that professional athletes and dancers have flocked to yoga for years.

Yoga

Yoga is accessible at all levels of physical fitness and can range from very basic meditative poses to extremely challenging postures that take years to perfect.

Yoga newbies need knowledgeable instruction. Some of the postures can cause back pain or injury to the ligaments if done improperly or if attempted before the body is sufficiently flexible. If you already suffer from back or joint problems, consult your doctor first. Researchers at the University of Washington have found that when done properly, with good instruction, yoga can be surprisingly effective for reducing chronic lower back pain.

Studies have reported lower blood pressures, lower rates of anxiety and depression, and decreased levels of the stress hormone cortisol in yoga practitioners. Remember Dr. Ornish and his vegetarian high-carb, low-fat diet, in chapter 7 (see page 108)? The participants in his program also followed a strict regimen of yoga, aerobic exercise, and meditation. By five years in, they had half as many heart attacks and other heart events as did those who chose not to follow the program, as well as much less cholesterol buildup in their arteries.

There are numerous forms of yoga, some more spiritual, others purely physical. One school of yoga, known as Bikram Yoga, involves practicing in a room heated to more than 100°F with 70 percent humidity. This type of yoga should not be attempted by someone who is not physically fit. People on blood pressure medications may also react badly to the hot and humid environment and develop dangerously low blood pressure.

Pilates

Like yoga, the Pilates techniques, developed by Joseph Pilates in the early 1900s, are embraced by dancers, golfers, equestrians, and many other athletes. Pilates, who believed that physical fitness was essential for true happiness, derived many of his exercises from yoga. Symmetrically strengthening the core muscles of the abdomen, along with the muscles of the back and buttocks, the Pilates method enhances balance, flexibility, and posture.

Many Pilates exercises can be performed quite effectively with minimal to no props. But in traditional Pilates, a contraption known as the Universal Reformer helps to isolate various muscle groups so that the muscles can be used most effectively. Although this and other time-honored Pilates devices, with their pulleys, straps, and head rests, may look like medieval instruments of torture, they really do work. By using this equipment, you can develop a sense of proper body alignment and learn to use each specific muscle group to its best advantage.

The best way to learn yoga or Pilates is through an accredited teacher who can help you learn proper body positioning. Once you have the basics, you can use DVDs at home to supplement your practice. Leisa Hart of *Buns of Steel* fame has some terrific yoga DVDs accessible to all levels (try *Leisa Hart: Fat Burning Yoga*), and I highly recommend Ana Caban's DVDs for Pilates, including her *Pilates for Beginners and Beyond* boxed set.

BEST PRACTICES:
EXERCISE

* Exercise reduces your risk of heart disease, dementia, diabetes, high blood pressure, erectile dysfunction, osteoporosis, colon and breast cancer, gallstones, depression, and insomnia. It also helps burn up belly fat, raise good cholesterol, and lower triglycerides and CRP.

* Try to do at least 2½ hours of aerobic exercise weekly. Aerobic exercise includes walking, running, swimming, and biking.

* Shoot for 20–30 minutes of anaerobic exercise (weight training) 2 or 3 days per week.

* To stretch and add suppleness to the body, calm the mind, and improve balance and coordination, try yoga or Pilates. A session once or twice per week can have lasting effects.

Because there are so many choices when it comes to exercise, it helps to define your goals. If your main objective is to prevent heart disease, then any brisk aerobic activity for thirty minutes, five days per week, is perfect. For body sculpting and fat burning, add a twenty-minute workout with weights two or three days per week. To help develop serenity, balance, and flexibility of mind and body, a thirty- to sixty-minute session of yoga or Pilates at least once per week can work wonders. Or you may find that a combination of all three forms of exercise creates the perfect balance of heart, body, and mind.

Use Your Common Sense

THERE COMES A TIME in our lives when the truth hits us like a ton of bricks: It just doesn't have to be so complicated! Whether it's getting a good night's sleep, keeping those pearly whites gleaming, or making time for your friends, there is strong medicine in the daily wisdom that we learned as children. Whether it came from a teacher, a trusted friend, or good old Mom or Dad, we've all heard the adage that a positive approach to life helps to keep you on the road to good health.

It's comforting to know that, old-fashioned or not, this down-to-earth advice never goes out of style.

11

Mother Knows Best—
Are You Listening?

M AYBE YOU HEARD the advice in this chapter from your mother every day growing up (if she's told you once, she's told you a hundred times!)—and maybe you didn't. Perhaps your Mom could benefit from some of this advice herself. But regardless of whether we learned them from Mom, Dad, Mrs. Brady, or Hallmark, we all know a Mom-ism when we hear one: "Walk the dog!" "Eat your breakfast!" "Hold on to your friends!" And deep down, we all know it . . . she's usually right. Although maternal wisdom may be mysterious in its origin, it is practical in its application.

DRINK UP

Your body is an expert at monitoring and maintaining fluid balance. The problem is that we often don't listen to what our body is telling us. Crazy as it might seem, oftentimes we misinterpret our thirst as hunger, and snack when we should be sipping.

Although the 64 ounces of water per day paradigm has been challenged, if you are active, this amount is usually sufficient to maintain good hydration and heart health. People who drink at least five glasses of water per day are less prone to heart troubles than are those who drink very little, probably because the fluid keeps the blood flowing smoothly.

Juice or other drinks, including sports drinks, run a distant second to water, and not only because of their higher calorie content. Some scientists suspect that they can be counterproductive to good hydration, by pulling fluid into the digestive tract and out of the bloodstream. There is an exception for marathon runners and those who spend long hours out in the heat of the day: In these conditions, electrolytes (including sodium, potassium, and magnesium) can become severely depleted, so it's important to replenish with low-sugar sports drinks, watered-down fruit juice, or healthy snacks such as fruit and veggies.

Certain medications, including diuretics, can predispose you to dehydration and electrolyte abnormalities, so be sure to have regular blood testing if you take these drugs.

It is possible, although rare, to literally go overboard, drinking water to excess and diluting the natural balance of electrolytes. This problem is more apt to happen in the elderly, people with psychiatric illness, and those with kidney failure.

DON'T FORGET BREAKFAST

Breakfast is not optional. Your brain and body need healthy fuel for peak performance. Both adults and kiddos who eat breakfast tend to have a more positive mood, and they perform better on tests of memory and attention span. Compared with people who eat a nutritious breakfast, breakfast skippers fare worse on tests of physical endurance, even though they often believe that they are working harder. Adults and kids who eat breakfast are also less likely to become overweight.

Don't be fooled by the fast-food siren song. A sausage patty on a pasty white English muffin with cheese does not constitute a hearty breakfast, nor does an icky-sweet doughnut or toaster pastry. A whole-grain-based breakfast boosted with a side of protein provides nutrients and fiber, and helps to control cholesterol, especially when it includes soluble fiber such as oat bran. It takes less than a minute to pour yourself a bowl of heart-healthy cereal, add some soy milk, and sprinkle on a few berries or a spoonful of dried fruit—and not much longer to eat it. Treat your body well, and you'll make your mother proud.

BRUSH THOSE PEARLY WHITES

You know your mother was right about this one, although she may not have known that poor dental health is associated with a measurably higher risk of cardiovascular disease and stroke. Periodontal disease, or disease of the gum tissue, is often caused by poor hygiene. People with this condition are up to 70 percent more likely to develop heart disease. The risks of carotid artery disease (which may lead to strokes) and disease of the leg arteries are also higher with poor dental habits.

Periodontal disease is associated with higher levels of CRP, indicating chronic inflammation. The theory is that this inflammatory condition may also cause inflammation in the heart arteries, making cholesterol plaques less stable and more prone to rupture, and setting the stage for a heart attack. Adults who are obese and those with diabetes are more likely to have gum disease than are individuals of normal weight.

Keeping your gums and teeth clean and shiny is not rocket science. See your dentist at least every six months, floss daily, and brush at least twice a day for two minutes, preferably with an ultrasonic-type electrical brush. Don't cheat. Two minutes can seem like a long time when you've got a toothbrush in your mouth, but a healthy smile is worth the effort.

PLAY NICELY WITH OTHERS

Above my desk hangs a small framed cross-stitch panel I received from a dear friend and medical school classmate. My little keepsake declares: "A true friend is the rarest of all blessings." I know this to be true. Together my friend and I survived gross anatomy lab and the rigors of our first nerve-jangling nights on call. I feel fortunate that we have been able to maintain this friendship, forged in fire, across the years and miles. A friend is a lifeline, both figuratively and literally.

When you are under stress, having a friend by your side will help keep your blood pressure and heart rate in line and lower your body's production of stress hormones. Perhaps not surprisingly, this effect is most powerful when the friend is a woman, regardless of whether you are male or female.

Many women are gifted with a natural ability to nurture and support their friends and family through good times and bad. For many men, and some women, this role does not come easily, yet we all need love and acceptance.

Male or female, people with poor social support are more than twice as likely to die in the first year after a heart attack as are people with a caring community of friends and family. People with larger social networks tend to be healthier and to live longer than do those who are more solitary. For example, individuals who describe themselves as lonely are much more likely to suffer from high blood pressure and the associated health problems that come with this condition.

Elderly people who are lonely and socially isolated are more prone to develop Alzheimer's-like dementia, although their brain tissue may appear normal. This finding suggests that loneliness might actually alter our brain chemistry.

Marriage is an intriguing situation. By and large, marriage seems to promote better health for men, but not so much for women. Married women tend to have higher blood pressure and stronger physical reactions to stress than do their single counterparts, whereas married men have lower blood pressure than single men do. Married or not, women stay healthier longer when they have supportive female friends. But for men, marriage can make all the difference. Single men are twice as likely to die after a heart attack as are married men and are two to three times more likely to die prematurely from any cause. This does not necessarily hold true for women, whose health does not appear to benefit substantially from tying the knot, with one notable exception. Married women or women in a long-term relationship with a man who shows his affection with hugs and (yes!) massages tend to have lower blood pressure and a less intense physical reaction to stress. Very little is known about the health effects, good or bad, of same-sex partnerships.

Compared to women in bad marriages, women who are happily married are less likely to develop the metabolic syndrome (see chapter 13, page 235). And though healthy disagreement and even heated discussions with a spouse can be constructive, married people who respond to arguments with downright hostility are more likely to build up cholesterol plaques. This is particularly true for women, especially those in marriages where both partners are hot-tempered; this effect seems to be less significant, although still important, for men.

In later life, cohabitation and marriage seem to help protect against cognitive impairment and dementia, especially for men. For either gender, the risk of Alzheimer's dementia appears to be as much as seven times greater for those who are widowed in middle age and remain single, compared to those in a long-term marriage or domestic partnership. Men who lose their wives in middle age and never remarry appear to be particularly hard hit.

GIVE A HOOT, DON'T POLLUTE

It is easy to see how air pollution might contribute to asthma, lung cancer, and chronic lung disease, but what many people don't know is that air pollution will also increase the risk of heart attacks, heart failure, heart rhythm disturbances, strokes, and dangerous blood clots in the legs. It probably does so by triggering inflammation within the blood vessels and by stepping up production of fibrinogen, a blood product involved in clotting.

Pollution is powerfully tied to the foods we eat. Emissions from coal-burning power plants dump tons of mercury into our air and oceans each year, contaminating much of the fish we consume. Our country's voracious appetite for meat also has environmental implications. According to a 2006 United Nations report, the livestock industry is responsible for nearly 20 percent of greenhouse-gas emissions worldwide.

Pollution should concern us all. Children who live close to a freeway have substantial reductions in normal lung development. It has been estimated that people living in highly polluted cities lose an average of one to three years of life due to the effects of pollution. The good news is that we are already turning this grim statistic around. In 2009, *The New England Journal of Medicine* published evidence that improvement in air quality over the past thirty years has added over half a year of life expectancy in communities where high pollution levels have diminished.

Limiting emissions and supporting research into alternative energy sources will not only help the environment, it will have a direct effect on your cardiovascular and neurological health. It makes sense to do what you can to contribute to a solution.

ROLL UP YOUR SLEEVE AND SAY "OUCH"

Everyone knows that a case of the flu is a recipe for pure misery, but most people are unaware of the true devastation the virus can cause. The influenza virus, which strikes 25 to 30 million people in the United States each year, attacks the respiratory system, causing fevers, chills, body aches, cough, and a sore throat. Although most people recover from the illness, in the United States, more than 200,000 people are hospitalized and about 36,000 people die from the flu and its complications each year.

The flu can leave the lungs more susceptible to pneumonia. It is known to increase inflammation, raise the risk of blood clots, and to increase the heart rate, all of which can threaten heart health. In higher-risk individuals, the flu can actually trigger a heart attack. In fact, by some estimates as many as 30 percent of heart attacks are preceded by the flu or upper respiratory infections.

Not everyone who catches the flu is at the same high risk for a heart attack. Those who are more vulnerable include people over 50 years of age and folks with chronic medical illnesses, including heart disease and lung disease. For these people, studies show that getting a flu shot may cut the risk of a heart attack by 25 to 50 percent compared to those who choose not to get vaccinated. The risk of stroke also decreases considerably, and the overall risk of death declines by half. Tens of thousands of lives could be saved every year, and even more disability prevented, simply by vaccination.

Potential Problems with the Flu Vaccine

Many people refuse to be vaccinated. Some have an irrational fear of needles; others are worried the shot will cause the flu.

Because the flu shot now in use is a killed virus, there is no way that it can cause the flu, so you should put this fear to rest. (However, the intranasal form does contain live virus and is not recommended for heart patients and others with chronic conditions.) If you have a severe allergy to eggs, you should check with your physician before getting the vaccine, as you may be more likely to experience a reaction.

You might catch the virus if you are not vaccinated soon enough, but don't blame it on the flu shot. It takes about two weeks for the flu vaccine to work within your system to produce immunity.

Other people who sidestep vaccination cite years in which they were vaccinated in plenty of time, but still caught the flu. This is often not a failure of the vaccine itself, but a failure of the vaccine's developer to anticipate the specific strain of flu virus for that year. Because the virus mutates easily, there are a many different strains of influenza, some of which dominate more than others in any given year.

If the Bug Bites

Whether you catch the flu or just a nasty cold virus, stay home until the worst of it passes. People who work while they are sick are twice as likely to suffer a heart attack as are those who stay home, and they are more susceptible to other infections. They may also pass their uninvited germs on to coworkers, who in turn can spread the virus to family and friends. Do what your first-grade teacher told you: Keep your sniffles to yourself, cover your mouth when you cough or sneeze, and wash your hands frequently—everyone will be the better for it.

DON'T BURN YOUR FOOD

Although it is important to cook certain foods, particularly meat products, at temperatures high enough to destroy harmful bacteria, we know that cooking fruits and vegetables on high heat can rob them of their vitamins. Even more troublesome is evidence that cooking foods at temperatures of more than 212°F may produce high levels of a carcinogenic (cancer-causing) substance known as acrylamide. Starchy foods such as french fries contain acrylamide in abundance. It has been estimated that acrylamide may be responsible for up to one thousand cancers each year in the United States alone, although the issue is far from clear.

Cooking food at high temperatures may form other chemicals known as advanced glycation end-products (AGEs), which promote inflammation in the body, raising CRP levels. These substances are found in meats, fatty foods, breads, and other foods that are browned in the oven. They react within the body to increase damage to arteries, nerves, and kidneys. Diabetics are particularly susceptible.

AGEs can be reduced by using moist heat rather than dry, limiting cooking times and temperatures, and by using acidic ingredients such as vinegar and lemon juice. Exactly what AGEs mean for those of us who enjoy grilling outside on a sunny weekend is not clear, but this is an area of research that promises to heat up.

A DOG IS YOUR BEST FRIEND FOR LIFE

The first thing I see when I walk in the door after a long day at work is the joyful, goofy grin of my sweet greyhound. No matter what the day has brought me, Rosie makes me smile, and I can feel the stress begin to slip away. While you and I may know firsthand the healing powers of pets, scientists have just begun to discover the ways that our furry friends can enhance our life and improve our health.

Studies have found that older pet owners are more active and report a greater sense of well-being than those without animals. Adults of any age who have pets tend to experience less of an escalation in blood pressure and heart rate when exposed to mental and physical stress, especially when their pet is nearby. In fact, State University of New York researchers found that stress produced a milder physical reaction when a pet was close than when a spouse was standing by.

Even people who are already on medication for high blood pressure register lower readings when there is a pet around the house. Dog owners who suffer a heart attack are less likely to die in the first year afterward than are those without a dog. And there is no doubt that dogs are great exercise companions. Once you begin a daily walking routine, your dog surely won't let you forget it.

Of course, having a pet is an important responsibility, but for many people, this responsibility adds more meaning and purpose to life. I remember speaking to a stressed-out and lonely young law student who confided in me that if it wasn't for his cat, he probably would have contemplated suicide his first year of school.

THANK GOD FOR GOOD HEALTH

Central to many religious traditions is the tenet that it is the spirit—or the soul—that joins the mind and the body together. The word *spirituality* is commonly used in a religious context, but it may also refer to a sense of connectedness with life or an experience of transcendence. People with strong spiritual ties—whatever their faith or beliefs might be—need no convincing that their health is profoundly affected by their experience of the divine.

Older people who attend religious services regularly live longer than do nonchurchgoers. Simply listening to religious radio or watching a service on television doesn't appear to offer the same health rewards as actually being there. People who attend church tend to have lower blood pressure, whereas those who watch it on television are more likely to have high blood pressure. Perhaps it is the experience of the service itself, or it could be the community provided within the church, but there is no question that a rich spiritual life contributes to the well-being of the body.

YEARS AGO, I was on the medical faculty at the University of New Mexico, where there was a very strong Native American culture. When a member of one of the local pueblos fell seriously ill, the medicine man was often called to the intensive care unit for a healing ceremony. These ceremonies were very private and usually involved family and others close to the patient. I remember Joe, a 38-year-old father of two who came in with a severely weakened heart and respiratory failure triggered by a viral illness. Because he was so ill, he required a mechanical ventilator to do the work of breathing for him. Little by little, his heart condition improved, but despite our best efforts, he seemed to struggle, and only high doses of sedatives kept him calm. This made it very difficult to get him off the breathing machine, and increased his likelihood of serious complications such as pneumonia. His family decided to call in the medicine man, and that made all the difference. I never knew exactly what took place, but afterward, he was distinctly calmer, his heart rate was slower, and our medical care was much more effective. Ultimately, Joe made a full recovery.

While religion and spirituality can work wonders, on the flip side, a Cornell University survey found that Protestant men tend to carry more body weight than nonreligious men do. No one knows why this happens, but my guess is that it's all those prayer breakfasts and potluck dinners that pack on the pounds.

GET A GOOD NIGHT'S SLEEP

JASON IS A dynamic, hard-working man in his late 40s who sees me for high blood pressure. He is the father of a 2-year-old son and works in a high-intensity corporate environment. Jason was not happy about having to take medication, but his blood pressure was too high to go untreated. He was about 50 pounds overweight, so I encouraged him to work on weight loss and exercise, with the hope that tuning up his lifestyle might bring down his blood pressure enough to allow him to come off the medicine.

This usually immaculate gentleman showed up in my office one morning looking haggard and disheveled, his hair desperately in need of a good cut, his skin tone flat, and with dark circles under his eyes. With his typical over-achieving zeal, Jason had taken my advice to heart. He was starting his day an hour and a half earlier so he could fit in time to exercise while his family slept, but he still went to bed at his usual late hour. He hadn't lost weight, his blood pressure was higher than ever, and his work and home life were suffering. Jason was miserable.

We all need to balance our busy life with deep and restful sleep. We cannot adapt to less sleep, no matter how hard we try. Not only does lack of sleep make us sleepy, it can stifle creativity and memory and limit our ability to work at optimum levels. People who do not get adequate sleep are also more likely to suffer from depression, and are more susceptible to colds.

Women and men in their 30s through 50s who sleep less than an average of six hours per night have a twofold risk of hypertension and a greater risk for stroke and heart disease. Their blood vessels often fail to respond normally to stress, and blood tests may show higher levels of inflammatory CRP. Palpitations, or irregular heartbeats, are more common when we're sleep deprived, probably due to higher levels of stress hormones.

With a few exceptions, most of us do best with seven to eight hours each night. Sleep only six hours and you increase your odds of obesity by 23 percent. Those who sleep just four hours bump that obesity risk up by 73 percent.

Even short-term sleep deprivation may increase hunger pangs and result in cravings for starchy carbohydrates and sweets. Not surprisingly, poor sleep habits may be an important contributing factor for diabetes.

Is there such a thing as too much sleep? Possibly. Some studies have found that people who routinely sleep nine hours or more are at increased risk of cardiovascular disease. However, people who nap for at least thirty minutes three times per week may actually decrease their risk for cardiac death substantially. Even occasional catnaps may help.

Sleep Apnea, Obesity, and Snoring

Obese people are at high risk for a condition known as obstructive sleep apnea (OSA), in which the airway becomes partially blocked during sleep. The thicker your neck, the more likely you are to suffer from OSA. People with OSA tend to snore heavily, followed by periods of not breathing at all, known as apnea, and experience frequent awakenings during the night. The quality of sleep suffers tremendously. It is estimated that at least 2 percent of women and 4 percent of men over 50 suffer from OSA, but many experts suspect that number is even higher.

People with OSA tend to suffer from overwhelming fatigue during the day and, consequently, fall into a dangerous and vicious cycle of overeating and inactivity. OSA is associated with high blood pressure, elevated pressures in the lungs, weakening of the heart muscle, abnormal heart rhythms, and even heart attacks and strokes.

Fortunately, OSA is easy to diagnose with an overnight sleep study and can usually be effectively treated with a special mask that is worn at night. If the mask is not tolerable, dental devices are a second option. In severe cases, surgery may be required. Often, once OSA is controlled, weight loss and exercise become much easier.

Off to Dreamland

So how do you ensure a peaceful night's sleep? Avoid caffeine within six hours of bedtime. Exercise regularly, but not too late in the evening, or you may find yourself too wired to sleep. Stay away from late-night snacks, especially if you suffer from gastric reflux. Avoid drinking too much water before bedtime, and try to go to bed at around the same time every night.

Don't watch television or catch up on office work in bed. Treat yourself to a relaxing bedtime ritual, such as soaking in a warm tub, reading a mindless magazine, or writing in a journal, and make your bedroom a place of tranquility and peace.

One glass of wine may be a pleasant way to end the evening, but for some people, alcohol can disrupt sleep. So can many over-the-counter sleep aids, particularly diphenhydramine (also known as Benadryl). The supplement melatonin works well for some people, but we don't yet know much about its long-term safety. If you are a true insomniac, see your doctor. If everything checks out normally, a temporary prescription for a short-acting sleep medicine can sometimes help to reset your internal clock.

BEST PRACTICES:
MATERNAL WISDOM

* Although there is no hard-and-fast rule, aim for 64 ounces (eight 8-ounce glasses) of water every day; more if you're exercising.
* Don't skip breakfast.
* Brush your teeth for 2 minutes, at least twice a day—preferably with an ultrasonic toothbrush.
* Play nicely with others. Make good friends and keep them, and cultivate a loving relationship with your spouse or partner.
* Try not to contribute to pollution. Avoid exercising in polluted air whenever possible.
* Stay away from burned or scorched food, particularly if you are a diabetic.
* Get a flu shot each year, and avoid spreading cold and flu germs.
* A dog is your best friend. Or maybe a cat.
* A healthy dose of spirituality can do wonders for your physical well-being.
* Sleep for 7–8 hours every night, and squeeze in a nap when you can.

12

Attitude and Stress: Don't Let It Break Your Heart

ON A BUSY Monday morning, I opened the exam room door to meet Tiffany, a slim and girlish 35-year-old with a swinging red ponytail, sent to my office by her family doctor for symptoms of chest pain.

Tiffany looked so healthy and young that I doubted that I would find anything wrong. Her blood pressure was perfect and her cholesterol levels were normal. But as her story unwound, it was clear that my first impression was way off the mark.

A mother of two, Tiffany had been devastated when she caught her husband in an affair a year earlier. She was now in the middle of a contentious divorce. Her financial affairs were a mess, forcing her to work a low-paying cashier's job to support her kids. At night, she attended a local community college to earn a degree in the hopes of providing a better future for her family.

Overwhelmed with stress, Tiffany had recently taken up smoking, a habit she had quit ten years earlier. Despite all of this, she still found time to work out on her elliptical trainer at home after the kids were tucked in for the night. Recently, she had noticed a deep, nagging ache in her chest when she exercised. It was annoying, but she would try to power through the feeling, determined to finish her workout.

"I'm embarrassed to even be here," Tiffany told me. "I'm sure that there are people who need you more than me, and I know I must be wasting your time." I reassured her that her concerns were important and scheduled a stress echocardiogram, an exercise test that includes imaging the heart with ultrasound. The study results were extremely abnormal—so much so that I sent her straight to the hospital.

There was an 85 percent blockage in one of Tiffany's major coronary arteries. Two stents (small, flexible metal tubes) were required to open the vessel to restore normal blood flow. Thankfully, no permanent damage was done to her heart muscle, and a combination of medical therapy, smoking cessation, and stress reduction helped to get Tiffany back on track.

Tiffany's case illustrates the harm that stress can inflict. She was loaded down with a burden of anxiety and tension that was nearing the breaking point. She had a couple of strikes against her already— smoking and a family history of heart disease. Unlike many younger women who develop heart disease, she was not on birth control pills, which can dramatically raise the heart attack risk in smokers; but her decision to smoke, even a couple of cigarettes a day, more than doubled her risk.

Stress made Tiffany feel as if life was spinning out of her control. As much as I would have liked, I could give her no magic bullet to vaporize her stress. But, with some insight and understanding of the impact of the competing pressures in her life, she reached out to others— a vital step toward easing anxiety.

Tiffany learned to ask for help from her family, to choose foods for health rather than convenience, and to add yoga to her exercise routine. A financial planner at her community college helped Tiffany create a manageable economic roadmap, which gave her valuable peace of mind. With these important changes, along with a lifelong commitment to medical treatment, Tiffany will probably do well for years to come.

Just as stress can trigger a heart attack, increased life stressors following a heart attack are associated with a greater threat of subsequent death and serious illness. Depression and stress may both play a role in destabilizing cholesterol plaques, increasing the heart's vulnerability. Tiffany's is a case in point.

MOST STUDIES HAVE shown that stress alone is not enough to cause a heart attack. Take my patient Andrew, who first met me in the emergency room when he rolled in with a full-blown heart attack that struck right after he was handed his divorce papers.

Andrew insisted I call his soon-to-be-ex immediately to tell her the heart attack was all her fault. I respectfully declined and explained to my unhappy patient that this heart attack was the outcome of a long series of events brought about not only by stress, but also by smoking, high blood pressure, and a lifetime of fast food.

BROKEN HEART SYNDROME

A relatively rare condition, broken heart syndrome, also known as takotsubo cardiomyopathy, typically occurs as a result of severe and intense emotional stress. The condition is much more common in women over 50 than in any other group. In this disorder, the heart acts just as if it is in the throes of a heart attack. Severe chest pain, marked abnormalities of the electrocardiogram (a recording of the heart's electrical pattern), and characteristic blood test findings all suggest a major arterial blockage. The heart appears enlarged and weakened. In fact, the word *takotsubo* is a Japanese term that refers to a type of fishing pot with a wide base and narrow neck, with almost a balloon-like contour. This is very similar to the shape of the affected heart.

Usually women (or men) with this syndrome will be taken urgently for a cardiac catheterization, or angiogram, to look at the heart arteries, in anticipation of finding a blockage. In most cases of broken heart syndrome, there are no blockages at all. Exactly why and how this happens is not well understood, but it is probably related to a massive and toxic outpouring of stress-related hormones and chemicals. Fortunately, the condition usually resolves with medication, and in most cases the heart muscle eventually returns to normal function.

THE SCIENCE OF STRESS

Job issues, family problems, financial worries, you name it—most of us, on any given day, are just trying to cope with what life throws our way. In a survey from the U.S. Department of Labor, more than 60 percent of working women, regardless of job or income, described stress as their number one problem. Men are not far behind. Nearly 30 percent of all Americans describe their daily stress levels as "extreme," a statistic that has risen sharply in recent years.

As tension builds, stress may lead to a wide range of physical ailments, triggering the body's natural fight-or-flight mechanism, which is designed to protect us in times of extreme danger. These stress-driven systems work to protect us in the event of an emergency, but it is easy to see how chronic and recurring stress may be harmful to your heart.

Your endocrine system doesn't know the difference between your angry boss and a marauding saber-toothed tiger; all your body knows is that you are in trouble and so it does its best to prepare you to fight back or run away.

Adrenaline is one of the stress hormones your body releases in response to acute anxiety. It causes a sudden surge in heart rate and blood pressure, which helps you to make a swift escape, but adrenaline can also irritate your heart muscle, causing irregular heartbeats that may feel like an uncomfortable pounding or fluttering sensation in your chest.

Cortisol is another hormone that is released in response to physical or emotional stress. People who suffer from depression and anxiety tend to overproduce this hormone. Excessive cortisol production may also be triggered if you drink more than three cups of coffee in a day.

A product of the adrenal glands, cortisol raises blood sugar, preparing your body for increased energy needs. As a result, your blood sugar may rise precipitously if you are diabetic or prediabetic with glucose intolerance. At the same time, your blood pressure and heart rate may soar to dangerous levels. People over 60 are especially vulnerable to such surges in blood pressure. Cortisol can even help to make you fat, because it boosts your cravings for high-fat foods.

Cortisol, along with other hormones, has a diurnal variation, meaning that levels rise and fall throughout the day in a fairly predictable pattern. These levels tend to be highest around 6 AM and lowest at midnight. It is thought that the early-morning rise in cortisol may account for the fact that heart attacks frequently occur first thing in the morning.

Is Stress Always Bad?

Anxiety, apprehension, and worry, particularly in women, often lead to overeating both during and after the stressful parts of the day. Highly stressed people are more resistant to the effects of medications used to treat blood pressure and heart conditions, and their beneficial HDL cholesterol levels tend to be lower. And stressed-out people tend to sleep poorly, which can lead to a plethora of mental and physical ailments.

Yet stress is a natural part of life, and not all forms of stress are harmful. What it all boils down to, it seems, is control.

Men and women who work in positions of responsibility in which they experience stress, yet maintain control of their work and reach their goals successfully, are much better off, heart-wise, than are those who have demanding work with low levels of control. Such high-demand, low-control jobs may include clerical, manual labor, manufacturing, and health-care jobs, but any sort of job can qualify. Not surprisingly, homemakers with emotionally distant or unreasonably demanding husbands also tend to be less healthy than are working women in positions of responsibility.

Chronic stress at work, with high demands, low control, and minimal social support, more than doubles the odds of developing the metabolic syndrome, a cluster of risk factors that includes high blood pressure, unhealthy levels of cholesterol and triglycerides, insulin resistance, and obesity (see chapter 13, page 235). Heart attacks and strokes are more common when people are required to work under these conditions day after day.

Long working hours can take a serious toll on your health. For instance, a Japanese study found that men who work more than sixty hours per week have twice the risk of heart attacks as do those who work less than forty hours per week. And a British study of civil-service employees reported that heart disease risk jumped by sixty percent in those routinely working three to four hours of overtime beyond a typical eight-hour day.

No matter what your occupation, stress in the workplace may be a fact of life for you. Often, management can make all the difference, by supporting and empowering you to be directly involved in decision making and in improving the workplace. If you are a procrastinator, know that it is your responsibility to take control of your schedule and to manage your life so that you have the time and space you need to get the job done on time, whether it is at home or in the workplace.

By the same token, marital counseling can help turn an unhealthy marriage around before the stress and resentment become intolerable. Feeling good about what you do, whatever that may be, and being supported and empowered to do it well, will tend to balance out job stress and reduce the harm that it can inflict.

If you believe that your stress stems from post-traumatic stress disorder (PTSD), get help immediately. Violence, suicide, and toxic relationships, as well as accelerated heart disease, are all consequences of this very dangerous form of stress. This is not something that you can conquer on your own.

Grannies and Stay-at-Home Moms

Not surprisingly, studies have found higher cortisol levels in mothers in the workforce, indicative of greater emotional stress.

Yet stay-at-home moms who spend more than twenty hours a week caring for their kids have a higher risk of heart disease than do women with no child-care responsibilities. Grandmothers who spend at least nine hours each week with their grandkids also carry a higher risk of heart attacks. So far, there are no good cardiac studies examining the interactions between work and child-rearing duties in men.

If you're a mom, accept that raising children is stressful, no matter how much joy the sweet things bring. Children are your most vital responsibility. Nurture them and guide them, but don't neglect yourself. It's important to allow yourself time out to be your own person. If you have a partner or spouse, make sure that he or she is carrying a fair share of the load. If you're feeling overwhelmed, check in with your friends or relatives to see if you can help each other by sharing childcare responsibilities. If the burden feels too great, talk it over with your doctor and be sure that you are not suffering from depression.

Managing Stress: The Mind-Body Connection

There is no doubt that stress affects the mind, body, and soul. Any sort of exercise can make a difference, but many people find that the more meditative disciplines are especially helpful. Yoga is a great way to learn how to control the way you respond to stress, allowing you to slow your breathing and to focus your mind. Meditation has a similar effect. Several mainstream medical studies of transcendental meditation, based on ancient Indian tradition, have found important cardiovascular benefits, including a reduction in blood pressure, improved blood glucose levels, and, in people with heart disease, fewer episodes of congestive heart failure. Quality of life and measures of depression also improved. Tai Chi, sometimes referred to as "meditation in motion," is another great option. Even listening to slower-tempo music will help calm the mind, reduce the heart rate, and slow respiration.

BEST PRACTICES:
MANAGING STRESS

* How do you cope with stress? First, recognize the problem and the factors that contribute to it.

* If you work, you may not be in a position to change jobs, but you can strive to improve your environment, or at least your mind-set.

* If you're a mom, stress is part of the job, but be sure you are managing it effectively and positively. Get help from your spouse or partner, and be sure to maintain healthy relationships with your friends and relatives. See your doctor if the stress becomes overwhelming.

* If your marriage is the problem, don't just accept the status quo. A credentialed counselor or trusted clergyperson can provide vital insight and guidance.

* Make time to exercise, even if it seems as if you have none to spare. Those who are aerobically fit feel less anxious and stressed, and their blood pressure and heart rate are much less affected by the day-to-day trials and tribulations we all face.

* Yoga, Tai Chi, or meditation may help to bring down levels of stress hormones and improve your physical reaction to the stress in your life.

* Sleep is a necessity, not a luxury. It is strongly linked to your mood and feelings of stress. People who get fewer than 6 hours of sleep are twice as likely to feel sad, stressed, and angry as those who sleep at least 8 hours.

* Recognize your stress triggers. Learn to tune in, to discover the sources of anxiety and stress in your life. Take ownership of the problem.

* Get help from an expert if you need to get organized, either from within your company or from an organizational consultant.

* Develop supportive social networks at work and at home.

- Eat well. A diet high in sugar, simple starches, and saturated and trans fats will ensure that you continue to feel sluggish, unmotivated, and overwhelmed. Instead, choose fruit, vegetables, whole grains, and high-quality protein to give you the energy you need to face your challenges.
- If you suffer from PTSD, get professional help without delay.

PERSONALITY AND HEART DISEASE

Although it's often a mistake to make generalizations, psychologists have recognized several distinct personality archetypes that shape an individual's response to stress.

Type A: Competitive and Impatient

If you are a type A personality, hard-driven, ambitious, quick to anger, and never satisfied, you may have the determination and competitive drive to get ahead and achieve great things, but the hostility and intolerance that often accompany these personality traits may be lethal.

When type A's get stressed out, their heart rate and blood pressure may climb dangerously. Those type A's who are highly irritable and impatient are at two to four times the risk for heart disease as their easy-going type B brethren. These personality traits do not necessarily cause atherosclerosis to develop, but they can make plaque that is already there more vulnerable to rupture, increasing the likelihood of a heart attack or stroke. This is why the risk of a heart attack escalates dramatically, up to nine times normal, in the first hour after an angry rage.

GREGG IS A highly successful and well-respected manager of a large grocery store. At work, he keeps an even keel, but at home, it is another story altogether. I met him in the emergency room late one night when he presented with chest pain and severely elevated blood pressure. It turned out that Gregg and his 16-year-old son, Darrell, had had a furious argument over Darrell's decision to quit the football team. Gregg loved his son desperately, but could not understand his lack of enthusiasm for the sport. Instead of calm acceptance, Gregg's reaction was destructive, divisive, and could very easily have cost him his life.

Being a type A isn't always a bad thing. If you can learn to focus your drive and competitiveness, and control your hostility and impatience, you are more likely than others to achieve healthy goals, such as exercise and weight loss, and to be professionally successful.

Type B: No Worries

Type B personalities are the original beach bums, the lighthearted, worry-free, noncompetitive spirits who prefer to "live and let live." Type B's in general have a lower risk for heart disease than do other personality types, but they often don't do as well after a heart attack occurs. This is probably because they frequently fail to take an active role in their recovery, assuming that everything will turn out all right in the end.

JULIE, A LOVELY woman with complicated high blood pressure and a leaky aortic heart valve, is a retired saleswoman whose penchant for entertaining is legendary. She is full of laughter and interesting stories, and it's always a pleasure to see her. Julie's easygoing attitude also extends to her health, and for years she rarely worried about taking her medications. She felt fine, so why lose sleep over it? Over time, her heart valve took the brunt of her medical apathy, and now she finds herself facing surgery. While we can't always prevent heart valves from deteriorating, in Julie's case, it's very likely that medical therapy could have made a difference.

Type C: Quiet Desperation

Type C's are the appeasers, deferring to the genuine or imagined desires of others. They have difficulty expressing any emotions, especially anger, and tend to bottle things up inside, preferring to maintain a neutral outward appearance. They are often lonely and feel a sense of despair and hopelessness that they prefer not to discuss with others. The type C personality may be at greater risk for cancer, but this personality type hasn't yet been studied much in regard to the risk for heart disease.

LILA, A 74-YEAR-OLD homemaker, spends her days caring for her spouse, 80-year-old Rick. Rick suffers from advanced dementia, and is often verbally and physically abusive to his wife. A thin and frail lifelong smoker, Lila uses inhalers for chronic lung disease and takes blood thinners for an irregular heart rhythm known as atrial fibrillation. It's hard to imagine this 105-pound lady bathing, dressing, and feeding an 180-pound man, but that is Lila's daily reality. Sadly, she refuses either to allow home health-care aides to visit, or to ask any of her four daughters to pitch in. Since she will not acknowledge that her health is suffering, there is very little that anyone can do to help.

Type D: Down

Type D's are pessimists. They are often irritable, anxious, and unhappy, and frequently suffer from depression. The Type D personality has a more dramatic physical response to stress, and is much more likely to do poorly than a non-D after a heart attack, particularly if younger than 55. Despite this, a type D is likely to delay visiting the doctor for serious health issues, waiting until the problem becomes critical. Type D's may convince themselves that it is not worth trying to live a healthy life, and may feel that they have no control over their future, making their poor health a self-fulfilling prophesy. Type D's are also more prone to dementia later in life.

JERRY'S HEART MUSCLE has been weakened by years of alcohol abuse. The 60-year-old retired airline mechanic is what we call a "frequent flyer" at the hospital, with numerous admissions for congestive heart failure, and is well known by the Intensive Care Unit staff. He would have a fighting chance at health if he were to simply come in for regular office visits. That way, I could monitor his progress and adjust his medications when necessary. Cutting out the booze would do wonders as well. Instead, despite the best efforts of his family and the hospital social workers, we only see Jerry when he is at death's door. I just don't know how much more abuse his poor heart can take.

DEPRESSION

We all get the blues from time to time, but people who suffer from true depression may be more prone to develop heart disease. Depression is characterized by feelings of hopelessness and worthlessness, and by an inability to experience pleasure and interest in activities of everyday life. In depression, the brain chemistry is altered, so it is difficult, if not impossible, to "just snap out of it." Nearly 12 percent of women and 6 percent of men will experience a major depression at some time in their life. It can come on without warning and last for months or even years.

Insomnia, low energy, and difficulty concentrating are hallmarks of depression. Studies of both women and men have found that depression may raise the risk of a heart attack up to twice normal. Depression will dramatically increase the likelihood of a stroke, with a fourfold risk in people under the age of 65. Depression is also linked to increased cholesterol buildup in the arteries and a greater probability of dying in the years following a heart attack.

People who experience anxiety along with depression may be especially vulnerable. Depressed people are less inclined to exercise, more likely to make unhealthy dietary choices, and less apt to take medications.

If you choose a heart-healthy Mediterranean-style diet, you'll be more likely to avoid or overcome a mild case of depression. However, it is not easy to beat depression alone. The first step toward recovery is recognition that there is a problem, and the second step is to seek help from your doctor. If you feel overwhelmed or even slightly suicidal, seek help immediately. (A good place to start is by calling the National Suicide Hotline at 1-800-784-2433.) Psychotherapy and medication, when appropriate, can be lifesaving.

LOOKING ON THE BRIGHT SIDE

Can a positive attitude save your life? Positive thinkers are less likely to develop chronic illnesses, probably because they are more apt to exercise, eat well, and cultivate other healthy habits. They may also cope better with stress than habitual pessimists. Once a serious disease develops, however, optimism will not necessarily prolong survival, although it may improve the quality of life.

Your attitude is a reflection of how you choose to live your life. Do your best to maintain a healthy optimism, but most importantly, follow through with a forward-thinking approach to your life and your health. Of course, if you need help, do not hesitate to turn to your doctor or other trusted professional who can help you. Allow yourself to experience the joy of a positive attitude.

BEST PRACTICES:
STRESS, ATTITUDE, AND DEPRESSION

* Stress can raise blood pressure, blood sugar, and heart rate; cause irregular heartbeats; and make you fat. The unhealthiest stress is stress you cannot control.
* If you have suffered a major loss or shock, make sure your physician takes any cardiac symptoms seriously. A

broken heart can be a genuine, although rare, medical condition, and is often caused by severe stress.

* If you're a "type A" achiever, try to keep anger in check and healthy living in mind: Your high-stress lifestyle can be tough on your heart, but your drive to succeed will serve you well if you make heart health your goal.

* If you're a "type B," don't neglect your heart: Your laid-back personality comes with a lower heart attack risk, but could lead you to take a passive approach to your health.

* If you tend to appease others and neglect your own needs, you may be a type C. People with this personality type often suffer from loneliness and may be more prone to developing cancer. Exercise and regular medical checkups can make a big difference.

* Type D's tend to be pessimistic and easily irritated. If this describes you, don't neglect the impact all this stress can have on your health. It's not unusual for a type D to have severe hypertension, raising the risk for stroke, heart disease, and kidney failure.

* If you are depressed, seek help: Not only is depression a serious condition in its own right, it can increase the risk of cardiovascular disease, including stroke.

* A healthy diet, exercise, meditation, and sleep can all reduce levels of stress, anxiety, and depression.

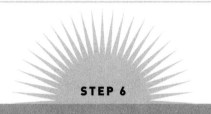

Know Your Options

IT'S A FACT of life that good health doesn't always come naturally. There is a world of options and alternatives available to help support, maintain, and protect your well-being. The challenge lies in learning how to make the right choices and knowing whom to trust. Learning to discern the truth from the myths will help you make the smartest choices for yourself and for those you love.

Vitamins and minerals are essential for a healthy heart, but recent medical research suggests that we need to be very careful when considering high-dose supplements. In most cases, when it comes to nutrition, fresh food in its natural state is your best bet.

Supplements and herbs are big business, and manufacturers aren't always the most reliable source of information about these products. There is good science behind many supplements, while others may just be a waste of your hard-earned cash, or worse.

Mother Nature is a master at prevention, but sometimes you need the care of a skilled practitioner. Whether the problem is simple or complex, it's important to choose someone you can depend on, and someone with your best interests at heart. Help may come in the form of a physician, a massage therapist, even a hypnotherapist. But while a good doctor is a valuable ally, for her to give you her best, you have to take your own health personally.

13

The Power of Preventive Medicine: Managing Risk, Preventing Consequences

THE WAY YOU choose to live your life can alter your destiny, protecting you from heart attacks, stroke, cancer, and dementia and granting you more time and energy to enjoy all that life has to offer. Wouldn't it be nice if simply choosing a healthy lifestyle was all it took? Unfortunately, many of us carry within our genetic makeup a natural inclination for high blood pressure, high cholesterol, and diabetes—among the most powerful risk factors for heart disease (see "Know Your Risk Factors," page 349). Some people have none of these risk factors, yet come from a lineage fraught with heart disease and stroke. In every instance, how we take care of our body makes a tremendous difference. Still, sometimes, healthy choices just aren't enough.

Thankfully, we live in an era of preventive medicine with unprecedented opportunities for treatment of these silent killers. One of my most important responsibilities as a cardiologist is the diagnosis and treatment of these common conditions. However, I cannot help you unless you take the first step. Get your blood pressure, cholesterol, and blood sugar tested. It is easy, and it just might save your life.

HYPERTENSION

People often confuse the word *hypertension* with the concept of being hyper or tense. However, hypertension is simply high blood pressure.

It is estimated that at least 68 million people in the United States—fully one third of the adult U.S. population—have high blood pressure. It is a major public health crisis that the number of individuals with hypertension has increased by more than 20 million since the early 1990s. Mounting obesity levels are a major contributor. Moreover, people are living longer, and the older you get, the more likely you are to have high blood pressure. After the age of 60, half of all men and women suffer from hypertension. In fact, older women are somewhat more likely than older men to have high blood pressure. If you live into your 90s, you will have a 90 percent probability of developing hypertension.

Although the condition itself is usually painless, hypertension is a major contributor to as many as 1 million heart attacks every year and is the most preventable cause of strokes. It taxes the heart, causing the heart muscle to become thicker and less efficient. It also injures the blood vessels of the heart, brain, kidneys, and other vital organs, making them more rigid and more vulnerable to cholesterol plaques.

People living with uncontrolled hypertension have a sevenfold increase in the risk of a stroke and are three times more likely to suffer a heart attack than people with normal blood pressure. Other devastating consequences include kidney failure, congestive heart failure, disease of the retina, and even dementia. Women with hypertension have a dramatically higher risk for preeclampsia, a dangerous complication of pregnancy that can threaten the lives of both the mother and the unborn child.

Many times, high blood pressure exists without symptoms, allowing years of silent and relentless damage to the heart, brain, and kidneys. Thirty percent of people with this condition have no clue that they are living with dangerously high pressure. Some do experience headaches when their blood pressure is excessively high, especially if they have what is known as labile hypertension, or erratic fluctuations in blood pressure, but many others have no warning signs when their blood pressure is high.

Of those who have been diagnosed with high blood pressure, only half actually take medication regularly. And even when medication is taken as prescribed, only two thirds of those people have their blood pressure adequately controlled. This is usually not because the blood pressure drugs don't work, but because either the patient or the physician chooses not to treat the condition aggressively.

It is easy to get frustrated with the process of controlling high blood pressure. Sometimes it's a matter of trying several different drugs before you hit on the right choice or combination. We are all unique individuals, and there is no "one size fits all" treatment. In the future, genetic testing may help to pinpoint which drugs would work best for an individual, but we're not there yet.

How Blood Pressure Is Measured

The only sure way to know whether your blood pressure is high is to test for it (see "Heart Health Checklist: What You Should Ask Your Doctor," page 348). If you've always had normal blood pressure, you should get checked at least annually. Those with high readings should be evaluated more frequently. Typically, your doctor's office performs this test, using a blood pressure cuff, or sphygmomanometer. You can also easily do it yourself, but some important nuances are worth understanding—so indulge me with this blood pressure primer.

Blood pressure is always given as two numbers, one above the other. The systolic, which is the first or top number, measures the pressure when the heart is contracting. The bottom reading, the diastolic pressure, represents the pressure in the arteries as the heart relaxes after the contraction. Both numbers are important.

Blood pressure readings should be taken after sitting quietly for about five minutes, feet on the floor, with your arm at heart level. The cuff is inflated briefly, preventing blood flow in the main artery that travels through the arm. As pressure in the cuff is slowly released, blood starts to flow in the artery, creating a pounding sound. The systolic blood pressure is the pressure at which this sound is first heard. The air is slowly emptied, and when the pulse is no longer audible, the diastolic blood pressure has been reached.

Generally, you should have at least three separate blood pressure readings on three different days before a doctor can make a diagnosis of high blood pressure. If your blood pressure is extremely high, however, this rule does not usually apply, and treatment is often started immediately.

What Those Numbers Mean

The ideal blood pressure is less than 120/80 mm Hg. (The abbreviation *mm Hg* refers to millimeters of mercury, which is the scale that is used to measure blood pressure.) Hypertension is defined as a blood pressure of 140/90 or higher.

A blood pressure between 120/80 and 139/89 is considered to be prehypertension. A blood pressure in the prehypertensive range is associated with a two- to threefold higher risk for heart disease. If you fall in this range, consider it a wake-up call to implement major lifestyle changes, including losing weight if appropriate, curbing salt intake, choosing a heart-healthy diet, and exercising.

Systolic pressures as low as 90 may be perfectly normal, especially in smaller people. However, excessively low blood pressure may cause dizziness and lightheadedness and is often due to dehydration, blood loss, or overmedication.

Both the systolic and diastolic blood pressures are important, but their relative importance changes with age. Below the age of 50, a high diastolic pressure is associated with a higher risk of heart disease and stroke. Over the age of 50, the systolic pressure becomes more of an issue. In general, each increase of 20 mm Hg systolic or 10 mm Hg diastolic above 115/75 doubles the risk of cardiovascular disease.

Many people suffer from "white-coat hypertension," or the phenomenon of higher blood pressure readings in the doctor's office. This problem is typically brought on by stress or anxiety. Often, the blood pressure can be rechecked a few minutes later, and it will be back in the normal range.

My patient Sylvia, an active 75-year-old who loves to travel, is a prime example of the trouble that white-coat hypertension can cause. Sylvia has had surgery to replace a defective heart valve, and her tests consistently show her heart to be functioning beautifully. Although normally a calm and rational person, Sylvia frets about her blood pressure reading as soon as she hits the waiting room. By the time my assistant checks her blood pressure, she is nearing panic mode, and, sure enough, her readings are almost always high. When we first met, my inclination was to add more medication to her list, but when Sylvia presented me with her home readings, they were absolutely perfect. We had her check her pressure at home at different times during the day. In addition, she brought in her blood pressure machine so we could confirm its accuracy. Everything checked out, and Sylvia's readings were well within the normal range. Had I prescribed medication based simply on our office measurement, it could have dropped Sylvia's pressure to a dangerously low level, putting her at risk of falling and seriously curtailing her very active lifestyle.

Measure Your Own Blood Pressure

If you want to monitor your readings, it's a good idea to obtain your own blood pressure cuff, as several measurements at different times and dates are much more helpful than a single pressure reading in a medical office. A home blood pressure machine is a great investment in your health, and most devices are easy to use. You can choose either an electronic or a manual cuff, but make sure you get it checked by your doctor to confirm that the readings are accurate. I recommend an upper arm cuff, because pressures measured in the wrist or finger are much less reliable. The cuff should fit properly, because a cuff that is too large or too small may result in false readings. Most obese people will need a large cuff.

Blood pressure is not a static number; it is normal for it to vary by about 20 percent throughout the day. Measure your blood pressure in the middle of the day, as well as morning and evening, so you can get familiar with the range of your numbers during your most stressful and most relaxing times of the day. Once you have a good representative sampling (usually across one to two weeks) you will not need to measure it as often, unless your doctor advises you to do so.

What Can Raise Blood Pressure?

- Stress and chronic pain can influence blood pressure, but are usually less important than other lifestyle factors.
- Drinking more than two alcoholic drinks a day or more than three cups of coffee may raise blood pressure.
- Seemingly innocent prescription drugs and over-the-counter medications may also affect blood pressure. Some women will find that birth control pills bump up the pressure, although this happens fairly infrequently. A wide range of prescription and over-the-counter anti-inflammatory medications, including ibuprofen and naproxen, may increase blood pressure and cause fluid retention.
- Over-the-counter decongestants and herbal stimulants are also culprits (see the table in "Supplements, Science, and Safety," page 279). And it is a little-known fact that an obsession with black licorice (only the genuine stuff) can raise blood pressure.
- Your doctor should exclude treatable and reversible medical causes of hypertension. A good screening evaluation includes a complete physical exam and a blood chemistry profile, which may uncover other associated problems, such as kidney disease or thyroid abnormalities.

Ways to Bring Blood Pressure Down

If your blood pressure is borderline or high, what should you do? Diet, exercise, and weight loss can help tremendously, especially in people below the age of 50 whose blood pressure is only mildly elevated. Up to one third of people with early-stage hypertension or prehypertension can bring their blood pressure down to the normal range with these simple lifestyle changes. If you are overweight, losing as little as 15 pounds can make all the difference. A diet high in fruit, vegetables, and low-fat dairy products is particularly effective, especially when combined with a low-sodium diet (see chapter 6, page 100, for more about salt and sodium).

Medical Treatment for Hypertension

Despite the long list of blood pressure offenders, the great majority of people with high blood pressure that is not easily controlled with diet and exercise have what we call *essential hypertension*. Essential hypertension refers to high blood pressure with no identifiable cause.

Unlike infections and broken bones, essential hypertension requires ongoing medical treatment and is usually a lifelong condition. Most of my patients are surprised when I tell them that the average person with high blood pressure requires two or three medications, and frequently more than that. If you have essential hypertension, you can often minimize the number of medications you need with a healthy diet, appropriate body weight, and regular exercise. Considering the high cost of most medications, this investment in your health will quickly pay dividends.

While it is beyond the scope of this book to review specific medications, it is helpful to go over the general classes of drugs that your doctor may choose to prescribe. There are scores of antihypertensive drugs, but most will fit into one of the following categories:

■ DIURETICS

Also known as "water pills," diuretic medications are often a great first choice to treat high blood pressure. Some women tend to retain fluid, often related to salt sensitivity, and diuretics can help. Most diuretics cause potassium loss, so a doctor may also prescribe a potassium supplement. If you take a diuretic, it is important to have regular blood work at least once or twice a year to monitor your electrolytes.

■ BETA-BLOCKERS

The term *beta-blocker* refers to the receptors in the heart and blood vessels that are blocked by these antihypertensive medications, resulting in lower blood pressure as well as reduced heart rate. This class of drugs is especially important for people with heart disease. They reduce the risk of a heart attack and are highly effective for the treatment of heart failure. Beta-blockers are also extremely helpful in people with palpitations due to a fast or irregular heartbeat.

Most people have no problems with beta-blockers, but these medications do have the potential to cause excessive slowing of the heart rate, depression, fatigue, and poor libido in a small percentage of people. As a result, the metabolism may slow a bit, and motivation to exercise may wane. These side effects are why beta-blockers are occasionally associated with weight gain in sensitive individuals, although we're talking an average gain of less than 3 pounds over about six months. Some beta-blockers can raise levels of triglycerides, although usually only to a mild degree. People who exercise vigorously may notice that their peak heart rate is somewhat constrained when taking beta-blockers. And beta-blockers can sometimes make asthma symptoms worse.

If you experience these or any other problems, it's important to discuss them with your doctor. In many cases, your doctor can substitute another drug for the beta-blocker.

■ CALCIUM CHANNEL BLOCKERS

Calcium channel blockers are medications that slow the flow of calcium into the cells of the heart and arteries, allowing them to widen and relax, thereby reducing blood pressure. Like beta-blockers, some calcium channel blockers also slow the heart rate, so they are sometimes used for this purpose as well. Don't let the name of this class of drugs fool you. A calcium channel blocker will not lower the calcium level in your bones or bloodstream.

Most people feel just fine on calcium channel blockers, but somewhere between 5 and 20 percent of people will experience side effects such as fluid retention and constipation. The drugs diltiazem and verapamil can also cause an excessive slowing of the heart rate in people who are sensitive to this effect, most notably in older folks.

■ ACE INHIBITORS

ACE inhibitors, or inhibitors of angiotensin-converting enzyme, block the production of a chemical that, among other things, causes arteries to constrict. ACE inhibitors are used to control blood pressure, treat heart failure, and prevent kidney damage in people with hypertension or diabetes. These medications help to relax your blood vessels, which improves the efficiency of the heart and lowers blood pressure. ACE inhibitors also increase blood flow, which decreases the amount of work required by your heart.

This class of drugs is a mainstay of heart disease treatment and has been proven to lower the risk of heart attacks and congestive heart failure. The most common side effect is a dry, itchy cough, which occurs about 5 percent of the time. Some individuals with kidney problems may be unable to take ACE inhibitors, which may worsen kidney function in a small percentage of people. It's easy to test for this complication with a blood test. ACE inhibitors should never be taken while pregnant, as they can cause birth defects.

■ ARBS

Angiotensin-2 receptor blockers (ARBs) work much like ACE inhibitors but are associated with fewer side effects. For instance, these drugs do not cause a cough. Like the ACE inhibitors, this type of medication is also a great choice for diabetics, as the ARBs help protect against kidney failure. A large Veterans Administration–based study suggested that the ARBs may be better than other drugs at preventing and slowing dementia. As with the ACE inhibitors, it is important to use blood tests to monitor kidney function in people with vulnerable kidneys. And like the ACE inhibitors, these drugs can also cause birth defects, so they should be avoided during pregnancy.

■ ALPHA-BLOCKERS

Alpha-blockers help to relax the blood vessels, thereby lowering blood pressure. They are often used to help men with an enlarged prostate, by improving urinary flow. Alpha-blockers are not especially beneficial to the heart, so they are not usually our first line of hypertensive therapy.

■ DIRECT RENIN INHIBITORS

A fairly new class of drugs targets an enzyme called renin, which is produced by the kidneys. High levels of renin contribute to high blood pressure by causing constriction of blood vessels. Kidney function should be evaluated with a blood test when one of these drugs is started, and these drugs should never be used during pregnancy.

BEST PRACTICES:
HYPERTENSION

* Know your blood pressure. For most of us, an ideal blood pressure is 115/75. Seniors and diabetics may do better with a systolic pressure of 120–140.
* For mildly elevated blood pressure, try dieting, exercising, and limiting salt intake. These lifestyle changes can often bring blood pressure back to normal without medication.
* If you need medication for hypertension, consult with your doctor about the best treatment for your situation. Available treatments include diuretics, beta-blockers, calcium channel blockers, ACE inhibitors, ARBs, alpha-blockers, and direct renin inhibitors. If you are pregnant or considering pregnancy, discuss this with your doctor before starting any medication.
* Take your blood pressure medication as prescribed, because most of these drugs wear off in 24 hours or less.
* If you experience side effects, let your doctor know. If your blood pressure is difficult to control, you may need

a referral to a cardiologist, kidney doctor, or other blood pressure specialist.

* Don't just give up and accept mediocre blood pressure control, or therapies that cause you to feel "not yourself." Many different medications are available, and your doctor can usually find one, or a combination, that will work well for you. Remember that the goal is to achieve not just a "number," but a blood pressure that will help to keep your heart, brain, kidneys, and the rest of your body safe, strong, and healthy.

CHOLESTEROL AND TRIGLYCERIDES: A RECAP

Chapter 3 explains the intricacies of the lipid profile (see page 26), but let's address the essentials here. LDL cholesterol (the "lousy" one) is influenced by genetics, but diet and smoking have a substantial effect. Trans fats and saturated fats are notorious for raising LDL cholesterol, whereas monounsaturated fats, from foods like olive oil and nuts, and soluble fiber from such foods as oatmeal and apples, can lower LDL. Dietary cholesterol itself plays a relatively minor but still important role in raising LDL. And adipose tissue (that is, body fat) increases LDL cholesterol levels.

In general, LDL should be less than 130 mg/dL; ideally, it should be below 100. If you have coronary artery disease or diabetes or are at very high risk for cardiovascular disease, your LDL should be under 70.

Fortunately, everyone also has HDL cholesterol, the good fairy. Exercise, moderate alcohol use (one or two drinks a few days a week), and a healthy diet will increase HDL. In general, higher HDL levels are better. Smoking, saturated and trans fats, and stress can lower HDL, as can a diet high in simple carbohydrates with a high glycemic load (see chapter 4, page 44, for more on this topic). When it comes to HDL, women tend to have an advantage over men, although menopause tends to level the playing field. HDL levels should be at least 50 mg/dL for women, and at least 40 mg/dL for men.

Triglycerides are also part of the lipid profile, and levels greater than 150 mg/dL are associated with a higher likelihood of heart disease, especially in women. Sweet, starchy, and fatty foods and heavy alcohol use (three or more drinks daily) will raise triglycerides, as will some medications and smoking. A diet higher in protein and lower in simple carbohydrates will help control the triglyceride level (see chapter 7, page 111).

BEST PRACTICES:
CHOLESTEROL AND TRIGLYCERIDES

* Know your profile: LDL is "bad" cholesterol; you want to lower this one. HDL is "good"; you want to keep it high. You'll also want to keep your triglycerides under control.
* Aim for an LDL level less than 130 mg/dL and ideally below 100. If you have coronary artery disease, diabetes, or are at very high risk for cardiovascular disease, your optimal LDL is less than 70. Weight loss, soluble fiber, and monounsaturated fats will lower your LDL.
* Keep your HDL above 50 mg/dL if you are female, or 40 mg/dL if you are male. Exercise, moderate amounts of alcohol, soy foods, and monounsaturated fats will raise your HDL. Avoid smoking, saturated fats, stress, and high-glycemic carbohydrates, which lower HDL.
* Keep your triglycerides below 150 mg/dL. Exercise and weight loss, when needed, will lower triglyceride levels. Avoid sweets, starchy foods, fats, heavy alcohol use, and smoking, which raise triglycerides. Be aware that some medications can raise triglycerides.

TREATING HIGH CHOLESTEROL MEDICALLY

The sooner high cholesterol is treated, the greater the opportunity to prevent heart disease and enjoy a life enriched by good health. In 2003, a group of British researchers published an analysis of more than two hundred studies and reported that by reducing cholesterol just 10 percent at age 40, the subsequent risk of heart disease could be lowered by 50 percent. Although it's never too late, at age 70, the same 10 percent cholesterol reduction translates to only a 20 percent lower risk.

If your heart disease risk is high or your numbers are substantially elevated, prescription drugs may be needed to improve your lipid profile enough to bring it into a safe range. It's important to remember that even if you do require medication to reach your lipid goals, diet and exercise are crucial to maintaining and supporting the health of your body. Taking a pill does not absolve you of your responsibility for your own health.

If you are pregnant, breast feeding, or considering pregnancy in the near future, be aware that you should not take cholesterol-lowering drugs, as these drugs may be harmful to the fetus or nursing baby.

Statin Drugs

Statins are truly modern miracles. When used appropriately, they reduce the risk of heart attack, stroke, and other life-threatening cardiovascular events by an average of 25 to 30 percent; with long-term use, the benefits may be even greater. This means not only a reduction in risk of death but an equally important reduction in the likelihood of disability due to stroke, congestive heart failure, and life-threatening heart rhythm abnormalities.

Statins are the most commonly used and most effective cholesterol-lowering drugs available. These drugs, which include such well-known brand names as Lipitor, Zocor, Pravachol, Lescol, Mevacor, Livalo, and Crestor, work primarily via the liver. The drugs help to prevent the manufacture of cholesterol, while also improving the liver's ability to clear LDL cholesterol out of the bloodstream. The amount of LDL lowering depends on the specific drug, the dose used, and the individual response, but reductions of 50 percent or more are typically achievable.

Statin drugs help to stabilize preexisting cholesterol plaques, making them less prone to rupture and cause a heart attack or stroke.

They also prevent formation of new plaques. At high enough doses, statins may even help to shrink cholesterol buildup. Statins also lower CRP, probably through antioxidant and anti-inflammatory mechanisms, although this has not been studied to the same extent as cholesterol. HDL is minimally affected by statins, although some can raise HDL by 5 to 10 percent.

The benefits of statin drugs may extend beyond heart health. There is good evidence of a lower risk of senile dementia in statin users. This stands to reason, because the brain is a vascular organ, and many cases of senile dementia are due to a series of tiny, almost imperceptible strokes.

A seven-year study from the Harvard School of Public Health also found lower rates of anxiety, depression, and hostility in long-term statin users, although the study could not definitively establish cause and effect. A Turkish study found improvement in erectile dysfunction in men who took a statin for one year. The average age of the men in the study was 45, and for most of them it took at least six months on the drug to see results. The researchers theorized that the lower cholesterol levels allowed blood to flow more smoothly to the penis, restoring normal function.

Who should take statins? Anyone who has suffered a heart attack or stroke or who has cardiovascular disease is a prime candidate. People with diabetes are at high risk for heart disease and often require a statin drug. Two thirds of people with high blood pressure also have high cholesterol; if the cholesterol cannot be sufficiently lowered with diet and exercise, a statin drug is an important preventive medication, as the combination of high blood pressure and high cholesterol can be deadly.

Talk with your doctor, and be sure that she or he has a firm understanding of the importance of prevention. Experts estimate that nine out of ten adults with high cholesterol are not adequately treated. Although it is never too late to start a statin drug (seniors aged 80 and up can generally use these drugs safely), the longer someone takes the drug, the greater the benefit.

If statins are all that, why don't we all take them? For people at low risk for heart disease, the potential benefits are small, so the costs and chance of side effects don't justify their use. When prescribed appropriately, statins save lives and are associated with a reasonably low risk of side effects. These drugs have been studied extensively for many years. However, some people are afraid to take a statin drug for fear of muscle or liver damage.

- Statins may raise liver enzyme blood levels in certain susceptible individuals. We can think of this simplistically as irritation of the liver. Liver test abnormalities will usually happen in the first three months of treatment, so it is important that your doctor check blood work during this time. It is routine to perform cholesterol and liver tests every six months thereafter.

- Liver test abnormalities are more common in women, people over 60 years of age, individuals with liver disease, and those who use alcohol regularly. Frequent use of acetaminophen, the active ingredient in Tylenol, will also raise liver enzymes. The higher the statin dose, the more likely you will have elevated liver enzymes. Less than 3 percent of people will need to discontinue treatment because of liver abnormalities, and the lab tests typically normalize by one to three months.

- Newer statins, such as Lipitor and Crestor, appear to be associated with fewer liver enzyme abnormalities than older statins. Because statins are all a little different, an alternative statin can be tried once the blood levels are back to normal, as long as blood work is followed closely.

- Liver failure is a completely different matter from liver enzyme elevations. Concern about liver failure is a fear that I address with my patients nearly every day. Although the media has done a good job of frightening people away from statins, the truth is that the odds of true liver failure in patients on statin drugs in the general population is 1 in 1.14 million people per year. The statistics for liver failure are the same, whether we take statins or not, and in all probability the odds have no relation to statin use at all.

- An extremely small percentage of people may experience problems with memory loss on statins, although, in general, statin drugs appear to reduce the risk of dementia.

- A more realistic concern with statins is the issue of muscle pains. Up to 10% of people who take a statin will experience aching muscles or joints. However, many people who take placebo pills in research studies of statins report the same thing, so it's not always clear if the statin is at fault. If you develop muscle pains on statin drugs, your doctor may order a blood test to determine if there is muscle injury.

- Note, however, that a blood test may not always detect the source of muscle pain. We develop aches and pains for many reasons, but if the discomfort begins after the introduction of the drug and stops when the drug is withdrawn, the statin is the likely culprit, regardless of the blood test results.

- If your vitamin D levels are low, you may be more prone to statin-related muscle aches. In that case, a vitamin D supplement might help. For relatively mild pain associated with statin drug therapy, it is worth considering CoQ10 supplementation. Creatine and L-carnitine might also help (see chapter 15, page 277, for more information on these supplements).

- Rhabdomyolysis is a very uncommon but dangerous side effect of statin therapy. This life-threatening complication is due to the acute breakdown of muscle tissue. The breakdown products can overwhelm the kidneys and cause kidney failure. Symptoms include profound weakness and severe muscle pain. The urine may appear brown, due to toxins from the damaged muscle tissue. Fortunately, this is a rare complication (affecting less than 5 in 100,000), and the risk of death is even rarer (less than one in a million).

- Symptoms of rhabdomyolysis can generally be caught early enough to avoid serious injury. To confirm the diagnosis, a blood test for CPK (creatine phosphokinase) should be ordered. Higher doses of statins are more likely to cause this problem, and some people are more sensitive to certain statins than others.
- Statin-related musculoskeletal problems, both mild and severe, are more common in women over 60, people with kidney or liver disease, and those taking other drugs that compete with statins for the same enzymes in the body.
- There is a small but real possibility of causing diabetes with any high-dose statin, although the reduction in heart attacks outweighs the potential risk of developing diabetes. If you need a high dose of a statin to control your cholesterol, it makes sense to work even harder on a heart-smart diet, exercise, and weight loss, when needed. By doing so, you're likely to reduce the amount of medication that you require.
- Grapefruit juice may interact with some statins but appears to be safe to take with Crestor (rosuvastatin), Livalo (pitavastatin), and Pravachol (pravastatin). If you have questions about potential drug interactions, be sure to discuss them with your doctor or pharmacist.
- Always be sure that your doctor and pharmacist know what other medications and supplements you are taking.

Fibrates

Fibrates, also known as fibric acid derivatives, are a class of lipid-lowering drugs that includes gemfibrozil (Lopid) and fenofibrate (Tricor, Lofibra, and Antara, to name a few). These medications are used to lower triglycerides, with typical reductions of 20 to 50 percent. Even greater declines may occur if the baseline triglyceride level is higher than 500 mg/dL. People with triglyceride levels of greater than 1,000 mg/dL are at high risk for pancreatitis, a dangerous inflammatory condition of the pancreas gland, which sits near the liver and stomach. In these cases, treatment of triglycerides is critical to lessen the risk of this dangerous condition.

A fibrate is generally chosen when a high triglyceride level is the principal lipid abnormality. Fibrates also have modest LDL-lowering effects and may raise HDL cholesterol by 10 to 35 percent. Despite their lipid-lowering effects, fibrates have not been consistently shown to reduce heart attack risk substantially. Diet and exercise are often much more effective at both lowering levels and preventing heart attacks.

In certain high-risk people with very elevated triglycerides and high LDL cholesterol, a physician may recommend combining a fibrate with a statin. This pairing can be highly effective, but depending on the specific statin and fibrate used, the combination may increase the risk for serious side effects, including muscle aches, liver enzyme abnormalities, and rhabdomyolysis, so careful monitoring is a must.

Niacin

Niacin, also known as nicotinic acid, is an important nutrient in your everyday diet. However, at high doses, prescription-strength niacin (Niaspan and Niacor) is also a drug that has powerful effects on HDL cholesterol and triglycerides and moderate effects on LDL cholesterol. It is also the only drug available to date that will lower Lp(a).

The results of medical studies are inconsistent, but prescription niacin on its own may reduce the risk of a heart attack by about 25 percent. However, adding niacin when your LDL is already successfully treated with a statin is not likely to reduce your heart attack risk any further, even when your HDL is low.

Dosage generally starts at 500 mg and increases to a maximum of 2,000 mg. The drug comes with a few caveats, the most important of which is the need for close monitoring of liver tests, just as with statin drugs.

People with uncontrolled diabetes may find their blood sugar more difficult to control if they take some forms of niacin, although prescription niacin generally does not cause much trouble. Just about everyone who takes high-dose niacin will experience flushing of the skin at some time, particularly if the drug is combined with alcohol, hot foods, or spicy foods. Red food coloring may also trigger this side effect. This side effect is why it is usually best to take niacin just before bedtime, preferably with a low-fat snack.

While it is easy to find inexpensive nonprescription high-dose niacin supplements, these products are problematic. Because they are sold as supplements, they are not approved for lipid lowering by the FDA and are not regulated like FDA-approved pharmaceuticals (see chapter 15, page 273, for more information about the FDA's approach to supplements).

Although "no-flush" niacin products may sound appealing, researchers from the University of Washington reported in 2003 that this form of niacin contains none of the active form of free nicotinic acid needed to treat lipids, even though it is the most expensive variety of nonprescription niacin.

Short-acting niacin is the least expensive niacin supplement available. Although it is less likely to cause liver problems than the long-acting niacin supplements, short-acting niacin tends to cause much more severe flushing and is usually not as effective as the prescription drug for improving the cholesterol profile. The longer-acting sustained-release supplements are associated with a significantly higher likelihood of liver toxicity than are the prescription forms, because they are metabolized primarily through the liver.

The prescription niacin known as Niaspan is in an intermediate-release form and is safer and more effective than any of the niacin supplements. Niacor is a prescription form of immediate-release niacin. Unlike supplements, both are regulated by the FDA.

Whether you take a prescription form of niacin or over-the-counter high-dose supplements, regular tests of liver enzymes (every three to six months) are important. Although niacin can be extremely effective when combined with a statin, the combination may increase the risk of side effects. As always, it is vital for your doctor to know what supplements you are taking, to give you the best care possible (see "Heart Health Checklist: What Your Doctor Needs to Know," page 347).

Bile Acid Sequestrants

Bile acid sequestrants (BAS) include cholestytamine, colestipol, and colesevelam (Welchol). They may come in a powder form, to mix up with liquid, or in a capsule.

BAS drugs bind to cholesterol-containing bile acids in the intestine, so the cholesterol cannot be reabsorbed by the body and put back into circulation. They are weaker than statin drugs, lowering cholesterol levels by 15 to 30 percent. In some people, BAS drugs will raise triglycerides, so they are not a good choice when high triglycerides are a problem.

BAS drugs often work well in conjunction with statins, but they have the unfortunate side effects of constipation, bloating, and flatulence. The powder forms should not be taken at the same time as other drugs, as they may interfere with intestinal absorption of those drugs. It is best to take most other medications either one hour before the BAS or four hours afterward. Because these drugs do not get into the bloodstream, musculoskeletal side effects are not an issue with them.

Ezetimibe

Ezetimibe, also known as Zetia, lowers LDL by inhibiting its uptake through the intestine. Unlike bile acid sequestrants, it does not "bind up" cholesterol, but works at the cellular level. By itself, ezetimibe can lower LDL by about 20 percent.

Because ezetimibe does not work through the liver, it won't generally cause the muscle pains that can occur with statin drugs. The lack of this side effect allows you to combine ezetimibe with a lower statin dose to achieve the same lipid-lowering results, potentially avoiding significant side effects. Studies of cardiovascular outcomes with ezetimibe are scarce, but it does not appear to be as effective as the statins at preventing heart disease; for that reason, it is not considered first-line therapy. The side effect profile of ezetimibe is quite low, although it may cause abdominal pains and allergic reactions in a few people.

Prescription Omega-3

Prescription fish oil, specifically the drug Lovaza, is used chiefly to lower triglycerides. It is refined and purified above and beyond the level of supplemental fish oil (see chapter 15, page 283, for more on fish oil supplements). Because it is considered a drug, the manufacturing process is regulated by the FDA, so the amount of active ingredient is standardized from one batch to another. The purification process renders Lovaza much more active than most supplements and also reduces the likelihood of side effects such as the "fishy burp" that is so common with many nonprescription fish oils.

At the usual dose of 4 grams daily, triglyceride levels are typically lowered 20 to 45 percent. HDL may increase with Lovaza, but usually less than 15 percent. If triglycerides are severely elevated, Lovaza may raise LDL cholesterol as the lipids rebalance. This drug does not interact with other lipid medications, making it a safe choice for people who are already on multiple prescription drugs.

BEST PRACTICES:
LOWERING YOUR LIPIDS MEDICALLY

* By choosing a heart-smart lifestyle and keeping your BMI in a healthy range, you can usually increase HDL cholesterol and lower your LDL, triclycerides, Lp(a), and CRP levels. This may help you avoid the need for medical therapy.

* If you have cardiovascular disease or diabetes, you will likely need a statin. These drugs can reduce your risk of a heart attack by 30% or more.

* Statins can be highly effective and are generally safe, but carry with them a small possibility of serious side effects, including muscle aches, muscle tissue injury, and elevated liver enzymes. If you are taking one, be sure you are routinely screened for liver abnormalities, and let your doctor know if you think you might be having a reaction to your medication.

- High doses of statins may raise blood sugar levels in some people.
- Other lipid-lowering treatments include fibrates, niacin, bile acid sequestrants, and ezetimibe, as well as prescription fish oil.
- Be sure that your doctor has an up-to-date list of your medications, including supplements, since there is a potential for some lipid-lowering medications to interact with other drugs, raising the risk of side effects.
- If grapefruit is a favorite food, ask your doctor or pharmacist if it will interact with your medications.

DIABETES

Twenty-six million Americans are diabetic, and about one in three are highly vulnerable to developing diabetes, mainly due to lifestyle factors including diet, obesity, and lack of exercise. The Centers for Disease Control and Prevention (CDC) estimate that the costs for treatment and management of diabetes and its complications, including lost productivity, surpass $174 billion each year. When we add the costs associated with prediabetes (when blood sugar is high, but not yet in the diabetic range), the charge jumps to $218 billion. Given the soaring costs of health care, these figures will likely continue to rise.

The Role of Insulin

Insulin is a hormone that allows your body to make use of the glucose that comes from the food you eat. Insulin also allows you to use the stockpiles of glucose (in the form of glycogen) that your body stores in its liver and muscle tissues. It holds your blood sugar levels steady and enables your cells to do their work safely and efficiently. But if you have diabetes, your body either doesn't make enough insulin or isn't able to effectively use the insulin it manufactures; oftentimes diabetes is a combination of both problems.

The hallmark of diabetes is a blood sugar, or glucose, level that is consistently high. Elevated levels of sugar in the blood can lead to serious problems with the cardiovascular system, eyes, kidneys, nerves, gums, and teeth, particularly when the problem continues unchecked over a long period of time.

There are two types of diabetes: type 1, which typically develops in childhood, and type 2, also known as adult-onset diabetes.

Type 1 Diabetes

The pancreas produces insulin and releases it when blood levels of glucose rise, typically after a meal or snack. When the insulin-producing cells in the pancreas are destroyed, the result is type 1, or juvenile, diabetes.

Type 1 diabetes usually begins in childhood and is thought to be the result of an immune response to a viral infection gone amok, causing the body to attack its own cells. Type 1 diabetics must take insulin shots, because there is no way for their body to produce its own insulin. Without insulin, a type 1 diabetic will die.

Type 2 Diabetes

In adult-onset, or type 2, diabetes, the cells of the body are unable to process the glucose that is circulating though the bloodstream, despite the fact that there is insulin available. We call this insulin resistance. Over time, the pancreas may begin to fail, compounding the problem by producing less and less insulin.

The vast majority (95 percent) of diabetics are type 2. Diabetes is an equal-opportunity disease, with at least as many women as men afflicted. Currently more than 11 percent of adults can count themselves among the ranks of diabetics, including over a quarter of folks over age 65. Black and Hispanic men and women are more likely to be diabetic than are Caucasians. Nearly one of every four diabetics doesn't know that he or she has the disease.

The prevalence of diabetes has more than doubled during the past forty years, and can be directly attributed to the effects of obesity and a downshift in our daily activity. Just between 1997 and 2004, the number of newly diagnosed cases of diabetes in the United States increased by more than 50 percent. Approximately 3 million new cases were diagnosed between 2006 and 2008. It has been estimated that at the rate we are going, of those born in 2000, a mind-boggling one in three will eventually develop diabetes.

Genetics can play a role, but obesity, lack of exercise, and a high-calorie diet are the major contributors to type 2 diabetes. Eighty percent of adults with type 2 diabetes are overweight or obese. In people over age 65, in whom diabetes is truly epidemic, nearly nine out of every ten cases are the direct result of an unhealthy lifestyle and obesity. Particularly troubling is the recent rise in type 2 diabetes in children, thanks to a toxic culture of fast food, television, and sedentary lifestyles.

People whose bodies store fat in the abdominal area are especially prone to type 2 diabetes. This type of fat tissue produces a variety of harmful substances, some of which increase inflammation in the body and contribute to insulin resistance. Because of this, even a modest weight loss of 5 to 10 percent of total body weight may substantially improve blood sugar control.

Many type 2 diabetics are undiagnosed and have no idea that they suffer from this slowly devastating disease. Some never experience the hallmark symptoms of excessive thirst and hunger, frequent but normal-volume urination, and unexpected weight loss; when they do, these warning signs often go unrecognized. The typical delay from type 2 diabetes onset to diagnosis is somewhere between four and seven years.

My father, who was a specialist in endocrinology (a branch of medicine that includes diagnosis and treatment of diabetes), did not, or would not, recognize that he was diabetic until his disease was far advanced. Many of the devastating health problems that plagued him in the last years of his life could have been avoided had his diabetes been treated early on. Like my dad, many people with type 2 diabetes are genetically susceptible, and sometimes despite a lifetime of good habits, diabetes just happens.

Diabetes and Your Heart

By far, the most serious problem caused by diabetes is heart disease. A man with diabetes doubles his risk of heart disease, but if you are a diabetic woman, you are up to five times as likely to suffer from cardiovascular disease or a stroke as is a woman who is not diabetic (see "Know Your Risk Factors," page 349). And even as deaths from heart disease are declining in diabetic men, there has been no such improvement in women.

Every year more than 230,000 lives are lost in this country to complications from diabetes. Fully two thirds of diabetics will ultimately die of cardiovascular disease, and about one in six will die from complications of a stroke. Despite these grim statistics, most diabetics do not realize that they are at risk.

The ravages of diabetes are not limited to the heart. Every year, 100,000 diabetic people go on dialysis for kidney failure. People with diabetes are at high risk for peripheral vascular disease, or disease of the blood vessels of the limbs, a condition that may ultimately lead to amputation. Blindness is yet another devastating complication of diabetes.

The best way to know whether you might be diabetic is to be screened with a simple blood test.

Diagnosing Diabetes

Adults should be screened for diabetes with blood tests at least once every three years, but more often if they are obese or have a history of borderline elevated blood sugar. A fasting blood sugar of more than 125 confirms a diagnosis of diabetes. Your doctor may order a hemoglobin A1c test to monitor your progress or to help to make this diagnosis. This blood test is like a crystal ball in reverse. It allows your doctor to assess your average blood glucose during the past ninety days.

Less commonly, your doctor might order a glucose tolerance test to evaluate your body's response to a sugary drink. If you do not clear the sugar from your bloodstream quickly enough, this would indicate either impaired glucose tolerance or diabetes. This test is used more typically to test for gestational diabetes (diabetes that develops during pregnancy).

Twenty percent of middle-aged adults and 35 percent of adults over 65 have glucose intolerance, also referred to as insulin resistance or prediabetes, with fasting blood sugar levels of more than 100 but less than 125. When tested with a glucose tolerance test, their blood sugar response is not normal, but it is not as impaired as that seen with full-blown diabetes. Most people with glucose intolerance are at least 20 percent overweight, and within five years, somewhere between 10 and 25 percent of them become true diabetics.

Diabetes in Pregnancy

Gestational diabetes is a condition that by definition occurs during pregnancy. It is more common in obese women over the age of 25. The incidence of gestational diabetes more than doubled between 1990 and 2004, reflecting our dangerously unhealthy lifestyles. Fortunately, gestational diabetes can often be controlled with diet, but it requires close monitoring throughout the pregnancy. Women who have gestational diabetes are more likely to become type 2 diabetics later in life. Babies of women with gestational diabetes are often born unusually large, increasing the likelihood of birth-related complications, and they are more likely to become obese kids.

Complications of Diabetes

How can a little extra sugar be bad for you? Sadly, "the sugar" is not so sweet. Elevated levels of blood glucose contribute to stiffness and damage of the artery walls and make blood vessels more susceptible to harmful free radicals. This damage then makes the arteries more vulnerable to cholesterol buildup, increasing the propensity for heart attacks, strokes, and kidney failure. When the blood sugar is high, the risk of blood clots goes up, as do the risks of high blood pressure and lipid abnormalities. The heart muscle itself may become stiff and nonpliable, sometimes leading to congestive heart failure. The typical diabetic has high triglycerides and low HDL cholesterol, further stacking the odds.

Insulin itself may be harmful in large amounts, although this is still open to debate. Many type 2 diabetics produce excessive amounts of insulin, in an attempt to overcome their cells' resistance to the hormone. Some scientists believe that excessively high levels of insulin may predispose the coronary arteries to spasm. Insulin may also stimulate the growth of the smooth muscle tissue that lines the walls of the arteries, making them more vulnerable to injury and development of cholesterol plaques. However, if you need insulin shots to control your blood sugar, it's important that you take them, as elevated blood glucose levels are clearly dangerous.

Diabetes commonly affects the small blood vessels, including those of the feet and hands, impairing the body's ability to heal itself. This condition may lead to skin ulcers, which often become deep and badly infected. Many diabetics suffer neuropathy, or nerve damage, so it's not unusual for a very nasty infection to go unnoticed when the pain receptors fail to fire normally. In the worst-case scenario, this can lead to gangrene, bone infections, and eventual amputation of a limb.

As a physician in training, I was taught to always examine the feet of my diabetic patients. Although it sometimes seemed like a nuisance to ask my patients to remove their shoes and socks at every visit, the importance of this part of the examination was driven home late one afternoon when Duong came in for his six-month checkup. A landscaper by trade, Duong was a hardworking gentleman with impeccable manners and neatly pressed khakis. I was shocked when I looked at the sole of his foot and saw a large ulcer that had eaten almost all the way to the bone. Duong had absolutely no inkling that his foot was so badly infected, and was stunned when I advised immediate hospitalization. Fortunately, we were able to save his foot, but had his appointment been a week later, it would probably have been too late.

Ignorance is not bliss. Because of poor nerve function, diabetics may not feel chest pain when they have a heart attack and may not recognize other symptoms of a troubled heart such as fatigue and shortness of breath. Once a heart attack happens, a diabetic person is twice as likely to die within a year as is someone without diabetes.

Diabetes, insulin resistance, and obesity can also contribute to a liver abnormality known as "fatty liver." This typically occurs when the fat content of the liver surpasses 5 percent. Most of this fat is in the form of triglycerides. Although fatty liver may not be harmful in and of itself, extensive testing is often required to rule out other types of liver problems. A small percentage of people with this condition will go on to develop cirrhosis of the liver and liver failure.

Treating Diabetes Medically

If you are diabetic, your doctor will probably recommend medical treatment. There are eight major types of medication prescribed to people with diabetes; most type 2 diabetics will ultimately require two or more medications. Several new classes of drugs are currently in the pharmaceutical pipeline, some of which may also prove to impact lipids and weight management. Blood sugar control is critical and has been proven to reduce the likelihood of such dreaded diabetic complications as heart disease, blindness, kidney failure, and amputation.

■ INSULIN

The body needs insulin to put glucose to work. Because type 1 diabetics are unable to produce this hormone, insulin shots are mandatory for this condition. However, many type 2 diabetics require insulin injections as well. This happens because either the pancreas produces an insufficient amount of insulin or, more commonly, the body is so resistant to insulin that higher levels of it are needed to push glucose into the cells, where it belongs.

Most insulin used in this country is human-type insulin, although older, less commonly used forms come from extracts of pig or cow pancreas and are referred to as "natural" insulin. Human insulin is generally made from a process using yeast (Novolin) or bacteria (Humulin). There are a number of varieties of insulin, classified according to onset of action, peak of activity, and duration. Usually two or more types of insulin are combined to create a custom fit for an individual.

Type 1 diabetics may use an insulin pump that injects insulin through a catheter and allows fine tuning. Although insulin must be injected under the skin to be effective, slow-release skin-patch forms of insulin are currently being studied, and may one day become available. Frequent finger-stick blood sugar tests are required to dose insulin appropriately.

One major drawback of insulin therapy is the possibility of overshooting by injecting too much insulin, leading to hypoglycemia, or low blood sugar. Hypoglycemia may cause lightheadedness, confusion, or even loss of consciousness. Changes in diet, exercise, and general health can alter insulin requirements, so regular glucose monitoring is essential.

SULFONYLUREAS

Sulfonylureas work by stimulating the pancreas to produce more insulin and by improving the body's ability to use insulin. Examples include glyburide (DiaBeta, Glynase, and Micronase), glypizide (Glucotrol), and glymepiride (Amaryl). Side effects may include an allergic rash, weight gain, and low blood sugar. There is also some evidence that glyburide and perhaps glypizide might increase the likelihood of abnormal heart rhythms in susceptible people. Other studies have suggested that these two sulfonylureas may lead to more complications after a heart attack. A review of over ninety-one thousand British diabetics published in 2009 found a significantly higher risk of death with all sulfonylureas when compared to other diabetic drugs, as well as a higher probability of heart failure.

MEGLITINIDES

Repaglinide (Prandin) works by stimulating insulin secretion. It is faster acting than the sulfonylureas, so is usually taken before a meal.

This type of medication allows more flexibility with mealtimes than do longer-acting drugs. Potential side effects include low blood sugar and weight gain.

■ ALPHA-GLUCOSIDASE INHIBITORS

Alpha-glucosidase inhibitors include miglitol (Glycet) and acarbose (Precose). They work by delaying the absorption of carbohydrates in the intestine, resulting in a slower rise of blood sugar after a meal. These drugs should be taken with meals. Side effects include diarrhea and flatulence, but not low blood sugar.

■ THIAZOLIDINEDIONES

This class of medication includes rosiglitazone (Avandia) and pioglitazone (Actos). Thiazolidinediones (TZDs) work by improving the cells' sensitivity to insulin. They generally do not cause low blood sugar.

Studies have found TZDs bring about improvements in CRP, HDL cholesterol, and triglycerides, in addition to lowering blood glucose. However, TZDs can cause fluid retention, which may lead to congestive heart failure. Rosiglitazone appears to increase the risk for heart attacks, especially when combined with insulin. Pioglitazone does not carry the same warnings and in fact appears to lower the likelihood of heart disease.

If you take a TZD, it is important to have regular monitoring of liver function blood tests, as TZDs can cause liver abnormalities in a small percentage of people. Anemia and weight gain may sometimes occur on these drugs, and they may increase the risk for bone fractures in women.

■ BIGUANIDES

Metformin (Glucophage) is the only biguanide currently available. This drug reduces the amount of glucose produced by the liver and increases sensitivity to insulin. (The body stores excess glucose in the liver and muscle tissue. In diabetes, there is a malfunction in the regulation of glucose release from the liver.) Unlike many other diabetes medications, metformin may actually cause a modest amount of weight loss.

Although highly effective, it has a range of potential side effects, most commonly gastrointestinal, including nausea and vomiting. Metformin may also cause a deficiency in vitamin B_{12}. More serious side effects include lactic acidosis, in which dangerously high levels of acid in the blood may result in kidney damage. This usually occurs in people with preexisting kidney damage or heart failure. Use metformin with caution if you drink more than moderately, because excessive alcohol may put you at risk for side effects.

Dehydration and acute medical illness will also increase the likelihood of problems with metformin. Iodine contrast dye and metformin do not play well together. If you have a radiology test using intravenous iodine contrast dye, such as a CT scan or cardiac catheterization, it is critical to avoid taking metformin for at least 48 hours following the procedure, to avoid potential kidney damage. The dye and the drug are both processed by the kidneys and in combination may cause harmful levels of metformin to build up.

Although the potential for problems with metformin clearly exists, life-threatening side effects are rare in those without contraindications, ranging somewhere between one and five cases per 100,000 people taking the drug. The elderly are more vulnerable to side effects. Your doctor should check your kidney function and blood sugar control regularly with a blood test to be sure that this drug is safe and effective for you.

■ D-PHENYLALANINE DERIVATIVES

Nateglinide (Starlix) stimulates the pancreas to produce more insulin and works quickly and for a short duration. It should be taken before a meal. Other than the potential side effect of low blood sugar, this drug appears to be very safe and well tolerated.

Dipeptidyl peptidase-4 (DPP-4) inhibitors increase the production of a group of hormones called incretins, which are produced in the gut. Incretins signal the pancreas to make insulin and tell the liver to stop producing glucose. In diabetics, levels of incretins tend to be low. DPP-4 inhibitors such as Januvia and Tradjenta are often used in conjunction with other drugs for diabetes. Side effects are not common, but can include headache and gastrointestinal problems. Typically, we don't see weight gain or low blood sugar with this class of drugs.

■ INCRETIN MIMETICS

Incretin mimetics including exenatide (Byetta) and lyraglutide (Victoza) are designed to mimic the effects of incretins, enhancing the body's own release of insulin in response to a meal and preventing the liver from overproducing glucose. What's more, these drugs can slow the emptying of the stomach contents into the small intestine, to reduce the rate that glucose is released into the bloodstream. These drugs are injected under the skin, and are almost always used in combination with other diabetic medications. Although they are injected, they are not a substitute for insulin. Side effects may include nausea and weight loss. In fact, it is the weight loss associated with these drugs that makes them so attractive to many doctors and diabetic patients.

BEST PRACTICES:
REDUCING YOUR RISK FOR DIABETES

* First, maintain your weight in the optimal range, by keeping your BMI less than 25 (see page 346). To do this effectively, it's going to take both diet and exercise. You've got to do both.

* Get moving to reduce your risk of diabetes. Exercise will improve your body's sensitivity to insulin, reducing the amount of insulin you require to process the food you eat.

Both aerobic exercise (including walking and jogging) and anaerobic exercise (weight training) can help.

* To help keep your blood sugar levels steady, try a Mediterranean-style diet rich in whole grains, fruits and vegetables, nuts, and unsaturated fats.
* Stay away from fast foods and convenience foods, as these foods are chock-full of the bad stuff. Those who eat typical burger palace or fried chicken meals more than twice a week are twice as likely to develop insulin resistance as are diners who rarely visit fast-food joints.
* Stay away from red meat and processed meats, including bacon and hot dogs, which will also boost your risk for diabetes.
* Drink moderately. People who drink too much alcohol (more than 2 drinks a day), as well as complete abstainers, are more likely to become diabetic than are moderate drinkers. (Of course, if alcohol gives you trouble, by all means avoid it.)
* Stay away from the smokes. For reasons that are not clear, smoking doubles the risk of becoming diabetic.
* If you have diabetes, work with your doctor to find the safest and most effective drug or drug combination to keep your blood sugar in an optimal range. There is a wide variety of medical options, including insulin therapy, sulfonylureas, meglitinides, alpha-glucosidase inhibitors, TZDs, biguanides, DPP-4 inhibitors, and incretin mimetics.

THE METABOLIC SYNDROME

The metabolic syndrome is a cluster of health risks, related in large part to lifestyle choices, which increase the odds of developing cardiovascular disease. Several definitions have been put forth; the strictest and most relevant criteria were developed in 2005 by the International Diabetes Federation. To meet the definition, you must have a waistline measurement of 37 inches or more if you are a white or black man

(35.5 inches for Asian, South Asian, and ethnic Central and South American men). For women of any ethnicity, 31.5 inches is the threshold. In addition, two of the following four criteria are required:

- A blood pressure of 130/85 mm Hg or higher
- A triglyceride level above 150 mg/dL
- A fasting blood glucose level greater than 100 mg/dL
- A high-density lipoprotein (HDL) level less than 40 mg/dL (for men) or under 50 mg/dL (for women)

Using these criteria, the metabolic syndrome affects about 25 percent of Americans, including a jaw-dropping 50 percent of those over the age of 60. If you have the metabolic syndrome but are not diabetic, you are nearly 40 percent more likely to develop heart disease (including heart attacks and heart failure) when compared to people without the syndrome. The risk jumps to more than 50 percent in those with diabetes.

Women are acquiring the metabolic syndrome at rates far greater than are men. Even more worrisome is a recent report that the metabolic syndrome may be found in one out of every seven young teens.

While cardiovascular disease risk increases over time, a study of people with the metabolic syndrome aged 55 and younger found that nearly 90 percent already had evidence of early cholesterol buildup in the carotid arteries, which supply blood to the brain. Because carotid artery disease is also a marker for vascular disease elsewhere in the body, it is likely that many of these folks also had significant but silent cholesterol buildup in their heart arteries.

The metabolic syndrome is widespread among obese people, nearly two thirds of whom meet the criteria, whereas less than 6 percent of individuals with normal body weight meet the criteria. Not surprisingly, most type 2 diabetics have the metabolic syndrome.

Watch Your Waistline

Notice that the definition of the metabolic syndrome does not include body mass index but, rather, waist circumference. The point is that not everyone with the metabolic syndrome is obese by BMI standards, and not all obese people meet the waist circumference criterion. The most dangerous fat in your body is your visceral, or deep abdominal fat. Think of the round-bellied "apple" shape, as opposed to the "pears" who carry more fat in the hips and buttocks. "Pears" are less likely to have the metabolic syndrome.

This visceral type of fat is dangerous because, unlike subcutaneous fat (fat under the skin), it is actually a functioning organ of the body. It manufactures a host of hazardous chemicals that promote inflammation, as well as other products that can trigger dangerous blood clots. Fat also produces chemicals that actually block the action of insulin and interfere with proper function of the insulin receptors in the body's cells, preventing insulin from being used effectively. The result is insulin resistance. Fat tissue raises LDL levels, lowers HDL, and raises triglycerides. Binge eating, a common problem in people who suffer from obesity, is also associated with high insulin levels and insulin resistance. For all these reasons, tackling the obesity problem is a major focus of efforts to prevent and treat the metabolic syndrome and diabetes.

To be sure, there is an inherited tendency toward storing fat in the abdominal area. Hispanic women, for example, have much higher levels of the metabolic syndrome, hovering around 35 percent, which is not entirely explained by diet or activity levels.

You Can Prevent the Metabolic Syndrome

Unlike many chronic diseases, the metabolic syndrome is highly preventable. Exercise combined with a healthy diet can reduce a thick middle, if you stick with it. And when it comes to diet, studies have found that the Mediterranean diet may be the best way to lower your risk of the metabolic syndrome. Flip to chapter 7, page 115, to learn more about this deliciously healthy way of eating.

Exercise and diet take time, and if you're in need of help, your doctor may choose to prescribe metformin, even if you're not quite diabetic. This drug helps to sensitize the cells to insulin so that they are better able to use it.

But your lifestyle is still the most powerful medicine. A 2002 study of more than three thousand people from the Diabetes Prevention Program Research Group showed a decided advantage of diet and exercise over drug therapy in treating the metabolic syndrome. In this study, people were followed for an average of three years; they were assigned to receive a phony placebo pill or metformin, or to follow a diet and exercise program.

The program included a modest weight-loss goal of at least 7 percent of body weight and an exercise commitment of thirty minutes five days a week. At the end of the study, 29 percent of the people who received placebo tablets had become diabetic, whereas 22 percent of those given metformin developed diabetes. That's a pretty significant response, but not earthshaking. The most exciting finding was the fact that only 14 percent in the diet and exercise group were diabetic by the study's end.

Put another way, taking on a few healthy habits cut the last group's risk of diabetes by 50 percent, without the use of potentially harmful and costly drugs. This was despite the fact that only half of the people studied actually achieved their weight-loss goal and less than three quarters were fully on board with the exercise recommendations. The benefits were there regardless of gender, age, or race.

BEST PRACTICES:
THE METABOLIC SYNDROME

* The metabolic syndrome is a prediabetic state associated with abdominal fat, high blood pressure, lipid abnormalities, and elevated blood sugar.
* If you are an "apple" shape, carrying your fat in your middle area, you are more likely to develop the metabolic syndrome than a "pear," who is bottom heavy.
* Exercise and diet are the most effective treatment for the metabolic syndrome.

POLYCYSTIC OVARY SYNDROME

Women who suffer from polycystic ovary syndrome (PCOS) are prime candidates for the metabolic syndrome. PCOS strikes about 5 to 10 percent of women of reproductive age and includes irregular menstrual cycles, infertility, ovarian cysts and, frequently, obesity. It turns out that fat tissue can manufacture estrogen, and this may interfere with normal functioning of the ovaries, where estrogen is usually produced. PCOS is not the same thing as run-of-the-mill ovarian cysts, which occur without the syndrome in 20 percent of women.

More than half of all women who suffer from PCOS are obese, and upward of 75 percent of obese women with PCOS have insulin resistance. About one in three normal-weight women with PCOS will also have insulin resistance. By the time of menopause, many women with PCOS will be diabetic, so if you suffer from this disorder, regular screening for diabetes is important.

PCOS is associated with other features that double or even triple the heart disease risk, including lipid abnormalities, which occur in most women with the syndrome. Thickening of the carotid arteries is also more common in women with PCOS and portends a higher likelihood of strokes and heart disease later in life. Obese women with PCOS also tend to have high levels of the male hormone testosterone, which is responsible for the acne and facial hair that plague women with this disorder.

Infertility, facial hair, and heart disease. You wouldn't wish it on your worst enemy, but the good news is that PCOS is treatable, and often preventable. The first and most important step is the heart-smart mantra: diet and exercise.

Losing even 10 to 20 percent of body weight may substantially improve all aspects of the syndrome. If that doesn't do the trick, the drug metformin is often used to treat PCOS. By lowering insulin levels, reducing testosterone, and improving rates of ovulation, metformin may be a real lifesaver. However, fertility rates may improve just as much, if not more, in women who choose to take control of their PCOS with diet, exercise, and weight loss.

BEST PRACTICES:
PCOS

* If you have PCOS, a weight reduction of 10–20% will improve your symptoms.
* If diet alone doesn't work, ask your doctor if metformin might help.

ASPIRIN: THE TRUE WONDER DRUG?

Aspirin has been in use, in one form or another, for more than two thousand years. In 1897, aspirin as we know it was created in the laboratory of the Bayer Company. By 1900, the drug had hit the market, and the rest is history.

As a blood thinner, aspirin works by inactivating platelets in the blood. These small, oblong-shaped cells are a vital part of the clotting process. Remember that a heart attack is usually caused by the rupture or fissure of an unstable cholesterol plaque in a heart artery. The body interprets this disruption as a wound, and platelets rush to the site to help close off the injured area by forming a clot. This clot, formed by the well-meaning platelets, is what ultimately blocks up the artery.

The loss of blood flow to the portion of the heart muscle that depends on that artery for its oxygen supply is what causes the heart attack, or what we doctors call a myocardial infarction. If blood flow is not restored quickly, then permanent damage follows. When we disable the platelets, this series of catastrophic events is less likely to take place.

If you think you might be having a heart attack, it makes sense to pop a full-strength chewable aspirin (for immediate release) in your mouth while waiting for help to arrive, because aspirin reduces the risk of a full-blown heart attack or death by nearly half in this time-critical situation.

In 1988, a remarkable finding emerged from a study of more than twenty-two thousand healthy male physicians aged 40 through 84: Just one 325 mg aspirin taken every other day for five years slashed the risk of a heart attack by 44 percent at the five-year mark. The benefits were seen chiefly in men over the age of 50. It is fair to say that this study profoundly changed the way we look at heart disease prevention, offering a simple, relatively safe, widely available, and cheap drug that could measurably save lives.

The statistics are a little different for women. In 2005, the Women's Health Study researchers found a 34 percent reduction in heart attacks and 30 percent drop in strokes in healthy women age 65 and older with no personal history of heart disease, who took 100 mg of aspirin every other day. Aspirin did not offer the same benefits in younger healthy women.

Aspirin users have other reasons to take heart. The drug may provide additional heart-healthy benefits, including antioxidant effects and the ability to protect the vulnerable lining of the blood vessels. Studies show that men with a high CRP reduce their heart attack risk by 55 percent when given aspirin, suggesting an important anti-inflammatory role. The risk of some forms of cancer, including colorectal cancer and prostate cancer, may also drop when people take aspirin regularly, although research is not definitive.

Is There a Downside?

In the Women's Health Study, aspirin increased the risk of severe intestinal bleeding, although this side effect was very uncommon, occurring in six out of every thousand women treated with aspirin for ten years, compared to five in one thousand of the women who received placebo pills. Nosebleeds, bruising, and other bleeding problems were also more common in the aspirin group. The risks of aspirin, including bleeding and ulcers, outweighed the benefits in healthy women aged 64 and younger. For men at low risk for heart disease, the risk for bleeding may also outweigh the potential benefits.

Should You Take Aspirin?

If you have already been diagnosed with heart disease or stroke, a daily dose of aspirin is generally an important component of your medical therapy. It will lower your risk of dying from cardiovascular disease by a full 25 percent. If you have a coronary stent, placed by a cardiologist to treat a blocked artery, long-term aspirin use is almost always required to keep the stent from closing. If you have two or more risk factors for heart disease, you may also benefit from aspirin. As always, it is important to discuss your treatment options with your doctor.

What Type of Aspirin Is Best?

Should your aspirin be coated or noncoated? Somewhere between 5 and 30 percent of people are resistant to the effects of aspirin. This aspirin resistance may be genetic in the way the body handles aspirin, but it also appears that 10 percent of normal-weight adults and more than 50 percent of those over 200 pounds simply do not absorb enough aspirin when it is given in low-dose (75 mg) coated form. In those cases, full-strength uncoated aspirin (325 mg) may be more effective. Smokers may also be resistant to aspirin, and may do better with a full-strength pill. If you weigh less than 200 pounds and you are not a smoker, low-dose aspirin (75 to 81 mg) usually works just as well, with a lower risk for bleeding and bruising.

If your stomach is sensitive, or you have a history of stomach ulcers, coated aspirin is a good idea. The coating keeps the aspirin from dissolving in the stomach and irritating the stomach's sensitive lining. However, if you are able to take aspirin without its causing stomach upset, it makes sense to take noncoated (chewable) aspirin with food in the morning. It's usually best to avoid taking it before bedtime, because there is a greater likelihood of the aspirin tablet's spending the night camped out in your stomach, which could cause ulcers. And bear in mind that acetaminophen (Tylenol), ibuprofen (Advil, Motrin), and other pain relievers are no substitute for aspirin when it comes to matters of the heart. In fact, ibuprofen and other drugs in its class may even increase the risk for heart complications.

When to Avoid Aspirin

If you've never had a heart attack, stroke, or blocked artery, how do you make the decision whether to take aspirin as a preventive drug?

First, check with your doctor to be sure that there are no medical reasons for you to avoid aspirin. If you have been diagnosed with any sort of bleeding disorder, or are about to undergo surgery, you should, as a rule, stay away from aspirin, unless directed to take it by your doctor. However, if you have heart disease, don't ever stop your aspirin without checking in with your cardiologist.

If you have problems with stomach ulcers, don't take aspirin unless the ulcers are healed and your doctor clears you to do so. People on other blood thinners and anti-inflammatory medicines are more prone to bleeding when aspirin is added, but depending on the situation, your doctor may decide that the benefit outweighs the potential risk. Some asthmatics and people with nasal polyps are sensitive to aspirin and may even suffer severe allergic reactions to the drug. And if you are pregnant, only take aspirin under the supervision of a doctor.

BEST PRACTICES:
ASPIRIN

* People with cardiovascular disease should usually take aspirin daily to lower heart attack risk.
* If you are male and over 50, or female and 65 or older, and you have risk factors, taking a low-dose aspirin tablet (81 mg) daily may help prevent heart attack and stroke.
* If you smoke or are obese, low-dose aspirin is less likely to be of benefit. You may need to take a full-strength, noncoated pill (325 mg) instead.
* Check with your doctor before starting any daily dose of aspirin, to be sure it's right for you. If your doctor has recommended aspirin, don't stop it without your doctor's approval.
* Take coated aspirin if you have a sensitive stomach. If you notice any signs of bleeding, contact your doctor immediately.
* At the first sign of a heart attack, take one noncoated, full-strength aspirin tablet—it may save your life.

PREVENTIVE MEDICINE: IT'S UP TO YOU

As VITAL AS medications are to those who need them, up to 20 percent of people who are hospitalized for a heart attack stop their medications within six months, often with dangerous consequences. I'll always remember Marguerite, a 68-year-old retired secretary who came to our hospital with a heart attack in progress and was treated with a cardiac stent to open a critically blocked artery. She was prescribed a regimen of drugs, including aspirin and another blood thinner, Plavix, which were essential to keep the artery open.

I sat down with Marguerite and her family before she left the hospital and reviewed with them the importance of taking her medications exactly as prescribed. Everyone seemed comfortable with the plan, and Marguerite assured me she would follow doctor's orders. But after a few weeks, Marguerite decided she was tired of taking her pills. They were too expensive, and, anyway, she felt just fine, so why bother? She also decided that she really didn't have the time to visit my office for her checkup and wasn't interested in cardiac rehabilitation, even though the cost was covered by her Medicare health plan. Unfortunately, three weeks after she stopped her medications, the paramedics rushed her back to the emergency room in severe distress, with a second major heart attack. Marguerite now suffers from congestive heart failure and from the knowledge that she could have prevented her condition had she just taken a little more responsibility for herself.

Whether you take pharmaceuticals for cholesterol, high blood pressure, or diabetes, it is vital to your health and well-being that you take your medications as prescribed. A study of statin drugs found that people who consistently took their medication were 45 percent less likely to die over a four-year time period than were those who were more lackadaisical.

If your doctor recommends aspirin, treat it with the same importance as you would any of your prescription drugs. People who stop taking aspirin in the first year after a coronary stent is placed for a blocked artery are nearly three times more likely to die or to have a major complication, including a heart attack.

Side effects can happen with just about any medication, so be sure to let your doctor know if you have concerns. There are often good alternatives.

Be honest with your doctor if you are concerned about the price of your medications. As a cardiologist, I want to help keep my patients' costs down, but sometimes I choose a specific drug for an individual based on its unique virtues that simply don't apply to the whole class of drugs. Although a generic may not always be the best choice, many times a similar drug can be substituted that will have a lower insurance co-pay. However, with hundreds of different health plans out there, your doctor often won't have that type of information at his fingertips. Make the effort to research the options yourself. If you are truly needy, many drug companies have programs to provide drugs at low or no cost, so be sure to ask if you need assistance.

BEST PRACTICES:
MEDICATIONS

* When your doctor recommends an over-the-counter product or prescribes medication, be sure that you understand why it is recommended, and discuss any concerns you might have about the drug at the time it is prescribed. Ignoring, skipping, or stopping these therapies on your own could have serious health consequences.

* Tell your doctor if you have any concerns about side effects. There may be other options available.

* If cost is an issue, discuss generic or other alternatives with your doctor and pharmacist.
* If you are financially needy, you may qualify for a drug company program that provides medication at low or no cost.

No matter how many medications you take, it is critical that you do all you can to reduce your risk of heart disease through diet, lifestyle, and exercise. Not only will you feel better, you will drastically reduce your personal cost of health care. Obesity and a sedentary lifestyle dramatically increase the risk of high blood pressure, high cholesterol, diabetes, arthritis, lung disease, and cancer. All of these diseases will cost you money, not to mention years of life and health. Take responsibility now, and it will pay off for the rest of your life.

14

Vitamins and Minerals
for a Healthy Heart

VITAMINS AND MINERALS are essential for keeping your heart, brain, and body healthy, happy, and in prime working condition. A vitamin is a chemical that typically cannot be made by your body (with the exception of vitamin D), but which is essential to your health. Ideally you should acquire vitamins from the foods you eat, as Mother Nature intended.

Although severe cases of vitamin deficiency are sadly common in the Third World, fortunately they are very infrequent in the United States. However, people with diabetes, alcoholics, and the elderly may be at higher risk for mild yet significant deficiencies of vitamins and minerals.

There are thirteen major vitamins, four of them fat soluble (A, D, E, and K) and nine water soluble. You store the fat-soluble vitamins in your liver and fatty tissues, whereas excess water-soluble vitamins are usually flushed out quite efficiently by your kidneys.

Provitamins are vitamin precursors that your body is able to convert into active vitamins. Two examples are beta-carotene (found in dark green, yellow, and orange vegetables), which is converted into vitamin A, and ergosterol (found in some yeasts and mushrooms), which becomes vitamin D.

Minerals are basically metallic elements, such as iron, calcium, and magnesium. At least twenty-two different minerals are essential to your health. Minerals are involved in just about every function of your body, including muscle contraction, normal operation of your cardiovascular and nervous systems, proper regulation of your hormones, and, of course, development and maintenance of your bones.

About half of us take vitamins regularly, but many people take these pills purely on faith. This chapter will walk you through the vitamins and minerals that keep your cardiovascular system humming happily, and show you how to make smart choices about these complex and vital chemicals. The following table gives a brief overview of the vitamins and minerals covered; please see the pages indicated for more detailed information.

VITAMIN OR MINERAL	RECOMMENDED DAILY MINIMUM INTAKE[1]	FOOD SOURCES	HOW IT HELPS	SUPPLEMENT SAFETY[2]
Beta-carotene (page 256)	No recommendation	Carrots, sweet potatoes, cantaloupe, dark green and yellow fruits and vegetables	Protects against heart disease and cancer; precursor to vitamin A	Supplements increase risk of lung cancer in smokers.
Calcium (page 264)	1,200 mg	Dairy, molasses, tofu, dark green leafy vegetables	May help lower blood pressure; protects and strengthens bones	Supplements may increase heart attack risk, while doing little to protect bone health.
Folic acid (page 260)	400 mcg	Dark green leafy vegetables, whole grains, brewers' yeast, liver	Works with vitamins B_6 and B_{12}; protects against heart disease; important for normal development of the fetal nervous system	Supplements may be recommended in pregnancy. High doses (over 400 mcg) may increase risk of heart attack, stroke, and cancer.
Iron (page 267)	8–18 mg	Red meat, turkey, shrimp, soybeans, lentils, leafy greens, dried fruits, enriched grains	Required for normal function of red blood cells	Deficiencies can be diagnosed with a blood test. Very high levels are harmful to the heart, liver, and other organs.

VITAMIN OR MINERAL	RECOMMENDED DAILY MINIMUM INTAKE[1]	FOOD SOURCES	HOW IT HELPS	SUPPLEMENT SAFETY[2]
Magnesium (page 268)	310–420 mg	Green leafy vegetables, nuts, wheat germ, avocados, chocolate	Supports heart and skeletal muscle function; maintains electrical activity in the heart; necessary for normal function of the nervous system; involved in bone health and immune function	Deficiencies can be diagnosed with a blood test. People on diuretics or chemotherapy often need prescription-strength supplements. Very high doses can cause dangerous heart rhythm abnormalities (especially when combined with certain medications and/or in patients with kidney failure).
Niacin (page 263)	14–16 mg	Meat, fish, peanuts, brewers' yeast	Minor impact on heart health at normal doses; very high doses (500 mg and up) can be used to treat high cholesterol	High-dose niacin for high cholesterol should be taken under a doctor's supervision. Side effects include flushing, itching, headaches, nausea, muscle cramps, and liver abnormalities.
Potassium (page 268)	4.7 mg	Fruits and vegetables	Supports heart and skeletal muscle function; maintains electrical activity in the heart; necessary for normal function of the nervous system	Deficiencies are common and can be diagnosed with a blood test. People on diuretics often need prescription-strength supplements. Very high doses can cause dangerous heart rhythm abnormalities (especially when combined with certain medications and/or in patients with kidney failure).

VITAMIN OR MINERAL	RECOMMENDED DAILY MINIMUM INTAKE[1]	FOOD SOURCES	HOW IT HELPS	SUPPLEMENT SAFETY[2]
Selenium (page 258)	70 mcg	Brazil nuts, whole grains, meat, fish	Protects heart muscle	Doses of 200 mcg or more may increase risk of diabetes.
Vitamin A (page 256)	700–900 mcg	Liver, egg yolks, fortified dairy	Supports skin health and immune function	High doses (3,000 mcg or over) increase bone fracture risk; doses over 7,500 mcg may harm the liver.
Vitamin B$_6$ (page 260)	1.3–1.7 mg	Fish, brown rice, whole grains, soybeans, organ meats	Supports arterial health; involved in the production of red blood cells and platelets; helps regulate blood sugar	Supplements may be recommended for alcoholics, people with kidney failure, smokers, and the elderly. Doses over 100 mg daily may cause nerve damage.
Vitamin B$_{12}$ (page 260)	2.4 mcg	Meat, egg yolks, poultry, milk	Supports heart health, the nervous system, red blood cells, and metabolism	A blood test can determine if there is a deficiency. Supplements are generally safe, but not usually necessary. Vegans typically require supplements.
Vitamin C (page 254)	75–90 mg	Citrus fruits, peaches, strawberries, broccoli, tomatoes, red peppers	Protects cells from free radicals; supports skin health and immune function; helps intestinal absorption of iron	High-dose supplements might increase risk of heart disease in diabetics. Extremely high doses may cause kidney stones and diarrhea.
Vitamin D (page 264)	600–800 IU	Sunshine (the skin manufactures vitamin D when exposed to sunlight). Food sources include fatty fish and fortified dairy	Protects heart and blood vessels; supports the immune system; necessary for bone and muscle health; may protect against cancer	Deficiencies are common and can be detected with a blood test. Doses of 1,000–4,000 IU are generally safe. Doses of 50,000 IU should only be taken under a doctor's supervision.

VITAMIN OR MINERAL	RECOMMENDED DAILY MINIMUM INTAKE[1]	FOOD SOURCES	HOW IT HELPS	SUPPLEMENT SAFETY[2]
Vitamin E (page 252)	22 IU	Vegetable oils, wheat germ, nuts, whole grains	Protects cells from free radicals; keeps blood cells flexible	Doses of 400 IU or more increase risk of prostate cancer, head and neck cancer, heart failure, and excessive bleeding. Supplements may interfere with muscle recovery after exercise and may block the effects of some cholesterol medications.
Vitamin K (page 266)	90–120 mcg	Green leafy vegetables, soy, cheese, whole grains	Integral to normal blood clotting; supports bone health	Deficiencies are very rare. In people on the blood thinner warfarin, high doses of vitamin K can make the drug less effective.

[1] The Recommended Daily Minimum Intake column is based in part on the Dietary Reference Intake established by the Food and Nutrition Board of the Institute of Medicine. The number listed is the minimum amount of a vitamin or mineral needed to meet the nutritional needs of 97 to 98 percent of adults.

[2] It's important to note that this safety information generally refers to supplements, and not food sources of these vitamins and minerals.

ALL-IMPORTANT ANTIOXIDANTS

Vitamins E and C, the provitamin beta-carotene, and the mineral selenium are antioxidants. This means that they help to neutralize free radicals, effectively disarming them. Free radicals are atoms and molecules with an unpaired electron. Because electrons like to be paired up, free radicals will try to steal electrons from other molecules, through a process called oxidation. It is the oxidized form of LDL cholesterol, for example, that is so damaging to the heart and blood vessels.

Free radicals come from many sources, including the food you eat and the air you breathe. Nitrite preservatives, often found in pork products, are highly potent sources of free radicals. When you eat fat, the process of metabolism (essentially breaking food down into its usable chemical components) churns out free radicals like a wicked little factory. Cigarette smoke and air pollutants are notorious free radical producers. Even exercise, particularly if you're out of shape and deconditioned, can produce free radicals, due to the breakdown of muscle tissue.

Antioxidants from the food you eat help to curb these constant assaults on the vital cells of your body. In the 1980s and 1990s, there was a lot of optimism that these nutrients, when taken in megadoses, might impact health and save lives. But recent well-done medical research has shown that sometimes more is just too much.

Vitamin E

Vitamin E, or alpha-tocopherol, is a fat-soluble vitamin that comes from plants. Vegetable oils, nuts, and whole grains are the best sources of vitamin E. Wheat germ oil is a vitamin E powerhouse. This vitamin has two major functions: the first is to defend our cells against oxidation, and the second is to help keep our red blood cells flexible. Vitamin E also helps counter the production of some of the factors involved in blood clotting and may lessen the amount of inflammatory CRP that flows through the bloodstream after a high-fat meal.

■ THE TRUTH ABOUT SUPPLEMENTS

Foods that are rich in vitamin E are also chock-full of other important nutrients, and in all likelihood, these other nutrients work in concert with vitamin E to help protect and strengthen our cardiovascular and immune systems. Supplements are a completely different matter.

The minimum amount of vitamin E required to support normal physical function is 22 IU (international units) daily, but dietary supplements are available in doses ranging from 100 to 1,200 IU and beyond. Both natural and synthetic vitamin E capsules are available. The synthetic form is less expensive, but natural vitamin E appears to be more accessible to the body.

Whereas foods high in vitamin E are clearly linked to improved cardiovascular health, scientific studies have found no net beneficial effect of supplemental vitamin E on heart disease, stroke, or cancer.

Although many people take the supplements in hopes of protecting their heart, one large study actually showed a slight increase in the risk of congestive heart failure in people taking high doses of vitamin E. In another, supplemental vitamin E was found to reduce the effectiveness of drugs designed to lower cholesterol, and under certain conditions, there was evidence that it might even promote a slight increase in cholesterol buildup.

Most studies of vitamin E have shown no benefit on cancer prevention; in fact, a large multicenter study published in 2011 found an increased risk of prostate cancer in men who took 400 IU of vitamin E daily. A Canadian study of people with cancer of the head and neck found that those who were treated with 400 IU of vitamin E daily increased their risk not only of a return of the original cancer, but also of developing a second cancer.

The most disturbing news about vitamin E surfaced in late 2004, when an analysis of nineteen studies involving more than 130,000 people concluded that those who took 400 IU or more of supplemental vitamin E every day had a 10 percent greater risk of dying than did people who took no supplement at all. Even doses of 150 IU were associated with a slight increase in mortality. Taking megadoses of 2,000 IU or greater raised the risk to 20 percent.

And daily doses of vitamin E of 400 IU or more are known to increase the risk of potentially fatal bleeding, particularly in the brain. That is one reason why people who take certain prescription blood thinners, such as warfarin, should avoid taking supplements of this vitamin.

Some athletes take vitamin E in the hopes that it will prevent muscle breakdown after an intense workout. A German study testing the effects of vitamin E and vitamin C after exercise found that the supplements were actually counterproductive, preventing the body's natural, and beneficial, antioxidant systems from coming into play, and reducing the sensitivity to insulin usually seen after exercise.

While it might appear that the supplement question is closed, there are still some legitimate questions being raised about the possibility that less common types of vitamin E supplementation might be useful in heart disease and cancer prevention. Although most supplements, natural and synthetic, contain alpha-tocopherol, this form is only one of eight different vitamin E compounds.

Gamma-tocopherol is actually the most common form of vitamin E in our diet. It is found in walnuts, peanuts, pecans, corn oil, sesame oil, and soybean oil. Some scientists believe that the difference could be important, particularly in the prevention of cancer and Alzheimer's disease. Another form of vitamin E is found in palm oil and may have promise in the prevention and treatment of breast cancer. So far, these are just interesting questions and speculation.

Vitamin C

Unlike vitamin E, vitamin C is water soluble. It works with vitamin E by functioning as an electron donor. What this means is that when vitamin E acts as an antioxidant, it transfers one of its electrons to a harmful free-radical molecule, rendering the dangerous molecule inactive. In turn, vitamin C (also known as ascorbic acid) generously donates one of its electrons to vitamin E, essentially reactivating the vitamin E. Vitamin C also supports the health of our skin and immune system, protects our nervous system, and helps us to absorb iron from plant-based foods.

Every school kid knows that vitamin C is found in citrus fruit, but peaches, strawberries, broccoli, and tomatoes are also excellent sources. Although some people fall short of the recommended daily value for vitamin C, true vitamin C deficiency, also known as scurvy, is very rare in this country.

To prevent deficiency-related complications, most women should get, at the very least, 75 mg of vitamin C each day; men, being generally larger, require a minimum of 90 mg. Smokers have been estimated to require 100 mg daily, and those who exercise vigorously should probably take in 100 to 500 mg each day from plant-based foods. Full saturation of the blood and tissue does not occur until you reach a daily intake of 200 to 400 mg. This amount of vitamin C is easily obtained from the foods you choose.

Whenever possible, enjoy your fruit and veggies at the peak of freshness, as the vitamin content may decline as much as 50 percent after just a week. Frozen fruits and vegetables are a surprisingly good choice, because freezing preserves the vitamins. Boiling vegetables can literally wash away the vitamins, so if you have to cook them, try a quick steaming or a brief spin through the microwave.

■ TO SUPPLEMENT OR NOT TO SUPPLEMENT?

Without a doubt, your diet is the best and safest way to get the vitamin C your body craves. Nature creates our food in an exquisitely balanced package, combining vitamins with hundreds of other phytonutrients. Science is only beginning to understand how these substances work in harmony, and in most cases, our clumsy attempts to thwart Mother Nature with mega-supplements have backfired, causing more harm than good.

If you eat your eight servings of fruit and veggies each day, you will never lack for vitamin C. In fact, you'll be way ahead of the curve. And they don't need to be citrus fruit or juice. For instance, just 4 ounces of red peppers will give you up to 215 mg of vitamin C, along with a tremendous infusion of important phytonutrients (another word for plant-based nutrients). Other foods, including cantaloupe, strawberries, and broccoli, supply on the order of 50 to 110 mg of vitamin C with each serving.

This sounds easy, but most people get less than 200 mg of vitamin C from the foods they eat. Obviously, it shouldn't take a vitamin pill to meet your body's needs, but when it comes to matters of the heart, a supplement is better than nothing.

High doses of vitamin C are another matter. There is no compelling evidence to justify the use of megadose vitamin C, either alone or in combination with other supplements, as a means to prevent heart disease. In fact, a multinational study found that diabetic women who took high doses of vitamin C supplements were even more likely to develop heart disease, although vitamin C from foods posed no such risk.

Evidence in favor of supplemental vitamin C as a cancer preventative is poor. And there is really no good data to support the use of vitamin C pills to prevent colds, although it is still possible that vitamin C might reduce the severity of cold symptoms.

Fortunately, vitamin C supplements rarely cause side effects, but kidney stones, anemia, and diarrhea may result from extremely high doses. Vitamin C doses in excess of 1,500 mg daily are essentially wasted, as your body will usually excrete surplus vitamin C through the urine.

Vitamin A and Beta-Carotene

Vitamin A is a fat-soluble vitamin. While it is not much of an antioxidant itself, one of its precursors, or provitamins, beta-carotene, is renowned as a powerful antioxidant. Beta-carotene provides the deep orange pigment to carrots, sweet potatoes, and cantaloupe but is also found in spinach, broccoli, and other dark green and yellow fruits and vegetables. Deficiencies of beta-carotene and vitamin A are rare in this country, but in the Third World, vitamin A deficiency is an all-too-common and easily preventable cause of blindness.

Beta-carotene is a potent antioxidant. Women whose diet is rich in beta-carotene have up to 26 percent less heart disease and a considerably lower risk of cancer when compared to those whose diet includes little or none of the nutrient. The same is likely true for men. Foods high in beta-carotene may even help to prevent diabetes.

If a little is good, shouldn't a lot be even better? You may have caught on by now that when it comes to supplemental vitamins, the answer is usually a heartfelt no. A study of nearly forty thousand women who were followed for two years and also given beta-carotene supplements found no effect on heart health or cancer risk.

That particular study was cut short when a large study of male smokers from Finland reported a chilling 28 percent increase in lung cancer in those who were given high-dose beta-carotene and vitamin E supplements. A similar increase in the risk of lung cancer was later reported in the *Journal of the National Cancer Institute* from a study of smokers in six different centers in the United States. (Despite these very compelling and sobering statistics, I was stunned to discover that a Web site selling beta-carotene supplements claimed that this very study actually reported a reduction in cancer deaths.)

How could it be possible that an antioxidant could increase the risk of cancer? Scientists are still studying the problem, but the theory is that once the beta-carotene becomes oxidized (i.e., after it donates an electron to neutralize a free radical), it becomes lodged in the lungs and bloodstream and now acts as a free radical itself, causing harm to the surrounding tissue.

High levels of vitamin A, although not beta-carotene, have been associated with other complications, including an increased risk of bone fragility and bone fractures. Extremely high doses of vitamin A taken in the form of supplements may even, over time, cause permanent liver damage. Beta-carotene obtained directly from food has not been found to have this effect. You can literally eat enough carrots to turn your skin orange, but your levels of vitamin A will remain normal, thanks to the body's remarkable ability to self-regulate.

The recommended vitamin A intake for women is 700 mcg (micrograms), or 2,300 IU; men require 900 mcg, or 3,000 IU. You have to take more than 3,000 mcg of vitamin A per day (or 10,000 IU) before it becomes harmful to the bones. Over time, daily doses of 7,500 mcg (25,000 IU) or more are known to cause liver damage.

Vitamin A is found in liver and other organ meats, egg yolks, and fortified dairy products such as milk and cheese, as well as in vitamin supplements. Someone who eats liver regularly could easily exceed the recommended amount, as 3 ounces of beef liver contains more than 30,000 IU of vitamin A. By comparison, 8 ounces of fortified milk supplies 500 IU, and an ounce of cheese provides about 250 IU.

Beta-carotene is not the only precursor to vitamin A. There are more than six hundred different dietary carotenoids, all of which have antioxidant properties and fifty of which have provitamin A activity. Lycopene, found in tomatoes and other red fruits and vegetables, is another example of a carotenoid that may help protect against cancer and heart disease. It is thought that the carotenoids work in conjunction with one another—as a team, so to speak—and that this may explain why taking one in isolation may have unintended, unbalanced consequences.

Although supplements may be dangerous, especially for smokers, there is no evidence that eating foods high in beta-carotene and other carotenoids is harmful; on the contrary, many studies have shown that these foods help to protect against heart disease and certain forms of cancer.

Selenium

Selenium is a trace element that is a vital element in many important antioxidant proteins in the body. Most of the selenium in our diet originates in the soil and comes to us not only through plants but also from the muscle tissue of grazing animals such as cattle and sheep. Seafood is also an excellent source of selenium, although mercury, a pollutant found commonly in the flesh of the fish we eat, can bind it up so that it is not available for our cells to use.

Brazil nuts and grains are potent plant-based sources of selenium, but it is possible to overdo it. Just 1 ounce of Brazil nuts supplies 840 mcg, or twelve times the required daily intake of 70 mcg. Three and a half ounces of tuna supplies more than 100 percent of the daily recommended intake, and two slices of whole wheat bread deliver about 30 percent. The Institute of Medicine recommends a maximal daily limit of 400 mcg, to avoid potential side effects such as intestinal upset, thyroid abnormalities, hair loss, and damage to the nerves.

When selenium levels are adequate, there is no special benefit to heart health in taking supplements. Extremely low dietary levels of selenium have been a problem in some European countries and may lead to weakening of the heart muscle, but low levels are rare in the United States. High blood levels of selenium have been associated with a possible slight increase in cancer risk.

At one time, selenium was thought to be protective against diabetes, but a seven-year study in which people were given a daily supplement of 200 mcg of selenium found the incidence of diabetes was more than doubled. Being that selenium deficiencies are extremely rare in the United States, it makes sense to get this mineral from the food you eat, unless you have a true medical need for a supplement.

BEST PRACTICES:
ANTIOXIDANTS

* Know your nutrients: Antioxidant vitamins and minerals, including vitamins E, C, A, beta-carotene, and selenium, neutralize many harmful substances in your body.
* It's best to obtain these nutrients via foods rather than supplements. Antioxidants in the diet are associated with a decreased risk of heart disease and stroke, but very high-dose supplements may actually increase heart disease and cancer risk.
* Aim for at least 22 IU of vitamin E per day. Good sources include walnuts, peanuts, pecans, corn oil, sesame oil, and soybean oil.
* Find vitamin C in citrus fruit, peaches, strawberries, broccoli, and tomatoes. Women require 75 mg per day; men, 90 mg per day; and those who exercise vigorously should probably take in 100–500 mg each day.
* For beta-carotene, one of the provitamins in vitamin A, look to carrots, sweet potatoes, and cantaloupe, as well as spinach, broccoli, and other dark green and yellow fruits and vegetables.
* Skip the selenium supplements: Chances are, you get all the selenium you need from your diet, and supplements could be seriously detrimental to your health.

THE B VITAMINS

The B vitamins are a family of water-soluble vitamins that help break down the food we eat into usable energy. Although all of them are essential for heart health, folic acid (B_9), B_6, B_{12}, and niacin (B_3) merit special attention for their important preventive properties.

Folic Acid, B_6, and B_{12}

Also known as folate or folacin, folic acid works in combination with vitamins B_6 and B_{12}. Folic acid is found in a wide variety of foods, including dark green leafy vegetables, whole grains, brewers' yeast, and liver, so a healthy diet will usually net you plenty of this nutrient.

Alcoholics, who may get most of their calories from alcohol, are vulnerable to deficiencies, as are people with serious gastrointestinal illnesses. Certain prescription drugs may counteract folic acid, in which case supplements may be required to maintain normal levels. During pregnancy, folic acid is vital for the healthy development of the fetal nervous system, so pregnant women are routinely supplemented with this vitamin. Most pregnant women do not require B_{12} supplements, but vegans should check their B_{12} levels with their obstetrician.

In 1998, the Nurses' Health Study reported that women with the highest intake of folic acid and B_6 had about half the risk of heart disease of women with diets deficient in these vitamins. Women whose diet included 500 mcg of folic acid and 3 mg of B_6 daily appeared to benefit the most. The same study also reported that greater daily intake of folic acid was linked to a lower likelihood of high blood pressure.

■ FOLIC ACID IN FOODS

In 1998, the FDA mandated fortification of food grain with folic acid, largely to help prevent birth defects caused by inadequate folic acid in pregnant women's diets. This boosted the average American's daily dose to about 300 mcg. Although this is still less than the daily 500 mcg dose that seemed to offer the most benefit in the Nurses' Health Study, a major study reported by the Centers for Disease Control and Prevention estimated that simply enriching flour and other grain products with folic acid might prevent forty-eight thousand strokes and deaths every year.

Years ago, there was some evidence that high-dose B vitamins might help prevent blockages from coming back in people who have undergone a coronary balloon angioplasty (a procedure in which a balloon is inflated inside a heart artery in order to open up a blockage). That led to an enthusiastic flurry of folic acid prescriptions for doses ranging anywhere from 1,000 to 5,000 mcg. Subsequent research showed that people with heart disease who take these megadoses of B vitamins are actually *more* likely to suffer a second heart attack or a stroke. For those who have had coronary stents placed (tiny metal mesh tubes that are used to open up blockages in the heart arteries), high-dose folic acid supplements increase the chances that the stent will close up over time.

In these high doses, the supplements may even raise the risk for cancer, because folic acid appears to enhance the growth of all cells, both healthy and malignant. In one study from the University of Southern California, folic acid supplements appeared to increase the likelihood of prostate cancer, whereas folic acid from foods actually lowered the risk.

If your diet is heart healthy, you won't need to worry about getting enough of this nutrient. If you're pregnant, your doctor may recommend a supplement, as pregnant women need at least 600 mcg.

■ THE BUZZ ON B_6 AND B_{12}

In combination with dietary folic acid, vitamin B_6 supports healthy arteries and is important in the production of red blood cells and platelets. B_6 also helps to keep blood glucose levels normal, although there's no advantage to taking high doses of the vitamin.

The recommended daily intake of B_6 is 1.3 to 1.7 mg, depending on age and gender (elderly men need the most), but research studies have used 5 to 50 mg daily with no evident adverse effects.

B_6 is found in fish, brown rice, whole grains, soybeans, and organ meats, and true deficiencies are uncommon in otherwise healthy people, with the exception of alcoholics. Smoking, advanced age, and kidney failure are all associated with a reduction in levels of B_6. Interestingly, low B_6 levels are associated with high levels of CRP, a marker of inflammation discussed in chapter 3 (see page 39). The National Institute of Medicine recommends that doses of B_6 should not exceed 100 mg daily, as higher doses may cause permanent nerve damage.

Vitamin B_{12} is critical to many of your body's functions, including your heart health, normal function of the nervous system, and metabolism of carbohydrates, proteins, and fats. It is also important in the maintenance and production of DNA, the genetic blueprint of your cells. The U.S. recommended daily allowance of B_{12} is 2.4 mcg, although most research studies have included 400 to 1,000 mcg of B_{12}.

In order for dietary B_{12} to be absorbed and utilized by the body, it must combine with a special protein in the stomach known as intrinsic factor. People who cannot absorb B_{12} can suffer serious consequences, including anemia, numbness of the extremities, and weakness. As people age, less intrinsic factor is produced, which is why deficiencies are much more common in the elderly.

The form of vitamin B_{12} that is found in vitamin pills is usually crystalline B_{12}, which does not require gastric acid for absorption, so it is generally effective even for those who are deficient in intrinsic factor. Nevertheless, people who are unable to absorb B_{12} from the stomach are often treated with injections, usually monthly. Symptoms of B_{12} deficiency in elderly people can be very vague, including just a general sense of malaise. Fortunately, a simple blood test can easily determine if you are deficient in this vitamin. Most people will not need routine testing of B_{12} levels, but if you suffer from anemia or neurological symptoms, your doctor may recommend testing.

B_{12} is produced by bacteria in the intestines of grazing animals. It is found in all manner of animal products, including meats, egg yolk, poultry, and milk. It makes sense for vegans to add B_{12} supplements to their diet, as it is not found in plants. Most vegans have not gotten the message, and up to 92 percent of them have been reported to be B_{12} deficient. Because it may take twenty to thirty years to fully deplete the body's stores, a B_{12} deficiency may not show up right away in a recent convert to veganism.

When taking folic acid supplements, it is critically important, regardless of diet, to add B$_{12}$, because high doses of folic acid in someone who is B$_{12}$ deficient may increase the likelihood of nerve damage. Norwegian researchers have reported a higher risk for cancer when 800 mcg of folic acid were combined with 400 mcg of B$_{12}$, so it's important to avoid these supplements unless you clearly need them.

Niacin

Niacin, also known as vitamin B$_3$, nicotinic acid, and nicotinamide, is important in regulating metabolism and maintaining healthy skin, nails, and gastrointestinal functions. Good sources include protein-rich foods such as meat and fish, as well as peanuts and brewers' yeast.

At the usual dietary doses of 14 to 16 mg per day, niacin really doesn't play a major role in heart health. However, at much higher doses (500 to 2,000 mg) niacin morphs into a powerful cholesterol-altering drug that can lower LDL, raise HDL, and reduce triglycerides. Niacin in this prescription-strength range should never be taken without a doctor's supervision, as it can cause such side effects as flushing, itching, headaches, nausea, and muscle cramps. Liver abnormalities are an uncommon but potentially serious side effect of high-dose niacin, so routine blood tests to evaluate liver enzymes are mandatory.

Prescription-strength niacin may also interact with other drugs. High-dose niacin is discussed in detail in chapter 13 (see page 220).

BEST PRACTICES:
B VITAMINS

* Aim for 500 mcg of folic acid per day. It's found in a wide variety of foods, including dark green leafy vegetables, whole grains, brewers' yeast, and liver.
* Avoid high-dose folic acid supplements (more than 400 mcg), which may increase the risk of heart attack, especially if taken after a coronary stent has been placed, and also of cancer.

- You need at least 1.3–1.7 mg of B_6, depending on your age and gender. B_6 is found in fish, brown rice, whole grains, soybeans, and organ meats.
- Unless you are vegan, you will likely obtain your daily recommended dose of 2.4 mcg of B_{12} from animal products: meats, egg yolk, poultry, and milk. However, over 90% of vegans are deficient in B_{12}, as are many elderly people. Low B_{12} levels can be diagnosed with a simple blood test.
- You need 14–16 mg of niacin per day. Good sources include protein-rich foods such as meat and fish, as well as peanuts and brewers' yeast.
- Prescription-strength niacin may help improve cholesterol levels but should be taken only under a doctor's supervision.

OTHER VITAMINS AND MINERALS

Beyond the A through E vitamin palette are other nutrients vital to heart health.

Calcium and Vitamin D

You need calcium and vitamin D to keep your bones healthy and strong, but both nutrients are also essential for good cardiovascular health. The two work in harmony, with vitamin D helping the body to maintain optimal levels of calcium.

Vitamin D is unique in that it is manufactured in your skin, when you are exposed to ultraviolet (UV) rays. While sun worshippers may end up with sun-dried skin and troublesome skin cancers, they hardly ever have to worry about missing out on vitamin D. Those who shun the sun, or who cover up with clothes or sunscreen when out of doors, are much more apt to be lacking. Obese people are also more likely to be deficient, because the vitamin D may be sheltered within the fat tissue, rather than going out into the bloodstream to do its work.

Using a cutoff blood level of 30 mg/mL, anywhere from 50 to 75 percent of Americans are deficient in vitamin D. The darker your skin is, the less efficient it is in converting sunlight into vitamin D, so people of African, Native American, Asian, and Latin ancestry are particularly likely to have lower levels of the sunshine vitamin. It's easy to test for blood levels of vitamin D, although it is not yet considered part of a standard blood panel.

Vitamin D plays important roles in immune function and inflammation, and receptors for this vitamin are found throughout the heart and blood vessels. Low levels of vitamin D have been linked to a higher risk for cardiovascular disease, especially in people with hypertension. However, definitive proof of the impact of supplements on heart health is still lacking, and several large studies are currently under way to help clarify the question.

Vitamin D deficiency may be associated with colorectal cancer, muscle weakness, and even cognitive decline in older folks. But too much vitamin D can be harmful as well, and can lead to dangerously high levels of calcium in the bloodstream. This in turn can cause mental confusion, abnormal heart rhythms, and deposits of calcium and phosphate in the soft tissues of the body.

As we age, our vitamin D requirements increase. Until we reach our 50s, adults need about 600 IU daily, including pregnant and lactating moms. After age 70, our daily requirement jumps to 800 IU.

The maximum safe daily dose of vitamin D is considered to be 4,000 IU, although higher doses are sometimes prescribed for people with serious deficiencies. Supplements may come in the form of vitamin D2 or D3; in general D3 is considered more potent. Very high-dose prescription-strength supplements of 50,000 IU taken on a long-term daily basis may cause side effects such as nausea, kidney stones, and heart rhythm abnormalities, and may even increase the risk of bone fractures. Such doses should only be taken under a doctor's supervision. Supplements and a sunny day are not the only way to boost your stores of vitamin D. Fatty fish, including salmon and tuna, are excellent sources of vitamin D, and also offer healthy omega-3 fatty acids. Milk and soy milk are usually fortified with vitamin D, as are many breakfast cereals, so getting a healthy dose of this vitamin can be as easy as fixing yourself a bowl of whole-grain cereal with milk.

A cup of milk supplies about 100 IU, and 4 ounces of salmon will buy you 400 IU. Fish oil capsules generally do not contain vitamin D. But for those who choose to take old-fashioned cod liver oil, 1 tablespoon of the slick stuff provides 1,360 IU of vitamin D, leaving little wiggle room for more.

Calcium can also be overdone. Most people need about 1,200 mg daily. Until recently, doctors routinely advised their patients over the age of 50 to take a calcium supplement in the hopes of reducing bone fractures. However, beginning in 2010, several large analyses of the effects of calcium on heart health have put a damper on our enthusiasm for calcium supplements. Once again, our attempts to trump Mother Nature have backfired, as evidence has surfaced that calcium supplements (but not calcium from food) may actually increase heart attack risk by as much as 30 percent. At the same time, the supplements only cut the risk for bone fractures by a measly 10 percent.

It's best to get most of your calcium from the foods you eat, as dietary calcium maintains bone density better than calcium supplements. Dairy products are a great source of calcium, but molasses, tofu, and dark green leafy vegetables also supply reasonable amounts.

A diet high in calcium (1,000 to 1,500 mg/day) may help to lower blood pressure modestly (about 1 to 3 mm Hg). When low-fat calcium-rich dairy foods such as yogurt are included, cholesterol levels may drop, and diabetes risk may lessen.

Vitamin K

Vitamin K is found in virtually all leafy green vegetables and in soybeans, cheese, and whole grains. This vitamin is also made by bacteria living in your intestines, so true deficiencies are rare. The major importance of vitamin K is its effect upon four critical clotting factors, all of which are manufactured in your liver.

If you take the blood thinner known generically as warfarin (the trade name is Coumadin), wide fluctuations in daily vitamin K intake can cause rather serious problems. This is because warfarin inactivates these vitamin K–dependent clotting factors, reducing the ability of your blood to clot. Warfarin is prescribed for people with a high risk of blood clots, such as those with an irregular heart rhythm known as atrial fibrillation, with implanted mechanical heart valves, and with a history of life-threatening blood clots.

For these individuals, consistency in vitamin K levels is extremely important. As long as vitamin K intake is kept steady, the dose of warfarin can usually be adjusted to accommodate it. That just means that some people may need to take higher-than-average doses of warfarin to overcome the effects of vitamin K. Given the tremendous health benefits of green leafy vegetables, the advice physicians used to give to warfarin patients years ago to limit these foods really does not make good medical sense. Of course, if you take warfarin and are planning to make changes to your diet, it's important to let your doctor know, so your blood levels can be monitored. Other blood thinners, including Pradaxa, aspirin, and Plavix, are not affected by vitamin K.

Iron

An essential mineral, iron is an integral building block of hemoglobin, a protein found in all red blood cells. Through hemoglobin, iron helps oxygen to flow throughout your body, right down to the tiniest capillaries, keeping all your cells oxygenated and invigorated.

Your body is very good at squirreling away a little extra iron to use in case of a temporary shortage, so if you don't get enough iron every day, you can still get by, at least temporarily. Your body is also incredibly efficient at self-regulation and can crank up absorption of dietary iron when your stores are running low and back off when supplies are plentiful. However, excessive amounts of iron can overload your system. In extreme cases, too much iron may even be fatal to young children.

Before menopause, women require about 18 grams of iron daily, since iron is lost through menstrual blood flow. Men and post-menopausal women need about 8 mg daily. Lean red meat, turkey, and shrimp are good animal sources of iron (supplying 3 grams or more per 4-ounce serving); and soybeans, lentils, leafy greens, dried fruit, and enriched grains provide similar amounts of plant-based iron per serving. And just in case you don't eat enough of these naturally iron-rich foods, many cereals are fortified with iron.

Whereas iron from animal sources is easy to absorb, plant-derived iron takes a little more work. Vitamin C assists with the process, so as long as vegetarians get enough vitamin C along with their iron, this does not pose much of a problem. Vitamin A is also important in maintaining a safe level of iron, because it helps to release stored iron during times when iron intake is low or when the body's demand for it is high.

Hemochromatosis is an inherited disorder associated with extremely high iron levels, which can cause severe damage to the heart muscle, liver, and other organs. Joint pains and diabetes are also common in hemochromatosis. A simple blood test can usually detect this condition, which affects at least one in every three hundred people. Screening is not considered part of a routine examination, but if you have a family history of the disorder, or if a blood test picks up high levels of iron, then testing is appropriate. Hemochromatosis is more common in men and in Caucasians. Treatment often involves what is known as a therapeutic phlebotomy; in essence, this is modern-day bloodletting, with blood removed through a vein to draw down iron levels.

Potassium and Magnesium

Potassium and magnesium are critical to maintaining heart health. Normal heart and skeletal muscle function, normal electrical activity of the heart, and proper functioning of the nerves and nervous system depend in large part upon potassium and magnesium. In most people, the kidneys keep these elements in a delicate equilibrium, as too much or too little could have disastrous effects. However, diuretics ("water pills") and some other medications can upset this balance, as can kidney failure.

Diuretics are often used to treat high blood pressure and can be very effective, but monitoring with blood tests is important, as diuretics can lower potassium, sodium, and magnesium. In people who take diuretics and develop extremely low potassium or magnesium levels, the risk of serious heart rhythm abnormalities may rise dramatically. Treatment with prescription supplements usually corrects the problem. Mildly low blood levels of potassium may even contribute to high blood pressure. Potassium levels on the high end of the normal scale may decrease the risk of stroke and improve glucose tolerance, reducing the chance of diabetes.

Most Americans take in about half of the recommended 4.7 grams of potassium per day. Fortunately, it is very easy to remedy this. Fruits and vegetables are potassium dynamos. Your granddaddy may have eaten a banana with his breakfast every morning, but just about every fruit is chock-full of potassium. If you are not on diuretic medications, and you eat your eight to ten servings of fruits and vegetables daily, it is unlikely that you'll ever lack for potassium.

■ DON'T DOSE YOURSELF

Although there are a few important medical causes of low potassium, if you are not on diuretic drugs, there is usually no reason to take a supplement. Potassium may be bought over the counter, but it is really pretty dangerous to try to dose yourself. Some prescription medications, including blood pressure medications and certain birth control pills, may increase potassium levels, and the body may be unable to effectively rid itself of the excess. This becomes especially problematic in diabetics and those with kidney disease, who may actually need to limit their potassium intake. Your doctor can easily check your potassium levels and kidney function, as well as your blood sugar, with a routine blood test known as a "basic metabolic profile." This test is often done as part of a yearly checkup.

Magnesium works closely with potassium, and oftentimes low magnesium levels make it difficult to attain a normal blood level of potassium. Magnesium is involved in normal functioning of muscles and nerves, as well as energy metabolism and bone health. While magnesium has been shown to be involved in the health of the immune system, supplementation above and beyond normal levels does not improve immunity.

Green leafy vegetables, nuts, wheat germ, and avocados are good sources of magnesium; as luck would have it, so is chocolate. Refined and processed foods tend to be relatively deficient in magnesium.

People with diabetes often have lower blood levels of magnesium and may require supplementation under a doctor's supervision. Excessive alcohol, diuretics, and chemotherapy may deplete magnesium stores, leading to heart arrhythmias, muscle dysfunction, and nerve impairment. Although it is not routinely measured, your doctor can run a simple blood test to check for a magnesium deficiency; if your magnesium is low, it's a good bet your potassium is as well. If supplements are needed, regular blood tests are important to be sure the dose is adequate, but not excessive.

BEST PRACTICES:
OTHER VITAMINS AND MINERALS

* Strive for 600–1,000 IU of vitamin D daily. Fatty fish, including salmon and tuna, are excellent sources, as are fortified whole grains, vitamin D–enriched dairy or nondairy milks, and cod liver oil.

* Dairy products are a great source of calcium, but molasses, tofu, and dark green leafy vegetables also help to achieve a dietary total of 1,200 mg daily.

* Vitamin K is essential to clotting, and is found in all leafy green vegetables and in soybeans, cheese, and whole grains. If you take warfarin, work with your physician to adjust its dosage, rather than avoid these heart-healthy foods.

* Iron helps to transport oxygen to your cells, so it's important to maintain normal levels. Find it in lean red meat, turkey, and shrimp, as well as plant sources such as soybeans, lentils, leafy greens, and enriched grains. If you are vegetarian or vegan, be sure you are getting enough vitamin C, which aids in the absorption of plant-derived iron.
* Most of us require about 4.7 grams of potassium per day; it's easily obtained from a variety of fruits and vegetables (not just bananas). Magnesium, which is essential to the processing of potassium, is found in green leafy vegetables, nuts, wheat germ, avocados, and dark chocolate. Low levels of potassium and magnesium can contribute to high blood pressure and trigger irregular heart rhythms.
* Don't take supplemental magnesium or potassium without your doctor's approval. Blood tests can easily determine whether you are deficient in these minerals.

There is no convincing evidence that a multivitamin supplement is necessary for most people. In fact, the Iowa Women's Study of over thirty-eight thousand women found a small increase in the risk of death for women who took multivitamins regularly, although the reason for this finding was not clear. Your first line of action should be to balance out specific deficiencies with heart-smart dietary choices, rather than a magic pill.

15

Supplements and Herbs

CAN ALWAYS COUNT on José, an energetic 67-year-old marketing executive and road biker with high blood pressure and elevated cholesterol, to arrive for his appointments balancing a stack of file folders brimming with the latest "breakthrough research" on supplements and herbs. José always seems a little apologetic about his forays into self-care, but he is good humored and respects my advice and medical opinion. I admire his initiative. Indeed, it was questions from inquisitive patients like José that helped to motivate me to research and write this book.

Nutritional supplements can be found in the medicine cabinets of at least one in five Americans. They account for out-of-pocket expenses of more than $18 billion each year, with an annual growth rate estimated to be on the order of 20 percent. Another $5 billion or more is spent on herbal products. We're talking big business. More important, the widespread use of supplements and herbs highlights a desire that many of us have to take control of our own health, in terms that make sense to us and in a way that seems more in tune with nature.

I applaud the active participation in and commitment to preventive health care. But all too often, supplements and herbs are taken on faith. Many times when I ask my patients why they are taking a particular supplement, the reply is simply: "It's supposed to help my heart." If I prescribed a medication for you and could give you no better explanation for it than this, you would probably be pretty skeptical. To help you become your own health advocate and choose supplements wisely, I want you to have some basic knowledge of dietary supplements as well as an understanding of the system that produces and markets them.

Let's be honest. Most doctors don't know much about herbs and supplements. In defense of the medical profession, there are many good reasons for this. First, it is not usually a part of our training. But also, we are trained as scientists. This is a good thing. We demand proof of efficacy and assurance of safety before we prescribe a medication to our patients. That means that I am not going to recommend a supplement strictly based on hearsay, advertising, or tradition.

What many doctors don't know is that there is actually very legitimate, peer-reviewed research available on a good number of supplements, with many new studies currently in the works.

SUPPLEMENTS, HERBS, THE FDA, AND YOU

We Americans depend on the Food and Drug Administration (FDA) to monitor and regulate the drugs that our physicians prescribe. While it is not perfect, the system now in place is designed to ensure both the effectiveness and the safety of the prescription and over-the-counter medications that we take. The FDA requires numerous well-controlled and scientifically sound research studies before it gives approval for a drug. These studies must include detailed assessment of risks and benefits, as well as potential drug interactions.

Despite the tremendous amount of time and resources a company may devote to bringing a drug onto the market, many are never approved. A perfect example is torcetrapib, a drug developed by the pharmaceutical giant Pfizer to raise HDL cholesterol. The company spent more than $800 million and many years developing and testing this very promising drug but, in the end, found an unacceptably high risk of side effects and withdrew the product from the FDA review process.

Once a drug manages to make it through, the FDA requires manufacturers to report all possible side effects that might be related to the use of the drug. Too many problems and a drug may be pulled from the market. By this process, the FDA does its best to ensure that the medications we take are as safe as possible and that they do what they are supposed to do.

Is the FDA infallible? Of course not. Occasionally a medication will be approved that is later found to have serious unanticipated interactions with other drugs or dangerous side effects that take many years to become evident. An example is the class of COX-2 inhibitors, including Vioxx, Bextra, and Celebrex. These drugs are associated with a higher risk of heart attacks, but that did not become apparent until several years, and millions of prescriptions, after their introduction.

To be sure, many drugs are known to have potentially serious side effects, yet approval is given because the benefits to a specific group of patients are important enough that they offset the possible risks.

Although it's far from foolproof, ours is arguably the best system in the world, and some drugs that are approved in other countries do not pass the FDA's muster. This lack of approval is not necessarily because the drugs do not do what they are claimed to do, but because the research to support the claims is not up to the FDA's high standards.

A DIFFERENT STANDARD FOR SUPPLEMENTS

The FDA does not apply the same standards to dietary supplements as it does to prescription and over-the-counter drugs. Manufacturers of dietary supplements have a measure of latitude and autonomy not available to pharmaceutical companies. Supplements are broadly defined by the FDA as "any product that is intended for ingestion as a supplement to the diet," with a few exceptions. This definition encompasses vitamins, minerals, herbs and other plant-derived products, amino acids, and extracts from certain animal organs and glands. Although these products may look like drugs, they are not considered by the FDA to be medications. As a result, they are not allowed to be marketed with the terms *diagnose*, *treat*, *prevent*, *cure*, or *mitigate*.

TRUTH IN LABELING

It is fine for supplements to be sold with a type of health claim known as a "structure-function" claim, as long as a clear relationship has been established between a given food product and health maintenance. For example, higher intake of fruits, vegetables, and fiber has been associated with a lower risk of heart disease, so this claim could apply to a supplement that contains these elements. Likewise, a product high in calcium could offer information regarding calcium's effects on bone protection. Manufacturers are required to include a standard disclaimer: "This statement has not been evaluated by the FDA. This product is not intended to diagnose, treat, cure, or prevent any disease." Nevertheless, these rules are frequently flouted, particularly on the Internet, where imposing regulation is very difficult.

By federal law, all products on the market must be considered safe, but specific information does not have to be provided to the FDA regarding any individual supplement product, and the FDA does not review or approve dietary supplements. The only exception to this rule is something known as a "new dietary ingredient" that is not already commercially available in some form. In that case, the manufacturer must prove only that its product is safe if used as stated on the product's labeling.

It is very important to understand that the FDA does not ensure the purity, composition, or quality of dietary supplements. This lack of regulation has created a wide-open market for these products and taken away a great deal of security for consumers. Recognizing that some companies had failed to follow even the most basic quality assurance standards, in 2008 the FDA began to require companies to confirm the safety of their products by testing for purity and authenticating the ingredients listed on the label. Realistically, given the wide range of companies and products, and the costs of performing inspections, the agency's ability to enforce good manufacturing processes is extremely limited.

Federal law requires manufacturers of supplements and over-the-counter drugs to notify the FDA of any reported side effects. However, because there are so many manufacturers, there is no way to monitor the accuracy of reporting.

WHAT YOU SEE MAY NOT BE WHAT YOU GET

When it comes to supplements, investigations have exposed an abysmal amount of misinformation and mislabeling of these products. The amount of active ingredient stated on the label is frequently incorrect, sometimes drastically so. In fact, one Department of Health investigation found that 32 percent of Asian "herbal" medications actually contained measurable amounts of prescription drugs, including steroids, hormones, and anti-inflammatory medications. More than one in ten included dangerous heavy metals such as lead, mercury, and arsenic.

Indian Ayurvedic medicine has become popular in the United States for its emphasis on traditional healing. But just because a practice has been around for centuries does not make it safe or even effective. A 2004 study of Indian Ayurvedic herbal medicine products bought in the United States, published in the *Journal of the American Medical Association*, found that 20 percent of these products also contained heavy metals. A follow-up study in 2008 found similar amounts of lead, arsenic, and mercury, regardless of whether the Ayurvedic supplements were made in the United States or India. Not surprisingly, it is estimated that about half of Indian children and nearly as many Indian adults test high for blood lead levels.

Some so-called herbal medicines from Japan have been found to be full of thyroid hormones, excessive amounts of which can cause tremors, life-threatening heart arrhythmias, and even heart failure. And up to half of all imported supplements marketed for erectile dysfunction are really bootlegged versions of prescription drugs known to interact dangerously with other commonly prescribed medications.

Although it is the responsibility of the Federal Trade Commission to regulate advertising, there are simply too many products out there and not enough funding for enforcement, making supplements an industry that is nearly impossible to police. Perhaps even more important is the explosion of Web sites offering dietary supplements for sale.

As many of these sites are not based in the United States, governmental oversight is nigh impossible. This is truly a case of "buyer beware."

A study from Johns Hopkins reviewed Web sites that offered herbal weight-loss products for sale. Of thirty-two different sites offering thirty-two different products, 41 percent did not disclose potential adverse effects, drug interactions, or conditions in which the supplement could be harmful, more than half did not include dose information, and a third contained incorrect or misleading statements including claims of "100 percent safety" and "no harmful side effects," even when the supplements were known to be potentially harmful.

In 2009, the FDA issued consumer warnings for over 140 contaminated supplements, many sold as natural weight-loss products, which contained a wide range of prescription drugs or prescription drug analogues. Most of the time, the labeling of these products gave no indication that these drugs were present. This was clearly just the tip of the iceberg, as there was no feasible way for all the available products to be tested at taxpayers' expense.

THE SPECIAL PROBLEMS WITH HERBS

Herbs in their natural state are notoriously tricky, as a single herb may contain hundreds of chemical compounds. Just which of these compounds is responsible for the purported benefit of the herb is often unknown. Adding to the confusion, the active compounds in the herbs can vary more than a hundredfold from one batch to another or from one brand to another. Different parts of the plant, different growing conditions, and different formulations can make an enormous difference. And just because a plant is an herb doesn't guarantee it is safe for humans to consume. For example, aconite, used historically to treat heart palpitations, can be fatally toxic.

It's important to be up front with your doctor about supplements and herbs (see "Heart Health Checklist: What Your Doctor Needs to Know," page 347). Many supplements will interact with prescription medications, either by raising drug levels and increasing the risk of drug toxicity or by inhibiting the drug from working properly.

FACTS TO KNOW ABOUT THE FDA, SUPPLEMENTS, AND HERBS

* Prescription and over-the-counter drugs are strictly regulated, and many new drugs that are developed are never approved for sale.
* Government oversight of supplements is minimal due to the Dietary Supplement Health and Education Act of 1994 (DSHEA).
* Supplements cannot claim to treat or cure a problem but are allowed to include "structure-function" claims.
* Supplement labels are often inaccurate, especially when it comes to herbs.
* Although illegal, some supplements, especially those from overseas, may contain heavy metals, hormones, or other health-jeopardizing ingredients.
* Make sure your doctor knows what supplements you're taking, because they can interact with prescription medications.

SUPPLEMENTS, SCIENCE, AND SAFETY

Following are some of the more commonly used supplements marketed for heart health. Although the scientific data may be scant for some, for others, a substantial amount of legitimate medical research is available. As a physician, I found many of these reports to be eye opening. Some theories that many of us accept as gospel have been debunked long ago, whereas others offer exciting new possibilities for prevention. The following table gives a brief overview of the supplements covered; please see the pages indicated for more detailed information.

SUPPLEMENT	WHAT'S IT FOR?	USUAL DAILY DOSE[1]	DOES IT WORK?	SUPPLEMENT SAFETY[2]
Bitter orange (also sold as sour orange, citrus aurantium, zhi shi, kijitsu, and neroli) (page 303)	Marketed for weight loss	Varies by product	Yes, but it's not worth the risk.	Dangerous and potentially fatal side effects include high blood pressure, heart attack, and heart rhythm abnormalities. Bitter orange may interact with prescription drugs.
Chitosan (page 295)	Marketed to lower cholesterol and promote weight loss	1,000–5,000 mg	No	Possible risks include abdominal cramps and constipation.
Chromium picolinate (page 301)	Marketed for weight loss	200–1,000 mcg	No	Doses over 1,000 mcg have been linked to kidney failure, blood abnormalities, and liver damage.
Coenzyme Q10 (page 296)	Marketed to strengthen and protect the heart and lower blood pressure, and also used to prevent muscle aches from statin drugs	50–200 mg	Possibly: Its strengthening effect on the heart muscle is minimal, and it may lower blood pressure, but this effect is unpredictable. It will help some people who have statin-associated muscle pain.	High doses may lower blood pressure too drastically.
Creatine (page 309)	Marketed to strengthen muscles	2,000–5,000 mg	Possibly: It may improve muscle strength in weight lifters (especially vegetarians).	High doses may harm the kidneys.
Ephedra (also sold as ma huang, country mallow, joint fir, Mormon tea, and heartleaf) (page 302)	Marketed for weight loss	100 mg	Yes, but it's not worth the risk.	The FDA has banned ephedra because of its dangerous side effects, which include stroke, heart attack, heart rhythm abnormalities, and death.

SUPPLEMENT	WHAT'S IT FOR?	USUAL DAILY DOSE[1]	DOES IT WORK?	SUPPLEMENT SAFETY[2]
Fruit and vegetable concentrates (page 310)	Marketed to protect the heart	Varies by product	Probably, but whole fruits and vegetables are even better.	Probably safe.
Garlic (page 291)	Marketed to lower cholesterol	600–900 mg (may vary by product)	No, although whole garlic has antioxidant properties.	Safe.
Ginkgo biloba (page 298)	Marketed as a memory enhancer	120–240 mg	No	Generally safe, but it may cause nausea, indigestion, headaches, rash, and, in rare cases, bleeding in the brain. Ginkgo interacts with some prescription drugs.
Ginseng (page 301)	Marketed to enhance energy and libido and improve the lipid profile	200–400 mg (ginseng extract); 1–2 g (ginseng root)	Possibly	May cause high blood pressure, nervousness, diarrhea, and increased risk of bleeding. Avoid Siberian ginseng, which is a different plant altogether.
Glucomannan (page 289)	Marketed to lower LDL cholesterol	500–1,200 mg	Yes	May cause intestinal gas, bloating, and liver toxicity.
Grape seed extract (page 299)	Marketed to protect the heart and help prevent cancer	100–300 mg	Possibly, although studies are limited.	Headaches or nausea may occur, and it interacts with some prescription drugs.
Guggul (page 294)	Marketed to lower cholesterol	3,000–6,000 mg	No	Guggul frequently causes a rash.
Hoodia gordonii (page 304)	Marketed for weight loss	Varies by product	Possibly, but most forms of "hoodia" available on the market are not actually Hoodia gordonii.	The risks are not well known, but may include liver toxicity.

SUPPLEMENT	WHAT'S IT FOR?	USUAL DAILY DOSE[1]	DOES IT WORK?	SUPPLEMENT SAFETY[2]
Hydroxycitric acid (also sold as garcinia cambogia, brindleberry, gorikapuli, citrin, gambooge, and Malabar tamarind) (page 304)	Marketed to improve energy and promote weight loss	1,500–2,500 mg	No	Risks may include liver toxicity.
L-arginine (page 306)	Marketed to improve blood flow and arterial function and to treat erectile dysfunction	400–6,000 mg	Probably not	Increases risk of congestive heart failure in people with heart disease and may increase risk of cancer.
L-carnitine (page 308)	Marketed to improve physical performance and to reduce muscle aches from statin drugs	2,000–3,000 mg	Possible improvement in muscle aches in people who take statins; possible improvement in leg pain from blocked arteries.	Increases risk of seizures in people with epilepsy.
Nattokinase (page 287)	Marketed for heart protection	50–200 mg	The food natto is probably as nutritious as other soy foods, but there's no evidence that taking nattokinase pills brings any greater benefit.	Natto is safe to eat, but the safety of nattokinase pills is unknown.
Omega-3 supplements (including fish oil, algal oil, and flaxseed oil) (page 283)	Marketed to protect the heart and blood vessels and reduce high triglycerides	1,000–2,000 mg	Yes (especially fish oil)	Generally safe at doses of 1,000 mg, but may increase risk of bleeding, especially at doses over 3,000 mg. High-dose flaxseed oil may also impair thyroid function.

SUPPLEMENT	WHAT'S IT FOR?	USUAL DAILY DOSE[1]	DOES IT WORK?	SUPPLEMENT SAFETY[2]
Plant sterols and stanols (page 290)	Marketed to lower LDL cholesterol	1,000–2,000 mg	Yes	Stanols may be safer and more effective then sterols. Both may decrease absorption of beta-carotene. People with homozygous sitosterolemia should avoid these.
Policosanol (page 294)	Marketed to lower cholesterol	10–40 mg	No	Probably safe.
Psyllium (page 288)	Marketed to lower LDL cholesterol	10–15 g	Yes	Generally safe, but may cause abdominal bloating and gas.
Pycnogenol (page 299)	Marketed to protect the heart and prevent blood clots	25–150 mg	Possibly, although studies are limited.	Probably safe, although gastro-intestinal discomfort and nausea may occur.
Red yeast rice (page 292)	Marketed to lower LDL cholesterol	2,400 mg	Yes	Like prescription statins, red yeast rice may cause muscle breakdown and liver toxicity. Blood work should be monitored.
Soy isoflavones (page 287)	Marketed to reduce cholesterol and treat menopause symptoms	40–90 mg	No	Safety is unknown, since many products contain other unidentifiable chemicals.

[1] Some supplements are taken in divided doses. See text for more details. Doses are based on common practice, and in many cases have not been thoroughly tested for safety.

[2] Always check with your physician before starting any supplements, especially if you are pregnant or breastfeeding.

THE OMEGA-3S: FISH OIL, FLAXSEED OIL, AND ALGAL OIL

Coldwater fish are loaded with the heart-protective omega-3 fatty acids known as EPA and DHA (eicosapentaenoic acid and docosahexaenoic acid), a topic we dove into in chapter 5 (see page 80). Omega-3 fatty acids support heart health on many fronts, including lowering triglyceride levels, limiting the harmful effects of LDL cholesterol, reducing susceptibility to blood clots, and perhaps even improving blood pressure. One of the most important benefits is the protection omega-3s appear to provide against life-threatening heart rhythms that can sometimes lead to sudden death.

A large Italian study published in 2002 included more than eleven thousand people who had suffered a heart attack within the preceding three months. The participants were randomly assigned to receive either 1 gram per day of highly purified, prescription-grade fish oil (currently marketed under the brand name Lovaza) or a placebo pill. After three months of treatment, there was a stunning 41 percent reduction in mortality in the fish oil group. The study was concluded after forty-two months, with the fish oil group still way ahead of the curve.

It's hard to argue with such great results, but a Dutch study published in 2010 found no added benefit with low-dose fish oil (about 375 mg of omega-3s) in people already on state-of-the-art heart medications, whose heart attacks had occurred several years before the fish oil was started. Some would argue that the dose prescribed was simply too low for a benefit to be seen.

Fish oil is often used to treat high triglycerides, and just 1 to 2 grams of purified fish oil daily will lower triglyceride levels by about 15 percent. In people who start out with high triglycerides (more than 150 mg/dL), it is not unusual to see reductions of 30 percent. Prescription-strength fish oil will lower triglycerides by up to 45 percent when taken at the recommended dose of four capsules daily (see chapter 13, page 223, for more about this FDA-approved medication).

Read the label to find the EPA and DHA content of an omega-3 supplement. The higher the sum of these numbers, the more potent the supplement will be. In a good-quality supplement, these two numbers will add up to about 300 mg, while prescription-strength fish oil weighs in at 900 mg of EPA and DHA per capsule. Although fish oil does not do very much for total HDL or LDL cholesterol, it does appear to reduce the number of harmful small, dense LDL particles and increase large HDL particles. Fish oil does not appear to affect CRP, even though it is known to have anti-inflammatory properties.

So Who Needs 'Em?

Who should take fish oil supplements, and how much is optimal? For most adults who don't enjoy salmon or other coldwater fish at least twice weekly, a daily 1,000 mg supplement (with 300 mg of EPA and DHA) may be beneficial, as long as there are no medical reasons to avoid fish oil. People who have had heart attacks might benefit from two or even three capsules daily, with a doctor's approval. By comparison, the average daily intake of DHA and EPA in the United States is estimated to be 180 mg per day.

Yet substantial amounts of omega-3 fatty acids can easily be obtained from the diet. For instance, just 3 ounces of wild salmon provides 1,800 mg, and there are 1,000 mg of omega-3s in 3 ounces of rainbow trout. Water-packed canned white tuna is also an excellent source, weighing in at 700 mg per 3 ounces, although the same amount of light tuna only provides 200 grams.

Someone who gets 7 grams (or 7,000 mg) of omega-3 fatty acids from fish each week probably will not benefit substantially from supplements. The exception is when triglycerides are too high, in which case pharmaceutical-grade fish oil (prescribed by a physician) may be helpful.

More than 3 grams of fish oil per day may be associated with a slightly higher risk of bleeding, so for most people the daily dose should not exceed 2 grams, unless recommended by a physician. Fish oil may also cause distasteful fishy burps, although the more purified the product, the less noticeable the taste. Freezing the capsules might help to reduce the fishiness, although it's not known what effect this could have on the potency of the product.

A study from the University of Washington, published in the *American Journal of Epidemiology* in 2011, linked high omega-3 blood levels to a greater likelihood of prostate cancer. This connection bears noting, but it has not been reported in other studies. In fact, there is good evidence that a fish-based diet lowers prostate cancer risk.

While many omega-3–rich fish are contaminated with mercury, it is reassuring that *Consumer Reports* magazine (July 2003) showed no significant mercury levels in the sixteen top-selling brands of fish oil supplements. This is because mercury is water soluble and is removed during the purification process. Due to the refining process, fish oil supplements tend to be low in other pollutants as well. This report also found that the labeling on these products was reasonably accurate, with most capsules containing the amount of omega-3 fatty acids claimed on the package. During pregnancy, omega-3 fatty acids are important to normal fetal neurological development. Expert panels from the World Health Organization and the National Institutes of Health recommend 300 mg of DHA daily for pregnant or lactating women. Because so much of our fish is contaminated with mercury and other pollutants, and mercury is harmful to the developing brain, fish oil is probably a better choice for pregnant women. Of course, if you're pregnant or breast feeding, it's important to check with your doctor before taking any supplement.

When Fish Is Just Too Fishy

Fish oil comes from fish, chiefly the lowly menhaden fish, a species that many larger fish rely on for their meals, and a great housekeeper for our oceans. The menhaden is a filter feeder, living on algae. When the population of menhaden is depleted, algae can grow unabated, contributing to environmental decline. That's why a new generation of environmentally neutral and sustainable omega-3 products made from calamari castoffs from the fishing industry have sprung up.

Although fish oil is the best source of omega-3s, vegetarians and the fish-averse have options, too. Algal-DHA is a form of DHA that comes from algae. It is not entirely clear whether DHA alone will provide the same benefit as the blend of EPA and DHA found in fish oil. Although the research is limited, DHA does appear to be most important for brain health. DHA is better for lowering triglycerides, but EPA is more effective for blocking the harmful oxidation of LDL cholesterol. A Japanese study of an EPA supplement found a 19 percent reduction in heart disease risk.

Plant sources of omega-3 fatty acids include walnuts and flaxseed oil. To put them to use, our bodies must convert the plant-derived omega-3 fatty acid, alpha-linolenic acid (ALA), into DHA and EPA. Alas, this biochemical process is quite inefficient and fairly unreliable. In fact, only about 6 percent of a given amount of ALA is converted to EPA and less than 4 percent becomes DHA. This cumbersome conversion process is further thwarted by the typical American diet, which is high in omega-6 fatty acids (from corn oil, safflower oil, and sunflower oil), because omega-3 and omega-6 fatty acids compete for some of the same enzymes. Nevertheless, preliminary research suggests that such plant-based omega-3 oils may indeed help to prevent cardiovascular disease, particularly in people who do not get omega-3 fatty acids from fish sources. Megadoses of flaxseed oil should be avoided, as taking more than 4 tablespoons daily can interfere with normal function of the thyroid gland.

BEST PRACTICES:
OMEGA-3 FATTY ACIDS

* Don't skimp on omega-3s: They're good for your heart, hair, skin, and brain, and may even support joint health and reduce inflammation. Three ounces of wild salmon supplies 1,800 mg of omega-3s, 3 ounces of rainbow trout provides 1,000 mg, and 3 ounces of water-packed canned white tuna will net you 700 mg.

* If you are getting less than 1,000 mg of omega-3s daily, if eating fish does not appeal, or you are pregnant or breast feeding, ask your doctor if a fish oil supplement makes good sense for you. Look for one high in EPA and

DHA. A daily dose of 1,000 mg of fish oil may protect your heart.

* Prescription fish oil, which is highly purified, can be used to lower severely elevated triglyceride levels; 1,000–2,000 mg of regular fish oil will lower your triglycerides by as much as 15–30%.

* Plant-based omega-3 oils, such as flaxseed oil, may help to prevent cardiovascular disease, but your body does not process these oils efficiently. Megadoses (more than 4 tablespoons per day) of flaxseed oil can interfere with the functioning of your thyroid.

SOY ISOFLAVONES

Soy is truly one of nature's wonder foods. It is no surprise that enterprising manufacturers have marketed soy isoflavones, or isolated soy extracts, as dietary supplements. But there is really very little data to back up the high-flying claims that often come with these products.

Most studies of soy isoflavone supplements show little or no meaningful effect on blood lipids. As we know that adding soy-rich foods to your diet may help to improve your cholesterol profile, it stands to reason that the improvement in lipids probably comes from the complete soy protein in combination with its related isoflavones, packaged with love by Mother Nature.

Isoflavone supplements are notoriously inconsistent. An analysis of thirty-three commercial isoflavone products, published in the *Journal of Nutrition* in 2001, found that many did not contain the amount of isoflavone reported on the package label; furthermore, no two supplements were the same. Of even greater concern was the discovery that a number of the supplements contained unidentifiable chemical compounds, the safety of which were unknown. Another investigation of fifteen different products found that the isoflavone content of these supplements varied up to two thousandfold.

Nattokinase is a soy derivative often sold as a heart-health supplement. Manufacturers claim a number of heart-protective attributes, including inhibition of harmful LDL oxidation and reduction in incidence of blood clots. Nattokinase is based on a fermented Japanese food called *natto*, delicately described by its fans as cheesy, with a strong smell and slimy texture. Although there are no well-done human studies on nattokinase, *natto* is a soy-based food, and thus a good source of soy protein and soy isoflavones. It is likely a fine addition to a heart-healthy diet for those strong enough to accept the challenge.

BEST PRACTICES:
SOY SUPPLEMENTS

* To improve your lipids, replace red meat and chicken with soy-rich foods. Don't bother with soy supplements, which have little to no effect.
* Although nattokinase is derived from *natto*, a soy-based food, there is no convincing evidence that it's effective as a supplement.

SUPPLEMENTS FOR CHOLESTEROL REDUCTION

Numerous products on the market tout their purported ability to lower cholesterol. Which are truly effective?

Psyllium

You may know psyllium as Metamucil, Konsyl, or Perdiem. This soluble fiber, which comes from the husk of the blond psyllium seed, is a bona fide multitasker. Not only does it promote bowel regularity, but psyllium can also lower LDL cholesterol by about 10 percent. (It has no real effect on HDL or triglycerides.) Psyllium contains an aptly named substance called mucilage that allows its volume to swell up to tenfold when exposed to liquids. This is one reason that it's such a great stool-bulking agent. It also helps the body to flush out cholesterol-containing bile acids through the stool and may directly interfere with the intestine's ability to absorb cholesterol and fat.

Studies of the effects of psyllium on cholesterol have focused mostly on a standard dose of about 10 grams daily. This is usually taken as two separate doses of 5 grams, but three 3-gram increments work just as well. Many forms of psyllium are available, including capsules, powder, and biscuits, all of which you can buy at the drugstore. Several high-fiber breakfast cereals are made using psyllium, including Kellogg's Bran Buds.

There are some unpleasant, and potentially embarrassing, drawbacks to psyllium, including increased intestinal gas, soft stools, and abdominal discomfort. If fiber has not been a big part of your diet, it makes sense to go slow. You can usually take psyllium along with prescription medications, including cholesterol-lowering drugs, but check with your doctor or pharmacist if you're not sure. In fact, by adding psyllium to a prescription cholesterol-lowering statin drug, the dose of medication required can often be reduced. If you have diabetes, psyllium may even help to lower your blood glucose. Psyllium does not appear to significantly affect absorption of vitamins or minerals.

Glucomannan

Glucomannan comes from the konjac root, an Asian tuber. Traditionally, it is used in jellies and noodles to give a rubbery texture, but it is indigestible, meaning it passes right through the intestinal tract. Although it has been peddled as a supplement for weight control, its real benefit appears to be in cholesterol reduction. Glucomannan is probably very similar to psyllium in the way that it absorbs bile acids in the intestine. It may lower LDL cholesterol by 7 to 22 percent, although reports of its effectiveness vary from study to study and, frankly, not a lot of research is available on this supplement. The greatest reduction in cholesterol was seen when people took it at doses of 0.5 to 1.2 grams three times daily with meals. Like psyllium, glucomannan also appears to help lower blood glucose levels modestly in diabetics.

Very little safety data is available on glucomannan. As with psyllium, the most common side effects are increased intestinal gas and bloating. However, a recent report of possible liver toxicity raises a red flag. Much more information and research are available on psyllium, so until we know more, psyllium is your better bet.

Plant Sterols and Stanols

Sterols and their derivatives, stanols, are naturally occurring plant-based products that bear a passing resemblance to cholesterol. As such, they compete with cholesterol in the intestinal tract, and by doing so, they limit the body's ability to absorb cholesterol from the foods we eat. Because stanols and sterols themselves are minimally absorbed, they basically just take up space on the special cholesterol receptors of the intestine, blocking the cholesterol molecules from getting in. As a result, LDL cholesterol drops by as much as 15 percent.

Dietary sources include fruit, vegetables, nuts, legumes, and vegetable oils. Although stanols and sterols can be potent cholesterol blockers, they occur in such small amounts in nature that it is unusual to eat enough to make a dent in cholesterol by diet alone. On average, we consume 250 to 500 mg per day of sterols and 20 to 60 mg per day of stanols. At least 1 gram (1,000 mg) per day is required to have much effect on lipids, and 2 grams per day seems to be optimal.

Sterols and stanols can be found in some fortified margarines, including Smart Balance and Benecol. However, to get enough of the active ingredient, you will need to use 2 to 3 tablespoons each day, so the calories can easily add up. And because some margarine products with plant sterols and stanols also contain trans fats, label reading is still important. Lighter forms are available that are trans fat free. If margarine is not for you, you can buy Benecol caramels, fortified with stanols, online. There is no detectable smell or taste, and there are no gastrointestinal side effects.

It has been reported that plant sterols (but not stanols) have been found in cholesterol plaques. Despite this, there is no evidence to date that sterols increase the rate of cholesterol buildup in most people. Products containing sterols and stanols can be used by people on cholesterol-lowering drugs, and the effects on cholesterol are additive.

That means that higher doses of prescription drugs might be avoidable if 2 grams per day of one of these products is added to the diet. (There is probably no benefit to taking more than 2 grams per day.) The effect appears to be greatest in people over the age of 50.

STEER CLEAR IF YOU HAVE HOMOZYGOUS SITOSTEROLEMIA

STEROLS AND STANOLS should be avoided by individuals with a very rare inherited disease known as homozygous sitosterolemia. This disorder occurs in about one in 6 million people and is characterized by cardiovascular disease occurring at a very young age. People who suffer from this disorder absorb sterols and stanols much more readily than most people, so theoretically their risk of heart disease could increase if they consume these products.

Stanols and sterols may decrease absorption of beta-carotene by up to 20 percent, with milder effects on vitamin E, lycopene, and alpha-carotene. If you are adding these products to your diet, it makes sense to eat more colorful fruits and vegetables, and many experts also suggest adding a multivitamin to be on the safe side.

Although no long-term studies have been done to specifically evaluate the effect of these supplements on the incidence of heart disease, it has been estimated that, based on their cholesterol-lowering effects, adding 2 grams per day of sterols and stanols to the diet might lower the risk of heart disease by as much as 25 percent. Several studies have reported that after a few months of regular use, sterols lose their effectiveness, whereas stanols continue to keep cholesterol levels down. Because of this, and because sterols can be found *in* cholesterol plaques, I suggest that you look specifically for products containing plant stanols rather than sterols.

Garlic

It stands to reason that something as pungent as garlic might affect the cardiovascular system as robustly as it does the nose. A "stinking rose" with the strength to deter vampires and the power to add character and passion to the cuisines of diverse cultures around the globe ought surely to discourage atherosclerosis. For centuries, potent health benefits have been attributed to garlic, and for the past thirty or more years, its effects on cholesterol have been studied in earnest. The disappointing verdict: When it comes to cholesterol, garlic just doesn't pack much of a punch.

Although many animal studies have suggested that garlic lowers cholesterol levels, these findings have not been borne out in humans. Of the six studies considered to be the most scientifically valid, none show a difference in lipids between garlic-takers and control subjects. Other studies have found no beneficial effect of garlic oil, powdered garlic, or garlic extract.

Garlic does have antioxidant properties, and so it might reduce the ability of LDL cholesterol to do harm. In combination with other nutritious foods, garlic no doubt contributes to good health, but there is really no compelling reason to take a supplement.

Red Yeast Rice

Red yeast rice is a type of fermented rice on which Chinese red yeast (*Monascus purpureus*) has been grown. What makes red yeast rice so fascinating from the standpoint of heart health is its remarkable chemical composition. Not only does it include a substance known as a monacolin, which is identical to the drug lovastatin (the original prescription statin drug for cholesterol), it also boasts a variety of other statinlike substances, sterols, isoflavones, and monounsaturated fatty acids.

To date, several small-scale studies of the proprietary brand of red yeast rice known as Cholestin have shown a significant reduction in LDL cholesterol of about 20 percent, when taken at doses of 2.4 grams daily. Some studies of red yeast rice have also found an improvement in HDL cholesterol and triglycerides, and at least one Chinese study has reported a reduction in heart attacks and strokes in people taking red yeast rice supplements.

The amount of lovastatin in the supplement is small: 5 mg as compared to 20 to 40 mg in the pharmaceutical strength. This small amount of lovastatin itself is unlikely to cause such a significant drop in cholesterol, so the sterols and isoflavones may also be important players. There are many different manufacturers of red yeast rice supplements, and because they are supplements, the FDA does not oversee or regulate the manufacturing process. An analysis by scientists at UCLA of nine different brands found dramatic variations in composition, with some containing virtually no monocolins at all. Consequently, the results seen with Cholestin and those in the Chinese study may not apply to other brands.

Most studies of red yeast rice have reported no serious side effects of this supplement. However, the majority have included less than one hundred people, which is not usually enough to detect uncommon side effects. In contrast, investigations of lovastatin and other statin drugs (see chapter 13, page 215) have enrolled thousands to tens of thousands of people.

RED YEAST RICE AND STATINS

IN SUSCEPTIBLE PEOPLE, red yeast rice can cause liver abnormalities. In fact, I have seen this side effect in my practice, in a gentleman who had previously experienced serious liver problems with prescription statins and who had no idea that the supplement he was taking could do the same thing. Although liver sensitivity is uncommon, if you choose to take this supplement, you should be monitored with blood testing six to twelve weeks after starting and every six months thereafter, just as is done for people on statin therapy.

Red yeast rice also has the potential to cause rhabdomyolysis—a rare but potentially life-threatening complication in which muscle tissues break down, potentially causing kidney damage. This is more apt to happen to people who are on medications that are known to interact with statin drugs, including certain antibiotics and antifungal drugs.

All in all, red yeast rice appears to be a relatively safe supplement, but one that should not be started without a doctor's supervision. If you are already taking a statin drug, you should not add red yeast rice. Although red yeast rice will not produce the dramatic lowering of cholesterol levels seen with more potent statin drugs, it may help bring mild to moderately elevated cholesterol down to a safe range.

Policosanol

Policosanol, often made from sugar cane, is another supplement that has been championed as a cholesterol reducer. For years, studies funded by its Cuban manufacturer claimed substantial benefits to the lipid profile. But in 2006, a rigorous study of policosanol from a respected German research institute revealed that the supplement had no effect on LDL, HDL, triglycerides, or Lp(a). On the bright side, no major safety issues were identified.

Guggul

An extract from the resin of the mukul myrrh tree, guggul has been touted for its purported cholesterol-lowering effect and is widely used in India for that purpose. In the United States, guggul is marketed as a dietary supplement, accounting for more than a million dollars in sales in 2002.

In 2003, a study by the University of Pennsylvania found that after eight weeks, there was no improvement in cholesterol readings in those who took guggul, regardless of whether they were on a high dose (2,000 mg three times daily) or a standard dose (1,000 mg three times daily). In fact, LDL cholesterol actually increased a little. Overall, there was no significant improvement in HDL, triglycerides, Lp(a), or CRP. Although no abnormalities in liver or kidney tests were reported, 15 percent of the high-dose guggul group and 3 percent of the lower-dose group developed a rash.

Chitosan

Chitosan, an indigestible substance derived from the shells of crustaceans such as shrimp, lobsters, and crabs, is used in treatment of waste water, as a coating for glass fibers, as an additive for paper and photographic film, and as a component of wound dressings, among other things. Since the mid-1990s, it has also been promoted as a weight-loss and cholesterol-lowering supplement. A positively charged substance, it is thought to bind negatively charged molecules like fatty acids. Theoretically, taking chitosan with a fatty meal might prevent the fat from being absorbed through the gut. In reality, studies show the effects of chitosan on fat absorption and cholesterol in humans to be minimal to none. At least two manufacturers of chitosan have been sanctioned by the FDA for making false claims.

BEST PRACTICES:
LDL-LOWERING SUPPLEMENTS

* If your LDL cholesterol is high, consider taking psyllium (sold as Metamucil, Konsyl, and Perdiem, among other brands). It may lower your LDL by 10 percent with a daily dose of 10 grams.
* Glucomannan, at doses of 0.5—1.2 grams taken 3 times daily, acts similarly to psyllium, but there is little safety information available.
* Plant sterols and stanols are another nonprescription option for high LDL cholesterol. They block intestinal absorption of cholesterol and can lower LDL as much as 15% in doses of 2 grams daily. Stanols may be more effective, and possibly safer, than sterols.
* Garlic is a heart-healthy food, but it does little for cholesterol numbers.
* Red yeast rice contains small amounts of naturally formed lovastatin (sold as the prescription drug Mevacor),

as well as sterols, isoflavones, and monounsaturated fatty acids. It may lower LDL by as much as 20% at doses of 2.4 grams daily. However, not all brands are the same, and composition may vary widely. Ask your doctor before starting this supplement.

* If you take red yeast rice, you must have blood tests for liver function at least every 6 months and be aware of the risk of muscle damage and drug interactions. Do not combine red yeast rice with a prescription statin drug.
* Policosanol does not do anything for cholesterol, despite manufacturers' claims to the contrary.
* Guggul does not lower LDL and may even raise it slightly.
* Chitosan neither lowers cholesterol nor blocks fat.

SUPPLEMENTS FOR HEART AND BRAIN PROTECTION

Some supplements promise to keep your heart healthy or ward off dementia. Do they really do any good?

Coenzyme Q10

Coenzyme Q10 (CoQ10), also known as ubiquinone, plays a vital role in energy production. It also has antioxidant properties. Your body already produces CoQ10 in the liver with the help of B vitamins, vitamin E, and vitamin C. Organ meats, salmon, mackerel, sardines, peanuts, and spinach are good dietary sources. (Maybe Popeye really was onto something.) CoQ10 has become one of the fastest-selling and most expensive dietary supplements in this country, bolstered by claims that it has the power to protect the heart against congestive heart failure.

In Japan and a number of other countries, CoQ10 is considered mainstream therapy. But a review of the supporting medical research is disappointing. Most of the studies on CoQ10 supplementation are poorly done, include only twenty or so patients, and do not include a control group, making the results questionable.

The most credible research on patients with heart failure shows minimal to no added improvement in those people already being treated with state-of-the-art twenty-first-century medical therapy. Heart muscle function, exercise duration, and patients' perceived quality of life did not generally improve in these studies despite doses of up to 200 mg of CoQ10 daily. This lack of improvement may well be explained by the fact that the prescription drugs we now have available do such a good job of treating heart failure that any extra impact provided by CoQ10 is fairly minor.

CoQ10 does appear to hold some promise for hypertension, although the peer-reviewed medical research to date only includes a few hundred people. Not everyone's blood pressure will drop when exposed to the supplement, but for those whose blood pressure does respond, there may be as much as a 16-point drop in systolic blood pressure. If you do choose to take the supplement, it's important to be aware of this effect. My patient Greg decided to start CoQ10 shortly before leaving for a tropical vacation, and ended up spending half of his holiday in a Caribbean hospital with dangerously low blood pressure.

Statin drugs, used to lower cholesterol, may reduce levels of CoQ10 by blocking the body's ability to produce it. CoQ10 is used by the mitochondria, which are the energy factories for our cells. This may explain the muscle aches that some people experience with statin drugs. Although these results remain somewhat controversial, most studies of statins (including red yeast rice) have found lower CoQ10 blood levels after a month of drug treatment. What we don't know is whether these reduced blood levels reflect what is going on in the muscle tissues.

It appears that some people are genetically susceptible to this statin side effect and therefore might benefit from supplemental CoQ10. Carnitine or creatine supplements, which I'll tell you about soon, may also be helpful. One small study from New York's Stony Brook University found a nearly 40 percent reduction in statin-related pain symptoms when 100 mg of CoQ10 was taken daily. Of course, if you develop muscle pains while on statins, it is important to let your doctor know right away. In rare cases, muscle breakdown can occur, which may be life threatening.

Although CoQ10 has been promoted as an energy booster for athletes, most studies, including an Australian study of endurance athletes, have shown no improvement in athletic performance.

CoQ10 is probably not harmful, and clearly some people may benefit from taking it. However, this is an expensive supplement, costing anywhere from $30 to $100 per month. As the body manufactures its own CoQ10, there may be a limit to how much extra CoQ10 it is able to put to use.

Ginkgo

We all want to hang on to whatever brain power we can. It's no wonder that *Ginkgo biloba*, purported to improve memory, cognition, and blood flow, is one of the best-selling herbs in the United States, accounting for nearly $18 million in sales in 2007 alone. In the laboratory, an extract of ginkgo leaves (which come from the maidenhair tree) has revealed antioxidant, anti-inflammatory, and anticlotting effects.

Unfortunately, most well-done studies of ginkgo in humans have failed to find any major effect on learning capacity, ability to concentrate, or improvement in blood flow to the brain. In 2008, the *Journal of the American Medical Association* published the findings of the Ginkgo Evaluation of Memory (GEM) group. The research was sponsored in part by the National Center for Complementary and Alternative Medicine and the National Heart, Lung and Blood Institute. This group, with members at five major academic medical centers in the United States, enrolled over three thousand seniors, and studied the effects of a high-dose (120 mg twice daily) standardized ginkgo supplement over the course of six years. After the data was analyzed, there was absolutely no reduction in the likelihood of dementia in those who took the supplement. In 2009, the same group reported that there was also no impact on cognitive decline, a milder and more subtle form of age-related mental impairment. The incidence of heart disease, stroke, and death was no different between groups.

Side effects of ginkgo may include nausea, indigestion, headaches, and rashes. Bleeding inside the brain has also been reported with ginkgo, although not in the GEM study. Ginkgo may interact with some prescription drugs, so check with your doctor or pharmacist before experimenting with this supplement.

Grape Seed Extract and Pine Bark Extract: The Proanthocyanidins

Proanthocyanidin is a million-dollar word that refers to the powerful antioxidants found in grape seed and French pine bark extracts. Similar antioxidants, including polyphenols, catechins, and flavonoids, are found in wine, tea, soy, chocolate, olive oil, and many fruits and vegetables. As there is very good evidence that antioxidants are protective against heart disease and certain cancers, grape seed extract and pine bark extract (also known commercially as Pycnogenol) represent an attempt to concentrate high-potency antioxidants into a pill-size package. Indeed, in the test tube, the antioxidant effects of these extracts far surpass those of vitamins E and C. But there are really very few studies in humans to support the use of either of these supplements.

Rat studies suggest that grape seed extract may help prevent fatal heart rhythms in the setting of a heart attack, probably via the protective antioxidant effects. One study of Pycnogenol indicated that this supplement might protect smokers from harmful blood clots. Animal studies suggest that both extracts may also improve the flow of blood through the arteries of the heart and the body. And a study of grape seed extract reported an improvement in the cholesterol profile in people whose fruit and vegetable consumption was relatively paltry, although there was no placebo group used for comparison. Some very preliminary research also points to a possible protective effect against cancers of the breast, lungs, and stomach, yet other researchers warn of a potential of these supplements to actually increase the risk of certain cancers.

As with most supplements, the potency and composition of the supplement may vary markedly from one manufacturer to another, and currently there is really no objective way to gauge the potency of any particular brand. Furthermore, we don't know which, if any, component of these extracts may be the most useful. The National Institutes of Health has expressed an interest in studying grape seed and pine bark extracts. Until more data is available, my advice is to choose a diet rich in whole foods, including fruits and vegetables, and get your antioxidants naturally.

BEST PRACTICES:
SUPPLEMENTS FOR HEART AND MIND

* Most people don't need a CoQ10 supplement, as it is produced in the liver. Organ meats, salmon, mackerel, sardines, peanuts, and spinach are good dietary sources. People already taking prescription medication for heart failure don't receive any appreciable benefits from additional CoQ10.
* At doses of 100 mg daily, CoQ10 might help prevent muscle aches in people on statin drugs and may lower blood pressure.
* *Ginkgo biloba* does not appear to help brain function and may have significant side effects.
* Get your antioxidants from a diet rich in polyphenols, catechins, and flavonoids, found in wine, tea, soy, chocolate, olive oil, and many fruits and vegetables. Although grape seed and pine bark extracts are high in antioxidants, there is very little valid research on these supplements.

SUPPLEMENTS FOR ENERGY AND WEIGHT LOSS

For optimal health, nothing can take the place of a heart-smart diet, regular exercise, and a healthy way of life. Although there really is no shortcut to wellness, drugstores, the media, and the Internet are rife with products claiming to boost your energy, improve your sex drive, or lower your weight. Are any the real deal? And are they safe?

Chromium Picolinate

For years, chromium picolinate has been breathlessly promoted as a weight-loss aid that will also lower cholesterol and improve insulin sensitivity, slashing the risk of diabetes and other chronic diseases. What the vendors of this supplement fail to mention is that for the past fifteen years, numerous studies, including one done by the United States Navy, have shown absolutely no benefit of this supplement.

Our body does need chromium, but it is found in abundance in a heart-healthy diet. Natural sources include fruit, vegetables, whole grains, and seeds. Research has consistently found no improvement in metabolism, body fat, weight loss, strength, lipids, insulin, blood sugar, or any other measure with the use of chromium supplements. And while no toxicity was reported in studies of 200 to 1,000 mcg daily, higher doses (1,200 to 2,400 mcg per day) have been linked to kidney failure, blood abnormalities, and liver damage. Some preliminary research has suggested that even at typical doses, this supplement may actually cause the formation of harmful free radicals, so my advice is to sit this one out.

Ginseng

More than 5 million Americans have experimented with ginseng, the root of plants of the genus *Panax*, for its legendary enhancement of longevity, energy, and libido. Ginseng may be purchased as a whole root, extract, tea, powder, or tincture. It comes in several species, including Asian, American, and Japanese. (So-called Siberian ginseng is actually of a different genus altogether and shares little in common with the *Panax* species; it is known to cause high blood pressure and has few if any well-documented beneficial effects.)

Ginseng has more than twenty potentially active compounds, but we still don't know which, if any, of these are beneficial. Many products that claim to be ginseng turn out to have absolutely none of these active ingredients.

Scientific studies on ginseng have yielded conflicting results. Ginseng does appear to have antioxidant properties and may even improve the lipid profile slightly. Most of the more favorable studies come from China and Korea, where ginseng is sometimes used to treat heart failure. Studies done in the United States have found relatively minor effects on aerobic capacity and reaction times. People over the age of 40 may be more apt to benefit from ginseng than younger people, and twelve weeks or more may be required to see any improvement. The standard ginseng dose is 200 to 400 mg daily of a 4 to 7 percent extract, or 1 to 2 grams of ginseng root daily.

Potential side effects of ginseng include high blood pressure, nervousness, and diarrhea. Ginseng may interact with blood-thinning drugs and cause an excessively high risk of bleeding.

Ephedra

An adrenaline-like stimulant, ephedra comes from the Chinese herb *ma huang*. Ephedra is touted as a "thermogenic," meaning that it is supposed to create heat in the body by speeding up metabolism and burning fat. Does ephedra work as a weight-loss aid? The answer is maybe.

An analysis of more than fifty studies published by the think tank RAND Corporation in 2003 revealed an average weight loss of about 2 pounds per month in people who took ephedra regularly for several months. However, this weight loss can come at a terrible price.

Ephedra has been associated with heart palpitations, high blood pressure, personality changes, anxiety, shakiness, and insomnia. Even worse, it has been implicated in a number of cases of permanent disability and death due to heart attacks, life-threatening heart rhythm abnormalities, and strokes. These catastrophic events have often occurred during heavy physical exertion. When it's combined with caffeine, as it often is, the risk of serious side effects escalates. A randomized study of a supplement containing both ephedra and caffeine showed potentially dangerous changes in the heart's electrical patterns after a single dose was given to healthy young adults.

More than 160 deaths have been attributed to ephedra, and thousands more users have reported serious side effects. In 2004, after reviewing the numerous studies of the supplement and evaluating the reports of adverse events, the FDA prohibited the sale of ephedra in the United States.

Small amounts of *ma huang* may still be sold by Chinese herbal practitioners for treatment of respiratory disorders, but ephedra is prohibited by the International Olympic Committee, the National Collegiate Athletic Association, and the National Football League, among others. Despite the ban, a quick Internet search reveals business as usual, with multiple Web sites continuing to hawk ephedra as a weight-loss and energy supplement.

Since ephedra and *ma huang* have earned such a bad name, and deservedly so, manufacturers of weight-loss supplements are increasingly turning to other sources of the chemical. Watch out for innocent-sounding ingredients such as country mallow, joint fir, Mormon tea, and heartleaf, all of which may contain ephedra. Always read the labels of any supplement you take and be sure to share that information with your doctor.

Bitter Orange

Bitter orange, also known as *Citrus aurantium*, is an extract of the Seville orange, a beautiful and aromatic plant native to southeastern Asia, now found around the world. The extract of the bitter orange peel is the next-generation thermogenic (or heat-producing) "ephedra-free" weight-loss supplement. It is sometimes referred to as "legal ephedra," and frequently combined with caffeine for a stronger kick. Although manufacturers and purveyors of bitter orange claim that it has none of the dangerous side effects of ephedra, the facts tell another story.

The active ingredient in bitter orange is synephrine, which is similar to epinephrine, also known as adrenaline. This chemical raises blood pressure, revs up the heart rate, and constricts blood vessels. Side effects are similar to those of ephedra and can include tremors, nervousness, anxiety, and headache. Bitter orange can also interact with prescription drugs, increasing the possibility of harmful drug reactions. Just like ephedra, bitter orange in combination with high doses of caffeine will shoot a double whammy to the nervous system.

Reports of life-threatening complications of bitter orange are becoming more frequent, including heart attacks, heart arrhythmias, and blackouts. Keep an eye out for ingredients such as *zhi shi*, *kijitsu*, sour orange, and neroli oil, all of which are alternative terms for bitter orange.

Hydroxycitric Acid

The key ingredient in a popular supplement, hydroxycitric acid is purported to burn fat and increase vitality. Hydroxycitric acid is derived from the rind of *Garcinia cambogia*, a yellow fruit native to India. It has been promoted as a weight-loss aid, although traditional Indian healers use it for joint and intestinal problems.

Studies in humans have shown no effect on fat burning with exercise, even when dosages of hydroxycitric acid used were more than ten times higher than the amount recommended by the manufacturer. What's worse, there have been reports of severe liver injury in people who took the popular supplement. In 2009, the FDA recalled one popular supplement, Hydroxycut, due to reports of at least twenty-three cases of liver failure, including one death. It was never absolutely clear what component of the supplement caused the liver problems, but subsequently, Hydroxycut was reformulated without *Garcinia* and put back on the market. Today, numerous supplements containing *Garcinia* are still widely available.

Hydroxycitric acid is also sold as brindleberry, *gorikapuli*, *citrin*, *gambooge*, and Malabar tamarind.

Hoodia

Hoodia gordonii has been a part of the culture of the San tribe of South Africa since time immemorial. Before the encroachment of a Western lifestyle, tribesmen chewed the succulent plant to stave off hunger during long hunting treks and times of famine. The active ingredient, a molecule tagged P57, apparently tricks the brain into thinking that the stomach is full. Presto! No more hunger.

The plant is extremely rare and very difficult to grow. There are other species of hoodia plants, but it is not known whether they have the same effect, or even if they are safe. It has been alleged that most, if not all, hoodia products on the market contain little, if any, of the active ingredient and that they are often adulterated with other weight-loss supplements.

Even more problematic are the lack of safety data and the scarcity of published studies of the plant. At one time, Pfizer acquired the rights to the active ingredient from the British company Phytopharm, which had a contract for developing the plant with the South African government. After investing more than $20 million, Pfizer dropped out of the project, citing difficulties extracting and synthesizing the active ingredients. Later, a Pfizer scientist also alluded to problems with potential liver toxicity. Hoodia rights were subsequently bought by Unilever, which manufactures Slim-Fast products, among others. However, Unilever ultimately relinquished its rights to hoodia due, in part, to safety concerns.

BEST PRACTICES:
ENERGY AND WEIGHT-LOSS SUPPLEMENTS

* Don't bother with chromium picolinate; studies have found no significant effect on weight loss, metabolism, muscle strength, cholesterol, or diabetes.
* Ginseng is an antioxidant. It might improve aerobic ability slightly but can raise blood pressure and cause nervousness and diarrhea.
* Ephedra might be slightly effective for weight loss, but it is illegal for good reason. Its dangerous side effects include heart attacks, heart rhythm abnormalities, and strokes. It is even more dangerous when combined with caffeine.

- Don't be tempted by bitter orange. It can raise blood pressure and heart rate and cause anxiety, tremors, and headaches. Like ephedra, it has been linked to heart attacks and heart rhythm disturbances.
- Don't use hydroxycitric acid supplements either; they don't help with weight loss and might hurt the liver.
- Hoodia may suppress hunger, but supplements on the market often contain little if any active ingredient. Hoodia may also cause liver toxicity.

Unlimited energy and easy weight loss are great marketing slogans, but in reality, your health depends on a daily commitment to a lifestyle that cultivates and nurtures wellness for body and mind. There is no pill or concoction that can do that for you.

AMINO ACIDS AND THEIR DERIVATIVES

Amino acids are the building blocks of protein, and are critical for good health. Most of us get plenty of these nutrients from the foods we eat, but amino acid supplements are widely available. As with other supplements, it's important to understand not only the potential benefits, but also the risks.

L-Arginine

A semi-essential amino acid, L-arginine is often promoted as a treatment for disorders of the vascular system. It is considered semi-essential because our body is able to manufacture enough L-arginine for most of our needs. However, during children's growth phases, the body requires more than it can produce, making a healthy diet crucial to normal development.

L-arginine can be found in many different foods, including soy and other legumes, fish, meats, poultry, dairy products, and nuts. Spirulina, a type of algae, is a rich source of L-arginine, providing 4 grams per 3.5-ounce serving. By comparison, 3 ounces of turkey has

1.8 grams, 3 ounces of salmon supplies 1.4 grams, and ½ cup of tofu has 1.3 grams. Most people get somewhere between 4 and 10 grams of L-arginine daily. Because our adult body can manufacture L-arginine, there is no official minimum daily requirement.

Several relatively small-scale studies of L-arginine have been carried out in humans. Some have shown modest improvements in blood pressure with L-arginine, and rat studies even suggest that L-arginine may mitigate the high blood pressure seen in salt-sensitive individuals when exposed to a high-salt diet. There is early evidence that this amino acid may also improve insulin sensitivity in adult-onset diabetes.

In the research lab, fairly high doses of L-arginine, generally on the order of 3 grams three times daily, appeared to improve blood flow in people whose arteries had already been affected by atherosclerosis. When researchers at Johns Hopkins University put this theory to the test in 2006, treating patients who had previously suffered heart attacks, they hoped to find improvement in heart function and reduced stiffness of the blood vessels. Instead, there was no improvement in heart or vascular function. In fact, the study was stopped early when more than 8 percent of those receiving the supplement died, compared to none of those taking the placebo pills. People taking L-arginine were also more likely to end up in the hospital with congestive heart failure.

Why did the facts of this trial not support the theory? The researchers noted that all the subjects involved already had normal levels of L-arginine, meaning that they were getting plenty from their diet and from their body's own production.

Researchers also raised the possibility that high levels of L-arginine could actually cause the body to produce free radicals, increasing the likelihood of harm to the artery walls.

While there are many manufacturers who tout their L-arginine products as a remedy for erectile dysfunction (ED), study results are mixed. Because many men with ED also have coronary artery disease, high-dose supplemental L-arginine carries the potential for significant risk.

There are some other important downsides to high-dose supplementation with this amino acid. A study of breast cancer patients given a whopping 30 grams of L-arginine daily or a placebo for several days prior to surgery found a disturbing increase in tumor growth and tumor activity. Doses this high have also been associated with weight gain, stomach upset, and excessive sleepiness.

L-Carnitine

L-carnitine is technically not an amino acid, although it is frequently marketed as such. (D-carnitine, which is structurally similar and sometimes sold over the counter, cannot be used by the body.) L-carnitine is nonessential, because our body is adept at manufacturing it, except in cases of very rare inherited deficiencies. People who are on hemodialysis for kidney failure may need to take L-carnitine supplements. For most of us, supplements are not necessary.

L-carnitine is abundant in meat, which supplies about 80 mg per 3-ounce serving, but is also found in poultry, fish, and dairy products. On average, most people get more than 100 mg of L-carnitine from their diet daily. Typical supplemental doses are 2,000 to 3,000 mg (2 to 3 grams) daily.

Because L-carnitine helps to transport fatty acids into the cells, and also plays an important role in muscle function during exercise, it has attracted a lot of interest. Studies, however, have been disappointing, indicating that the supplement is probably not taken up by the muscle tissue, and showing no improvement in physical performance.

Research is still under way to determine whether L-carnitine might help people who have had heart attacks. So far, there appears to be little or no benefit, although preliminary evidence suggests that it may help people who have pain with activity due to blocked leg arteries. There may also be a role for L-carnitine in the treatment of statin-drug-related muscle aches, because about a third of people who experience this side effect may have genetic abnormalities of muscle L-carnitine.

Drawbacks to L-carnitine include a fishy body odor when taken in doses of more than 3 grams daily, and an increased likelihood of seizures in people who have experienced seizures in the past.

Creatine

Creatine is a favorite of weight lifters and bodybuilders for its reputed effects on muscle strength. It is found naturally in meat and fish, but our body is able to manufacture it quite readily from essential amino acids obtained from other dietary sources. Even vegetarians make enough creatine for their body's usual needs.

Most studies of creatine have found that it does indeed appear to improve muscle strength for tasks like weightlifting, which require fairly short bursts of energy. Vegetarian weight lifters may benefit more than meat eaters. Creatine does not, however, appear to affect aerobic or endurance training.

A small study of people who experienced muscle aches on statin drugs reported significant improvement in some, but not all, patients when creatine supplements were taken.

The supplement appears to be safe when taken in reasonable amounts. Creatine is usually taken in doses of 2 to 5 grams daily. One study of college football players who were dosed with an average of 5 grams of creatine per day for up to 21 months found no evidence of harmful effects on blood tests of kidney, liver, or blood cell function and no urinary abnormalities. However, higher doses have been linked to kidney disease. Like many supplements, not enough is known about creatine, but it appears to be safe when taken in moderation.

BEST PRACTICES:
AMINO ACIDS AND THEIR DERIVATIVES

* L-arginine is important for normal function of your blood vessels. Adult bodies can manufacture plenty of L-arginine, and it is abundant in spirulina, turkey, salmon, and soy, so supplements are not usually necessary. Don't take L-arginine supplements. High doses might increase the risk for heart attacks and heart failure in people who already have heart disease, and may also increase tumor growth in women with breast cancer.

- L-carnitine keeps your muscles functioning normally, but supplements are rarely needed. Your body likely makes enough L-carnitine from scratch.
- Creatine is involved in muscle energy production. It is found in meat and fish, but your body can make it from other foods you eat.
- L-carnitine and creatine supplements might be beneficial if you get muscle pains with statin drugs.
- Daily doses of 2–5 grams of creatine appear to be safe and might be helpful for weight lifters; higher doses have been linked to kidney disease.

FRUIT AND VEGETABLE CONCENTRATES

A multilevel marketing phenomenon, capsules containing dried fruit and vegetable juice concentrates have been promoted as the latest in antiaging supplements since the 1990s. The proprietary product Juice Plus+ is marketed aggressively by laypeople as well as by some health professionals. Independent distributors of the product make money from their own sales as well as from the sales of the people they recruit. Because a year's supply of the product costs about $500, sales people are exceptionally motivated to acquire new customers. It is important to remember that although these salespeople may present themselves as medically savvy, most of them are not trained, educated medical professionals.

The idea behind juice and vegetable concentrates is not a bad one: Package the antioxidants found in fruits and vegetables in a form that can be easily taken on a daily basis. Because we know that the majority of Americans do not choose to eat enough fruits and vegetables, this is one way to at least obtain some phytonutrients, including antioxidants, albeit without as much fiber. Basically what you are getting is dehydrated, desugared fruit and vegetable juice, along with a bit of fiber and other nutrients, packaged in capsule form.

To its credit, Juice Plus+ has sponsored medical research, some of which has been published in reputable journals. *The Journal of the American College of Cardiology*, in 2003, published a study that demonstrated an improvement in blood flow after a greasy fast-food breakfast in people who took these supplements regularly. Arteries tend to constrict in response to high levels of fat in the bloodstream, which is one reason that a high-fat diet can be so harmful, and it appeared that Juice Plus+ countered this effect. This research study has been cited by Juice Plus+ salespeople as proof that their product works.

Although it probably is an important effect of the supplement, the same improvement in blood flow is seen in people who eat eight to ten servings of antioxidant-rich whole fruits and vegetables every day. Furthermore, eating fruits and vegetables in their whole forms supplies far more fiber and phytonutrients than does a supplement capsule and also curbs the appetite, reducing cravings for less nourishing foods.

If your diet is deficient in fruits and vegetables and you have no intention of changing, these products might be reasonable, though pricey, supplements to take. But if you truly want to support a healthy heart and body, it makes much more sense to eat the real thing.

BEST PRACTICES:
FRUIT AND VEGETABLE CONCENTRATES

* Fruit and vegetable supplements may improve blood flow after a fatty meal and appear to be safe and well tolerated; however, fresh fruits and vegetables clearly have the advantage.

Particularly because many of these products slip through the net of the FDA, it's important to be up front with your doctor about any supplements and herbs you wish to take. Just because a product is natural or comes with celebrity testimonials does not mean it's safe . . . or does what it promises to do. And many supplements will interact with prescription medications, either by raising drug levels and increasing the risk of drug toxicity or by inhibiting the drug from working properly. Just as with vitamins and minerals, often your most heart-smart choice is to ensure these healthy substances are simply part of your regular diet.

16

Complementary and Alternative Medicine: Hope, Hype, or Healing?

SOMETIMES MODERN HEALTH care can seem so complicated, and the technology and science supporting it far out of our reach. We want answers about our health that make sense to us. Overwhelmed by the vast and sometimes impersonal medical infrastructure, many people have chosen to take their search outside the realm of conventional medicine. We may seek treatments that will complement standard medical therapies, or perhaps even replace them with alternatives we hope will be safer and gentler. More than half of Americans have dipped our toes into the alternative healing pool at least once, and for many, it is truly a way of life.

As a physician, I take my responsibilities to heart. Your health and well-being are my utmost concern, and I work hard to earn your trust. So if a therapy has the potential to harm, or if it will cost you some of your hard-earned money, I want to be absolutely sure that my recommendations to you are as well researched and supported as possible. Yet I know that with or without the support of your physician, you may seek alternative care.

As trained scientists, we physicians are understandably skeptical of claims that lack sufficient scientific support. In general, complementary and alternative medicine (CAM) practices are not as thoroughly tested as most mainstream medical care. Over time, some have even been shown to be harmful. Now, spurred on by intense public interest, the scientific community is beginning to investigate some of these therapies with the same rigor it applies to traditional medicine.

The breadth of CAM is far too wide to address fully in one chapter, but here are some important CAM practices that relate specifically to the health of the heart.

MASSAGE THERAPY AND AROMATHERAPY

I am a great fan of massage therapy, but alas, its effects on the heart are fairly short lived. Although your blood pressure may drop during a session, the effect is not long lasting. However, a respected and valuable adjunct for certain conditions, it is known to temporarily reduce tension and stress, and when combined with physical therapy, may help injured muscles to heal. On the other hand, massage is not entirely safe for some people.

You should check with your doctor before signing up for a massage if you are prone to blood clots in your legs, have active inflammation or infection, or suffer from severe osteoporosis or thin and weak bones. If you are on blood thinners, be sure to tell your massage therapist, as some forms of massage involve strong pressure that could cause bruising in sensitive individuals. Choose a well-trained, certified therapist, and be honest about your medical history and about the benefits you hope to obtain from your session.

Aromatherapy, which uses volatile plant oils, is often used for stress reduction in conjunction with massage. Indeed, studies have shown that smell can affect mood and temporarily reduce anxiety levels. Aromatherapy may be beneficial for calming people with Alzheimer's dementia, and some find that it can even cut their cravings for food. But although a recent American Heart Association survey found that 26 percent of women believed aromatherapy could protect against heart disease, it simply does not hold that power. Most reputable practitioners of aromatherapy are careful to avoid making such claims.

CHELATION THERAPY

Chelation therapy is a specialized medical practice that involves infusing a chemical into the veins through a catheter to bond with and remove dangerous heavy metals from the blood. It is used primarily to treat heavy-metal poisoning, including lead, mercury, and arsenic. In these fairly rare cases, only a qualified physician should administer the medication, and only after the diagnosis has been confirmed.

Chelation therapy is not approved for other conditions. There is no reliable evidence that it has any effect on atherosclerosis. Promoters like to claim that it will bind up free radicals in the bloodstream, preventing damage to the blood vessel walls, but that has not been proven and does not seem biologically plausible.

Scientists in the United States, Canada, and Europe have carefully evaluated chelation therapy in heart patients, assessing both symptoms and vascular function. Multiple studies have shown that regular treatments for up to six months have zero cardiovascular benefits.

Chelation therapy is not benign. It may deplete the body of zinc, which is important to the immune system; it may seriously lower calcium levels; and it has the potential to cause life-threatening side effects.

Currently, a study of more than two thousand people is under way to objectively and scientifically determine once and for all whether chelation therapy is an effective treatment in coronary artery disease. The study will also look at the effects of high-dose vitamin infusions. For now, considering the cost (about $4,000 for thirty treatments) and the time commitment (three hours per treatment, generally twice a week), your time and money would be much better spent exercising, taking a stress-free vacation, or practicing healthy cooking with someone you love.

PATRICK IS A 63-year-old man who came to our hospital in full-blown congestive heart failure, gasping for air, with a major heart attack in progress. Ten years earlier, he had undergone triple bypass surgery. He had been cautioned to take his medications, exercise, and follow a Mediterranean diet, but he just wasn't interested in making such drastic changes. Although he trusted his heart surgeon, he was deeply suspicious of the medical profession in general and failed to follow up with his cardiologist. Instead, he trusted a chelation practitioner, and over the years had subjected himself to multiple rounds of chelation therapy. When all was said and done, Patrick's heart had been permanently damaged from years of neglect. Sadly, much of the damage might have been averted with a judicious medical regimen and a healthy way of life. Even sadder is the fact that Patrick's case is only one of many similar scenarios that I have treated over the years.

HYPNOSIS AND ACUPUNCTURE

Although hypnosis has not been studied rigorously enough to draw firm conclusions, it appears to be as effective as nicotine patches for smoking cessation, with about 20 percent of people who undergo hypnotherapy quitting for good. Some studies have reported success rates of up to 60 percent in motivated individuals.

Hypnosis may also help you lose weight, if it is included as part of an overall diet, exercise, and lifestyle modification program.

My advice to my patients is this: Hypnotherapy is safe, it may be more effective than doing nothing, and it could help you quit smoking or lose weight—but you must first be motivated to change your habits. Nobody else can do that for you.

Acupuncture is widely used in treating addictions, chronic pain, and other health conditions. Recent research hints at a possible role of acupuncture in heart health. Scientists at UCLA studying people with congestive heart failure have reported that acupuncture may decrease the intensity of the sympathetic nervous system's response to stress. Activation of the sympathetic system leads to the "fight or flight" response, raising blood pressure and heart rate. This can be harmful in those with weakened heart muscles, so blunting this reaction can be advantageous in heart failure.

Whether acupuncture can help lower blood pressure is debatable. A study of nearly two hundred people, funded by the National Institutes of Health, found no reduction in blood pressure after acupuncture, when compared to a sham procedure. However, a German study of 160 patients with high blood pressure reported modest reductions, on the order of a three- to five-point drop in pressure. For now, there is simply not enough definitive information available, but acupuncture appears to be relatively safe and is unlikely to cause you harm, as long as the needles used are sterile.

If you do choose to pursue acupuncture for treatment of high blood pressure or heart failure, it is important that you not discontinue any ongoing medical therapy unless you do so under your physician's supervision. As with any type of CAM, consider your doctor your ally and keep her fully informed about all aspects of your health care. It will help her take better care of you.

BEST PRACTICES:
COMPLEMENTARY AND ALTERNATIVE THERAPY

* Although both are relaxing, don't expect massage or aromatherapy to treat heart disease.
* Avoid chelation therapy. It is only recommended by physicians to treat rare cases of heavy metal poisoning. It is not likely to be beneficial for the heart and may cause harm.
* Don't dismiss hypnosis; it may help you quit smoking and lose weight, especially when combined with lifestyle changes.
* Acupuncture may relieve pain and suppress your body's "fight or flight" response, which will keep your heart calmer. It has not been proven to lower blood pressure, but may have a modest effect.

Be Hip to Your Hormones

FOR MEN AND WOMEN, hormones are an integral part of the fabric of life.

Women are intensely aware of the changing hormonal tides that affect their body and mind. Thanks to birth control pills and postmenopausal hormone replacement, they no longer have to be bound to the whims of their hormones. Women are fortunate to have these options, but taking control of their hormones may have some unintended consequences. Medical science has arrived to the party unfashionably late, and the risks and benefits of birth control pills, hormone replacement therapy, and alternative treatments for menopause symptoms are still being worked out.

Although men do not experience a change of life as dramatic as menopause, subtle and gradual changes in hormone levels may also impact a man's life as he ages. Erectile dysfunction is another dilemma that many men face, yet most are not aware that it is a harbinger of heart disease. Understand this connection, and taking charge of heart health may take on a whole new meaning.

17

Smart Talk
About Hormones

H ORMONES ARE THE chemical messengers for the body, and are vital for growth, metabolism, immunity, and reproduction. There are well over fifty different hormones, but it is arguably the sex hormones, estrogen and testosterone, that create the most havoc.

Estrogen is made primarily by the ovaries, so it is considered a "female" hormone. Progesterone is another important female hormone that works in concert with estrogen. Testosterone, the "male" hormone, is produced by the testes. However, the ovaries generate trace amounts of testosterone, and the testes manufacture a little estrogen and progesterone. Without the sex hormones, there would be no reproduction, and men and women would be difficult to tell apart. As aggravating as estrogen and testosterone might be, the world would be a much less interesting place without them.

BIRTH CONTROL PILLS AND YOUR HEART

Oral contraceptive pills (OCPs) were first introduced in the early 1960s. They were arguably a powerful force in the development of the women's movement, allowing women to control a part of their biology that was previously by definition uncontrollable.

Early versions of oral contraceptives, loaded with up to five times the estrogen and ten times the progesterone found in today's pills, clearly raised the risk of heart attacks and strokes in women who used them. Thankfully, times have changed, and most recent studies have shown no statistically significant increase in heart attacks and strokes in women who use modern lower-dose OCPs, with three important exceptions.

Risks with Today's Oral Contraceptive Pills

First, women with blood-clotting disorders should not take OCPs. Although OCPs do not appear to cause atherosclerosis, they do increase the likelihood of blood clots, particularly in vulnerable individuals. This affects a small minority of women, but unfortunately the clotting disorder is often not identified until a stroke or heart attack occurs while on the pill. Specific blood work can be ordered by your doctor to test for one of these disorders, but it is not standard practice to do so. If you have a family history of unexplained blood clots or a clotting disorder, it is critical that you let your doctor know this before OCPs are prescribed.

Second, some women will develop high blood pressure or high cholesterol while on OCPs, in which case it may be necessary to discontinue or change the dose or type of pill. When starting OCPs, it's important to get your blood pressure checked within a few weeks after your first dose.

The most important high-risk group is smokers. A woman on the pill who smokes, particularly if she is over 35, has a probability of a heart attack that is forty (yes, forty!) times normal. The risk for stroke is similar. As a cardiologist, I've seen both scenarios more times than I'd like to remember. Because up to 20 percent of women and nearly 35 percent of teenage girls smoke at least occasionally, the potential for harm is tremendous.

Taking any form of OCP increases the risk of deep venous thrombosis (DVT), even in women without a clotting disorder. The risk is low, but it is real. These blood clots in the veins of the legs are more common in women who are sedentary, overweight, or can't move their legs due to injury or illness. Women over 40 are more vulnerable than younger women are to DVTs. Of course, having a preexisting clotting disorder greatly increases the likelihood of this complication.

If you use the birth control patch, your risk for DVT is twice that of women on the pill. Although the number of women affected is small, about six out of every ten thousand who use the patch, there is a chance that the clots can migrate to the lungs, a potentially fatal condition called pulmonary embolus.

If you are taking OCPs, the composition of the pill will be listed on the package. Pills containing the specific progestins known as desogestrel, drospirenone, and gestodene are more likely to be associated with this problem, with an estimated sixteen to thirty extra DVTs per 100,000 women per year. With other progestins (norethindrone, levonorgestrel, or ethynodiol diacetate), the risk is lower.

Oral contraceptives can raise inflammatory CRP. Some studies have found a doubling of CRP in pill users. Because our understanding of CRP is still in its early stages, no one really knows yet what to do with this information. Aspirin lowers CRP, but it has not been studied in the context of OCPs.

OCPs may contribute to insulin resistance in some women, possibly increasing the risk for prediabetes; African American women are especially vulnerable to this effect. However, one retrospective study actually found less cholesterol buildup in the arteries of postmenopausal women who had previously taken OCPs, so the news is not all bad.

We still don't know for certain whether OCPs increase the likelihood of breast cancer, although most studies show little if any risk. Women with a strong family history of breast cancer should be extra careful to have close medical follow-up, as they may be at higher risk than are women with no such family history. On the other hand, it is well known that OCPs cut the risk of ovarian cancer in half.

Contrary to popular belief, the pill will not make you fat, although for some women it may cause water retention on the order of about 5 pounds. However, if you are overweight, the pill may not be as effective. Researchers at the University of Washington found that overweight women who took their pills faithfully were more than twice as likely to become pregnant as were women on the pill whose weight was in the normal range.

It is important to understand that what we know about OCPs does not apply to hormones used to treat symptoms of menopause. The doses and types of hormones are quite different, although both may include combinations of estrogen and progesterone.

AGING WITH GRACE

Women and men experience aging in different ways, but for all of us, aging brings challenges and changes, forcing us to confront our body's limitations and the natural drop-off of the hormones that may have ruled our youth. For women, menopause is a clear and sometimes abrupt transition, but for men, the natural decline of testosterone may be more subtle.

Menopause and a Woman's Heart

Thanks to good nutrition and high-quality health care, women are living a longer, healthier, and more productive life than ever before. Only one hundred years ago, our foremothers did not expect to live past 50, which dovetailed with the end of their childbearing years. These days, the average life expectancy for a woman is around 80; many women pass through menopause and thrive well into their 80s and beyond. Often, those extra thirty or so years are highly productive and rewarding, particularly when the body and mind are healthy and strong.

Menopause is a perfectly normal and natural stage of life, yet it brings with it challenges that can seriously rock a woman's world, escalating her risk of heart disease, stroke, and other unpleasantness. As a T-shirt declares, "Menopause is not for cowards."

Most women will suffer hot flashes, mood swings, and insomnia as estrogen levels decline; however, the majority will be rid of these annoyances after about five years, although vaginal dryness often persists. An unlucky 15 percent will struggle with menopausal symptoms for years. Without a doubt, hormone replacement therapy (HRT) will put the brakes on these troublesome symptoms, and for many women, it is the only effective treatment. At some point, nearly all women will face the dilemma of whether to start hormone replacement therapy.

MENOPAUSE

MENOPAUSE IS THE natural decline of estrogen production that usually occurs in women between the ages of 45 and 55, when the ovaries, women's principal source of estrogen, stop functioning. Menstruation will gradually become less frequent and eventually stop. It can also happen suddenly, if the ovaries are surgically removed (ovariectomy), or after some forms of radiation therapy or chemotherapy.

How you know: A woman has usually passed menopause when she has not had a period for twelve months in a row. Blood tests can help determine when menopause is beginning.

The downside: a cornucopia of physical symptoms—hot flashes, night sweats, irregular heartbeat, insomnia, irritability, mood swings, loss of libido, vaginal dryness, and fatigue.

The upside: No more periods—hooray! And no worries about getting pregnant.

Hormone Replacement Therapy: A Doctor's Dilemma

The study of estrogen and menopausal hormone replacement therapy (HRT) is still a work in progress. Although the effect of HRT on the heart is controversial, it is well established that HRT slows down bone loss caused by low levels of estrogen. However, because several other good medications to protect bone health are available, HRT is not considered to be the first choice to treat this condition. And while we worry about raising the risk for breast cancer, there is a possible small decline in the risk of colorectal cancer in women who take HRT.

There are two basic HRT regimens. If a woman has had a hysterectomy and chooses HRT, she will receive estrogen. However, if she still has her uterus, estrogen replacement puts her at risk for uterine cancer, so another hormone, progesterone, will be added to cancel out the risk.

The first HRT, Premarin, was introduced in 1942. By 2001, 42 percent of women aged 50 to 74 were taking some form of HRT. But, beginning in 1998, formal clinical trials began to reveal that hormone therapies, especially those that combined Premarin with the hormone progesterone, posed serious risks and might even increase the danger of heart attack and stroke.

In 2002, a landmark Premarin-progesterone study from the Women's Health Initiative was stopped earlier than planned because the risks to women in the study appeared to be greater than the benefits. These risks included heart disease, breast cancer, stroke, dementia, and blood clots.

Although most women would not experience a problem, the risks were substantial, given the number of women taking HRT. Researchers estimated that for every ten thousand women treated with combination HRT (specifically, Premarin plus progesterone), there would be eight strokes, seven new cases of heart disease, eight potentially fatal blood clots in the lungs, thirteen cases of blood clots in the deep veins of the legs (deep venous thrombosis, or DVT), and eight new cases of breast cancer. According to a Dutch study, there would also be one extra case of ovarian cancer. Although these numbers sound relatively small, let's put it in perspective. If 6 million women took combination HRT for five years, there would be as many as thirty thousand new cases of breast cancer. On the bright side, there was a significant reduction in the risk for colorectal cancer, and, as expected, a lower incidence of hip fractures. Women over the age of 65 who took combination HRT had a much higher risk for dementia, squashing the idea that HRT could help rejuvenate the aging brain. (Other studies have found no such risk in those starting HRT early in menopause.)

The story is somewhat different when we look at estrogen replacement alone. In women who received Premarin without progesterone, there was an increased risk of stroke and blood clots, but no significant effect on heart disease or breast cancer. These women also experienced fewer hip fractures, but had no reduction in colorectal cancer risk.

Many criticized the large HRT studies for the fact that only about 30 percent of the women studied in both groups began HRT before the age of 60, whereas in practice, HRT therapy is usually prescribed near the beginning of menopause. Doctors and women were stymied, stuck in a "damned if you do, damned if you don't" conundrum. And meanwhile, the hot flashes rage on.

JENNIFER'S STORY

THE RECENT SEA CHANGE in our understanding of HRT has shaken some women's faith in medical science. Take Jennifer, a patient who first came to my office in 1995 full of trepidation. At age 50, she was just beginning menopause. She had heard that estrogen might help to prevent heart disease—the scourge of her father's side of the family.

As a cardiologist, I never prescribe hormone replacement therapy myself. This is a decision best made by a woman with her gynecologist or primary physician. However, as Jennifer was interested in keeping her heart healthy, she sought my opinion because she was aware of my great interest in estrogen and its effects on the heart and cardiovascular system.

We know that the risk for cardiovascular disease begins to rise more sharply after menopause hits. In addition to the effects of aging, the natural drop off of estrogen levels may be an important factor. Women who have an ovariectomy before menopause hits are at particularly high risk, but even after menopause, an ovariectomy will increase heart disease risk. This is because the ovaries continue to produce small amounts of hormones that probably contribute to heart health.

At the time that I first saw Jennifer, the best information available to us, from both observational studies and laboratory experiments, suggested that by replacing estrogen after menopause, we could protect the heart. Although it was well established that HRT could cause harmful side effects, most studies before the mid-1990s indicated that the benefits outweighed the risks.

The problem was that none of those scientific studies was definitive, and the answers Jennifer was searching for that day in my office were still another five to ten years away.

By the next time I saw Jennifer, in 2002, the news on hormone replacement therapy was not good. The latest research suggested that hormone replacement therapy might not protect her heart, and the chance of serious complications, such as cancer, stroke, and blood clots, was higher than we once thought. Due primarily to these concerns, prescriptions for HRT fell by a third between 2001 and 2003.

My advice to Jennifer was this: to review her case again with her gynecologist or primary physician. As her cardiologist, I advised her that based on the most up-to-date research available, I could not recommend estrogen replacement for heart protection. The only clear-cut indication for estrogen replacement was for prevention of intolerable menopausal symptoms.

Fast-forward to the present, and we see the pendulum swinging back toward a potentially beneficial effect of estrogen replacement therapy for heart health, but only when started early in menopause. This is still a murky area, with evidence to support arguments on both sides.

Where Do We Go from Here?

It is clear that women who are on combination HRT remain at greater risk for complications than women who take estrogen alone; thus, women who have had a hysterectomy and can forgo progesterone may stand to benefit the most. Most large studies were done with Premarin, rather than with other forms of hormone therapy. There is still no clear consensus as to whether the harmful effects seen with Premarin and progesterone apply to other prescription forms of HRT. I'll tell you more about the differences among the various forms of HRT in the next section.

Just how long estrogen can be safely continued is unknown. Importantly, the risk of harm appears substantial in women over age 60, especially when the drug is first started more than five years after the onset of menopause; younger women are less likely to have problems. Diabetic women and women who have high cholesterol may also be more vulnerable to HRT complications.

Several large-scale studies are still in progress, but the picture is becoming clearer. The party line (admittedly a moving target) is this: Take HRT only if you need it for symptoms of menopause, and take it at the lowest possible dose for the least amount of time necessary. If your problem is primarily vaginal dryness, you have the option of a low-dose vaginal estrogen cream, which typically can be used without progesterone, as it will not raise blood levels of estrogen substantially.

Pill, Patch, or Cream—Smart Talk About Tough Choices

If you have decided to take prescription HRT, the next step is to consider the options and pick your potion.

▪ ESTROGEN PILLS

Most large research studies of HRT used the drug Premarin, so less is known about other forms of estrogen. All forms of HRT pills appear to raise triglyceride and CRP levels, although the estrogen patch does not. While these changes are potentially harmful, a moderate drop in LDL cholesterol and a bump in HDL are also common when women start HRT. Just how much these changes in blood levels contribute to the risks and benefits of HRT is still not clear.

Ironically, Premarin, the original and best-selling HRT, appears to be the prescription estrogen least like our own natural estrogen. Distilled from the urine of pregnant horses, it contains more than a dozen different varieties of estrogen. Small studies have found evidence that Premarin is more likely to cause heart attacks and strokes, and may even raise the risk of depression, when compared to other prescription forms of estrogen.

Several prescription forms of estrogen pills are plant derived, including Cenestin, Menest, and Ogen. Pharmaceuticals such as Estrace and the combination HRT product Activella contain a specific form of estrogen called 17-beta-estradiol, which women produce naturally.

Estratest is a combination estrogen-plus-testosterone product. It is used when estrogen alone does not restore libido. Because of the testosterone component, it may raise cholesterol and cause acne, hair loss, deepening of voice, breast pain, and leg swelling.

Some women and doctors prefer to use estrogen products termed "bioidentical." This means that the products are purported to be identical in composition to the hormones the body produces naturally. Bioidentical hormones are various combinations of estrogen, progesterone, DHEA (a hormone produced by the adrenal gland), and testosterone, usually concocted by a compounding pharmacy. They are often sold over the Internet, sometimes without a prescription (and typically without FDA oversight). Few well-designed studies have been done on these compounds, so there is no guarantee of safety. However, because they are hormone products, in all likelihood, the risks are similar to those of prescription HRT.

If you have not had a hysterectomy, you must take progesterone along with estrogen to reduce the risk of uterine cancer. Provera is the most commonly used progesterone prescription drug. Because progesterone appears to carry more risk than estrogen, studies are under way to try to determine the lowest dose and safest regimen. Although progesterone cream products are often sold as natural supplements, there is no evidence that they are any safer than prescription forms of the hormone, and, as they are not regulated by the FDA, the potency between products has been found to vary by as much as two hundredfold.

■ ESTROGEN PATCHES, CREAMS, AND VAGINAL PRODUCTS

Estrogen skin patches, creams, and vaginal rings release estrogen directly into the bloodstream, bypassing the liver. Because of this, there is no increase in triglycerides or CRP and no change in cholesterol levels. Small studies have suggested a lower risk for heart complications and strokes, when compared to estrogen pills. All but Premarin cream are derived from plants. The patches release estrogen gradually into the bloodstream, keeping blood levels fairly stable. Some women may be sensitive to the adhesive used on the patch, and if so, estrogen creams or vaginal products may be better tolerated.

These products should be used along with progesterone, unless you have had a hysterectomy. As with HRT pills, regular gynecological checkups and mammograms are essential.

Hope in a Bottle: The Search for a Natural Solution

The "change of life" is big business, and natural foods stores and neighborhood pharmacies alike stock a variety of products marketed as natural treatments for menopausal misery. But medical researchers, and most of my patients, have found little evidence that these treatments work. Moreover, the risks are largely unknown.

Common supplements include soy, black cohosh, red clover, evening primrose, and Mexican yam. Many of these products claim to provide nonprescription forms of estrogen, or to mimic the effects of estrogen. This sounds good, but we have no way of knowing if they are any safer than prescription hormone replacement.

Placing blind faith in prescription estrogen replacement can lead to disastrous consequences for some women. There is no reason to believe that other forms of estrogen might not be equally harmful. Furthermore, the products are not standardized and are not regulated by the FDA, meaning that you have no guarantee that the product actually contains the ingredients listed, or that it is consistent from one batch to the next.

Mexican yam raises some serious red flags. Its active ingredient, diosgenin, is used to make a synthetic progesterone cream that can be bought over the counter. Women sometimes use this instead of prescription progesterone pills when taking combination HRT. This cream may improve menopause symptoms, but its safety has not been carefully investigated.

Black cohosh may help some women, but although its short-term use may be safe, there are reports of liver toxicity. Studies have not shown either red clover or evening primrose to be useful in improving menopausal symptoms.

The bottom line: If you choose to take one of these products, it's important to have regular checkups so your doctor can look out for harmful side effects.

YOUR MAMMOGRAM: A KEY TO YOUR HEART

Most women are aware that mammograms are a vital link in the fight against breast cancer. But many, physicians included, are unaware that mammograms can also pick up early signs of heart disease.

About one in every six women will have calcification of the arteries that supply normal breast tissue. These calcifications indicate cholesterol buildup, and are a red flag that cholesterol is likely to be lurking in the arteries of the heart, brain, and other organs. They are unrelated to calcifications in the breast tissue itself. In a 2011 study of women undergoing mammograms in Hartford, Connecticut, researchers found that breast arterial calcifications were associated with a threefold increased likelihood of developing coronary heart disease over the ensuing five years, along with a fourfold risk for stroke.

Because many health professionals are still unaware of this link, it makes sense to review your own mammogram report. If arterial calcifications show up on your mammogram, it's time to take a serious look at cholesterol levels, blood pressure, and other risk factors, and to work with your doctor to do all you can to keep your heart healthy and strong (see "Heart Health Checklist: What You Should Ask Your Doctor," page 348).

WHAT TO DO NOW

If you are postmenopausal or getting close, you no doubt have many questions about what type of therapy, if any, is right for you now. The answers are still far from clear, but we are getting closer all the time. Keep yourself informed. Read the newspaper, talk to your doctor, and realize that the answers are slowly coming. In the meantime, exercise, follow a healthy diet, and get adequate sleep. As simple as it sounds, this will help you through the process.

BEST PRACTICES:
BIRTH CONTROL, HRT,
AND MENOPAUSE

* If you smoke, do not take birth control pills or use the birth control patch. Smokers who use these hormonal forms of birth control have a heart attack risk up to 40 times that of nonsmokers.

* If you are overweight, birth control pills will be less effective as a contraceptive.

* Hormone replacement therapy (HRT) for menopausal women decreases the risk of osteoporosis and helps with menopausal symptoms such as hot flashes and vaginal dryness.

* Estrogen without progesterone increases the risk of endometrial cancer in women who have not had a hysterectomy. If you still have your uterus and need HRT, you will need progesterone.

* The combination of estrogen and progesterone slightly increases the risk of heart attacks, strokes, dementia, blood clots, and breast cancer, especially in women over 60.

* Estrogen (without progesterone) slightly increases the risk of strokes, blood clots, and possibly dementia. It may be less likely to cause harm when started within a few years of menopause.

* Natural products sometimes taken for menopausal symptoms include soy supplements, black cohosh, and red clover. Although they may work for some, they are usually ineffective, and their long-term safety is unknown.

* If your mammogram image shows arterial calcifications, be sure to discuss your heart risks with your primary care physician.

DHEA—FOUNTAIN OF YOUTH OR JUST A WASH?

Dehydroepiandrosterone, or DHEA, is heavily marketed as a way to slow the aging process in both men and women. Whereas our adrenal glands produce DHEA from cholesterol, the pills sold as supplements are generally made from the same Mexican wild yams that are used to make supplemental progesterone cream for menopausal women. The body converts DHEA into estrogen and testosterone, but the process is inexact and may vary from person to person.

The use of DHEA can have unintended consequences. Increased aggressiveness and heart palpitations are potential side effects. Higher levels of testosterone generated by the supplement may cause acne, facial hair growth, and even male-pattern balding in women. There are also reports of serious liver damage with DHEA.

Prodded by industry estimates of $50 million in DHEA sales yearly, researchers at the Mayo Clinic decided to investigate the supplement for themselves. A two-year study of men and women over the age of 60 showed no major improvement in body composition, physical performance, or quality of life with DHEA.

TESTOSTERONE, AGING, AND THE MALE HEART

For decades, the male heart was the sole focus of researchers' efforts to understand and treat heart disease. Thus it is a bit ironic that while our understanding of estrogen and women's heart health has grown by leaps and bounds, research on testosterone and the heart is still in its infancy.

The popular term *andropause*, referring to a male version of menopause, is something of a misnomer. Although men do not go through a change of life as dramatic and unmistakable as menopause, testosterone levels do tend to drop by about 1 percent per year after the age of 50. In addition, the body tissue becomes less sensitive to testosterone over time. These changes can lead to fatigue, depression, changes in the skin and hair, weakening of the bones, decreased muscle mass, and erectile dysfunction.

Although it may be impossible to halt the decline of testosterone over time, physical activity on the order of 150 minutes of moderate exercise each week may give levels a lift. Obesity is known to lower testosterone levels, so weight loss can make a big difference as well.

Very few studies of testosterone and the heart have included more than a couple of hundred men, and all in all only a few thousand have participated in scientifically valid research on the subject. Because the numbers are so small, the conclusions are still somewhat speculative. Overall, in men with low testosterone at baseline, testosterone therapy sufficient to bring levels back into the normal range probably has minimal effect on cholesterol or blood pressure. However, some men treated with the hormone may retain fluid, which could potentially lead to congestive heart failure if the heart is already weakened. A 2010 study from Boston University of chronically ill men over the age of 65 treated with testosterone was stopped early because there did appear to be a higher risk of heart complications. However, the number studied was small (just a little over two hundred men), and the results were far from conclusive.

If you suspect you might have low testosterone, a blood test can be helpful. Testosterone levels are often higher in the morning, so it's usually recommended to have the blood drawn before noon. If you are deficient, your doctor will likely prescribe a gel or a patch, or perhaps an injection.

Testosterone pills are risky business, because they can cause liver abnormalities and may increase the risk of some forms of cancer. These pills are considered supplements, and because they are not prescription products, they are not regulated by the FDA. Androstenedione and other precursors of testosterone are often peddled over the Internet or by unscrupulous athletic trainers, including some who have gotten their pro-athlete clients into very hot water indeed. Ironically, these supplements may stimulate the growth of breast tissue, shrink the testicles, contribute to infertility, and increase the likelihood of baldness. They are also likely to raise blood pressure, and are well known to provoke hostility and rage reactions.

WHAT CAN ERECTILE DYSFUNCTION TELL YOU ABOUT YOUR HEART?

Erectile dysfunction (ED) affects as many as one in three men over the age of 50. It is often assumed to be caused by low levels of testosterone, but in many cases, the problem is related to the health of the arteries feeding the penis. That's why ED is so strongly connected to disease of the heart and other blood vessels. In fact, a study from the University of Texas Health Science Center in San Antonio found that men who have occasional or frequent bouts of ED are up to 45 percent more likely to develop cardiovascular disease, including heart attacks and strokes, compared to men with no ED problems at all.

That's the bad news. The good news is that ED can often be prevented, and can sometimes be reversed, with simple changes in diet, exercise, and lifestyle. The landmark Health Professionals study of over thirty-one thousand men found that physically active men were 30 percent less likely to develop ED when compared to couch potatoes, while obesity increased the odds of ED by 30 percent. Smoking, excessive alcohol, and too much time spent in front of the TV were all linked to ED. An Italian study of sixty-five men found that the Mediterranean diet appears to improve ED, although it may take a year or two for the arteries to recover normal function. There is also evidence that statin therapy for high cholesterol may benefit some men with ED, probably by reducing cholesterol buildup and improving blood flow.

A SUCCESSFUL LAWYER, Jason had always considered himself a "man's man," but as he hit his 40s, the weight began to pile on, and he let his workouts slip to nearly nothing. By the time he was 55, he weighed over 250 pounds, suffered from high blood pressure, and was pre-diabetic. Jason had also become dependent on Viagra to achieve normal erections, but unfortunately the pills seemed to become less effective as time wore on. After a heart attack nearly took his life, Jason resolved to get serious about his health. Because of the risk of drug interactions, Viagra was no longer an option, and Jason was certain that the drugs I prescribed for his heart condition would only add to his woes in the bedroom. Nevertheless, he followed doctor's orders, switched to a Mediterranean diet, and started working out as soon as I cleared him to do so. To his great surprise, six months later and 50 pounds lighter, Jason had his mojo back. His wife, who also got on board with the program, has lost 30 pounds herself, and never misses a chance to thank me for helping to get her marriage back on track.

BEST PRACTICES:
TESTOSTERONE, DHEA, AND ERECTILE DYSFUNCTION

* Exercise and a healthy body weight will help maintain testosterone levels.
* If your testosterone levels are low, your doctor may prescribe a patch, gel, or injection.
* Avoid nonprescription testosterone supplements, as they can harm the liver and cause unwanted side effects.
* DHEA is not an effective anti-aging supplement. Save your money.
* If you are experiencing erectile dysfunction, be sure to tell your doctor. It may be an early sign of heart disease.
* To lessen your chances of ED, exercise, maintain a healthy body weight, and try a Mediterranean diet.

Hormonal changes are complicated and affect each of us in different ways. Although medical therapy can help, it may also cause harm. As you enter your middle and later years, a heart-smart lifestyle, nutritious diet, and regular exercise are essential for a healthy, productive, and fulfilling life.

18

Kids Have a Heart, Too

THE FIRST TIME I met 16-year-old Katrina, I was charmed by her wide smile and sunny disposition. The teenager, with her mom in tow, came to see me because her blood pressure was dangerously high.

After other causes were ruled out, it became clear that Katrina's obesity and couch-potato lifestyle had put her on the fast track to hypertension. Tipping the scales at nearly 300 pounds, Katrina had spent her summer break eating pizza, playing video games, and watching TV.

Katrina did not have a summer job, because she preferred to sleep in. She had tried working at a pet store but shrugged that "it just wasn't for me." Her cholesterol was sky high, and her blood sugar was pushing the upper range of normal. It was clear to me that without serious intervention, Katrina was barreling headfirst toward a lifetime of high blood pressure, diabetes, heart disease, and arthritis. If the statistics were right, she was also destined to face a lifetime of personal hurdles and disappointments in employment and relationships brought on by her weight and her lifestyle choices.

If you think heart health is for mature audiences only, think again. Childhood is the springboard for a lifetime of habits and choices, nurtured and shaped by family, friends, and teachers. During these early years, atherosclerosis often takes a foothold in the arteries throughout the body, including the heart. This slow, insidious process may culminate decades later in a heart attack or stroke. Although cholesterol buildup in adults may have many causes, including genetics, in children, atherosclerosis is nearly always a direct result of an unhealthy diet and sedentary lifestyle.

The effects of diet and lifestyle are profound and far reaching. Kids who eat foods high in saturated fat and cholesterol tend to have lower levels of cognitive and social functioning, regardless of socioeconomic status. The heart size of obese kids is measurably larger, and their arteries respond poorly to physical stress. Many already have "middle-aged" conditions such as fatty deposits in their livers and high blood pressure. Up to 40 percent have the metabolic syndrome, a condition closely linked to diabetes.

There are more obese kids per capita in the United States than virtually anywhere else on Earth. Since 1976, childhood obesity has tripled. About 30 percent of our children are overweight, and nearly one in every six teens is obese. When it comes to gender, obesity is an equal opportunity player, although black girls are at especially high risk. If the rate of obesity continues on its present course, researchers at the University of California, San Francisco, predict that by 2020, a staggering 44 percent of women and 37 percent of men ages 35 and up will suffer from obesity and all of its attendant complications.

WHERE OBESITY STARTS

Young creatures, human or otherwise, are not naturally inclined to laziness or obesity. The truth is that we have allowed this to happen.

The stage for obesity may be set during pregnancy, as overweight moms (who are more prone to develop gestational diabetes) tend to give birth to larger babies. Obese moms are also up to twice as likely as moms of healthy weight to give birth to babies with serious birth defects, including abnormalities of the heart.

Even our very youngest have become victims of their parents' toxic lifestyles. Today, more than one in five children aged 2 to 5 are medically overweight, with more than 10 percent meeting the criteria for obesity. Because these kiddos are more likely to become obese and unhealthy as they grow older, it is vital that we recognize that good health begins with a healthy mother.

CAREGIVERS COUNT

Moms are important every step of the way. For instance, babies who are breast fed tend to have fewer chronic health problems as adults, including obesity, high blood pressure, high cholesterol, and diabetes. And women who breast-feed appear to be at lower risk for heart disease as they age.

Young children are absolutely dependent on their parents and caregivers for the food they eat. But in the United States, where fresh food is abundant, nearly one third of children aged 4 to 24 months eat no fruit or vegetables. It is a sad reflection on twenty-first-century parenting that by the age of 18 months, the most common "vegetable" consumed is the french fry.

It is way past time for parents to take responsibility for the heart health of their little ones. Let's be honest. It is not the kids pulling up to the drive-through on the way home from work. It is Mom or Dad, choosing the path of least resistance.

THE FAST-FOOD GENERATION

It's no surprise that the more often a kid eats fast food, the more likely he or she is to be obese. Eating out also raises blood pressure and lowers good cholesterol in kids, just as it does in adults. Preschool girls who are regularly fed french fries grow up to have a measurably higher risk of breast cancer later in life, with the risk rising 27 percent with each additional serving per week, compared to girls who eat no french fries at all. And it has been well established that a child will tend to eat more food when given larger portions. This is why "super-sizing" is such a harmful practice.

At least one in every three kids eats fast food every day. Don't expect big business to have your child's best interests in mind. As of 2011, McDonald's Web site claimed to "want the very best for your children." In fact, the company's "Happy Meals" supply between 380 and 700 calories per meal, with up to 27 grams of fat (for a small cheeseburger, small fries, and low-fat chocolate milk), including 9 grams of saturated fat, 1 gram of trans fats, and 45 mg of cholesterol. To put this in perspective, most healthy children between the ages of 4 and 8 do not require more than 1,600 calories and 20 grams of saturated fat daily. And at this rate, a child could easily reach the daily maximum for saturated fat in a single meal.

Research shows that active kids are less likely to overeat, probably because they do more to keep their mind and body engaged, and thus have less time for mindless snacking. Not surprisingly, kids whose parents habitually feed them meals from fast-food joints are much more likely to be sedentary than are kids who eat home-cooked meals.

TURN OFF THE TV

Marketing junk food to kids takes many forms. It is estimated that kids view a mind-boggling 7,500 food advertisements each year, most of which feature foods high in sugar and fat and low in nutritional value. A 2008 study from Yale University reported that two thirds of breakfast cereals marketed to children failed to meet basic national standards for nutrition.

According to the Henry J. Kaiser Family Foundation, American kids watch, on average, three to four hours of television every day and spend nearly two more hours on the computer or playing video games. A child spending this much time in front of the tube is not experiencing his or her own life, but living vicariously through make-believe characters and strangers. And although the American Academy of Pediatrics strongly advises against any TV for very young children, a recent report from Children's Hospital in Cincinnati found that 40 percent of 2-year-olds watch at least three hours of television per day.

Kids who watch two or more hours of TV daily tend to eat more high-calorie snack foods, including chips and caffeinated sodas. They are also more likely to start smoking, to be overly aggressive, and to have difficulty concentrating. Researchers at Columbia University found that kids who watched TV for three or more hours per day were more apt to struggle in school and less inclined to pursue higher education. Even an hour of TV every day put kids at a disadvantage, when compared to those who watched little to no television.

THE ROLE OF SMOKING

Like poor eating habits, smoking is a behavior that is often learned at home. About one in five teens smoke, and most believe they can quit whenever they want. Nearly all of my smoking patients started as teenagers, and most would do anything now to have never taken that first drag. Tobacco is highly addictive; perhaps more so than any other drug available. Kids who are exposed to smokers at home or in their community are up to four times more likely to smoke. And children of smokers are more likely to suffer from asthma and other diseases of the respiratory system.

OTHER FACTORS: LOVE AND MEDICINE

Love really does nourish a healthy heart. Children who are emotionally battered, those who come from families where substance abuse is commonplace, and those who grow up in crime-riddled homes are more likely to develop heart disease later in life.

A small percentage of overweight kids may have medical conditions that predispose to obesity, so it is important to check in with your pediatrician or family doctor. These conditions include genetic abnormalities, diabetes, thyroid problems, polycystic ovary syndrome (see chapter 13, page 239), depression, and eating disorders. Doctors can screen for most of these ailments.

Nearly half of all obese children have abnormal lipid levels. Because high cholesterol in childhood is clearly linked to atherosclerosis in young adulthood, many pediatricians recommend routine screening, on the order of every five years, for all kids. Kids with a family history of heart disease or high cholesterol are at higher risk for cholesterol problems and should have a blood lipid test at least once. Adopted kids should also be tested, because their family history is often unknown. In children, cholesterol can often be lowered with a healthy diet and exercise. However, severely elevated levels may require medical treatment.

KEEPING YOUR CHILD'S HEART HEALTHY

How can you ensure that your child will get the best possible start for a healthy heart? First, understand, and take to heart, that you are personally responsible for the food your youngster eats. It is not a toddler's decision to eat fries or drink a soda—that choice is made by the parent. If your child is exposed to these foods at school, it is up to you to effect change. Enlist other parents and make your voices heard. A German study found that simple changes such as substituting water for sodas in the schools can reduce the risk of a child's becoming overweight by as much as 30 percent. Even more important, don't depend on others to do the right thing for your family. It only takes a few minutes to pack a healthy lunch. You cannot just love your child passively; as a mom or dad, you must be your child's advocate and protector.

Second, limit snack foods, candy, and sodas to special treats, if you allow them at all. Teach your child to enjoy nature's wide bounty of fruit and grains, even if it does cost a bit more than a bag of chips. Watch out for liquid sugar in the form of high-fructose corn syrup, which is frequently found in popular fruit drinks and sodas. Americans, on average, gobble and slurp the equivalent of a whopping half a pound of sugar a day, and children may consume even more. The average teen drinks nearly a gallon of soft drinks each week, but kids who drink more milk tend to be healthier and leaner.

Third, be sure your child gets plenty of grains, dairy foods, and healthy proteins. Avoid prepared foods tainted with food coloring and preservatives, as these have been linked to attention-deficit disorders. And stay away from trans fats, which are found in many fast foods, snack foods, and bakery products. Don't be fooled by labels listing "no trans fats," as regulations allow serving-size levels of less than half a gram to be considered "zero." Look for the words "partially hydrogenated" in the ingredients list and avoid these products.

Fourth, control portion size. This is so easy to overlook, especially when eating out. Why not share your own restaurant meal with your child? That way you'll reduce your own portion, teach your child how to make smart choices, and save a little money in the process. If you choose to eat most of your meals at home, you'll not only have more control over how much your child eats, you can also steer clear of the excessive sugar, starch, sodium, and fat found in typical restaurant meals.

Fifth, divert your child from mindless nibbling and snacking. Avoid buying snack foods like cookies, candy, and chips, and keep only healthy snacks, such as fruits and vegetables, on hand. And don't let your family eat meals in front of the television—it is too easy to lose track of how much you've eaten.

Most important, teach your child to revel in the joy of good health. Maintaining a healthy weight and an active way of life cannot happen without motivation and support. Don't forget to take care of your own health, as you are your child's most important role model. Overweight and obese parents tend to raise overweight and obese kids. For a child or teen, it is critical that the whole family be involved in making smart choices and limiting dangerous temptations.

More than ever before, this is the time for tough love. Put your love into action, and stand your ground, even when your kids accuse you of being cruel, out of touch, even uncool. Join a gym together, boycott fast food and high-calorie snacks, and shop smart for food at the grocery store. Make a bike ride together a regular outing, or just take a walk or a hike. Enroll your child in a physical activity that she or he enjoys; there are so many options, even for kids who don't enjoy competitive team sports. Dancing, swimming, even yoga for kids are all possibilities. Limit everyone's TV and video time, your own included, to less than two hours a day (preferably much less), and keep computer and gaming screen time to a minimum. Help your child to know the joy of a strong, healthy body and a well-nourished mind. Resolve to get healthy and stay healthy together.

We all want the best that life can offer our children. It takes more than money and platitudes. A commitment to a heart-healthy lifestyle takes discipline, but for young people, like my patient Katrina, caring enough to make these changes is truly love in action.

BEST PRACTICES:
YOUR CHILD'S HEART

* Breast feeding helps reduce a child's risk of obesity, diabetes, and high blood pressure. It's also better for Mom's heart.
* Limit kids' total screen time (television and computer) to 2 hours or less per day. Kids who watch TV for 2 hours or more per day have higher levels of aggressive behavior, are more likely to be obese, eat more junk food, and are more likely to smoke.
* Do not smoke in your home or car; children are vulnerable to secondhand smoke.
* Encourage your children to be active—they'll reap the benefits of heart-healthy exercise, and be less inclined to overeat.
* Provide healthy meals for your kids. Avoid fast-food joints and advocate for heart-healthy meals in their schools. Pack healthier lunches yourself, whenever possible.
* Parents do make the difference. Teach your children well, and lead by example.

AFTERWORD
POWER UP YOUR LIFE

WRITING THIS BOOK for you has been a deeply satisfying experience for me. Through my research and critical review of the medical literature, I have deepened my understanding of the ways our small and seemingly trivial daily choices can profoundly influence our health and well-being.

Living is all about learning. No matter what your age, weight, or medical condition, I hope that I have helped to empower you to take control of your health and, in so doing, to create a more satisfying and joyful life for yourself and for those you love. Good health is truly a journey, not a destination, and it is my wish that this book will serve as a roadmap to help guide you along your way.

We are fortunate to live in a time of tremendous progress in medical science. As I write, new developments and discoveries are emerging, and I have no doubt that our understanding of heart disease, diet, supplements, hormones, and lifestyle will continue to evolve. It is an exciting time to be a cardiologist.

Despite all our advances, we are far from having all the answers. Life is tremendously complex, a rich and spicy gumbo of possibilities and permutations. If we were simply machines, our lives would be predictable, our breakdowns all repairable. But we are not. There are very few straight lines or absolutes for the human organism. A plus B does not always equal C, and that is why we, as a species, survive.

Yet despite the uncertainties, there is no doubt that the choices, big and small, that you make each day can have a tremendous influence on the quality and duration of your life. Choose wisely, and live well. You owe it to yourself and to those you love.

APPENDIX

BODY MASS INDEX (BMI)

The BMI uses your height and weight measurements to calculate whether you are at a healthy weight. The way to find your exact BMI is to divide your weight in kilograms by the square of your height in centimeters. This table makes it simple to see where you fall. Most people with a BMI below 18.5 are underweight. If your BMI is 25 or more, you are probably medically overweight, unless you are exceptionally muscular. A BMI of 30 defines medical obesity, and more than 40 is considered morbidly obese.

HEIGHT (IN)	WEIGHT (LB)													
58	91	96	100	105	110	115	119	124	129	134	138	143	167	191
59	94	99	104	109	114	119	124	128	133	138	143	148	173	198
60	97	102	107	112	118	123	128	133	138	143	148	153	179	204
61	100	106	111	116	122	127	132	137	143	148	153	158	185	211
62	104	109	115	120	126	131	136	142	147	153	158	164	191	218
63	107	113	118	124	130	135	141	146	152	158	163	169	197	225
64	110	116	122	128	134	140	145	151	157	163	169	174	204	232
65	114	120	126	132	138	144	150	156	162	168	174	180	210	240
66	118	124	130	136	142	148	155	161	167	173	179	186	216	247
67	121	127	134	140	146	153	159	166	172	178	185	191	223	255
68	125	131	138	144	151	158	164	171	177	184	190	197	230	262
69	128	135	142	149	155	162	169	176	182	189	196	203	236	270
70	132	139	146	153	160	167	174	181	188	195	202	207	243	278
71	136	143	150	157	165	172	179	186	193	200	208	215	250	286
72	140	147	154	162	169	177	184	191	199	206	213	221	258	294
73	144	151	159	166	174	182	189	197	204	212	219	227	265	302
74	148	155	163	171	179	186	194	202	210	218	225	233	272	311
75	152	160	168	176	184	192	200	208	216	224	232	240	279	319
76	156	164	172	180	189	197	205	213	221	230	238	246	287	328
BMI (KG/M^2)	19	20	21	22	23	24	25	26	27	28	29	30	35	40

HEART HEALTH CHECKLIST:
WHAT YOUR DOCTOR NEEDS TO KNOW

Your doctor will likely have other questions to ask you, but having this information handy will help the visit go more smoothly and allow more time for your doctor to focus on your concerns.

- What prompted you to make this appointment?
- If you are experiencing symptoms (pain, discomfort, or other concerns) of any kind:
  - What do the symptoms feel like?
  - How long do the symptoms last?
  - What triggers the symptoms?
  - What makes them better or worse?
  - Are there other associated symptoms?
  - How long have you been experiencing these symptoms?
  - Have you experienced similar symptoms in the past?
- What medications (including prescription drugs, over-the-counter drugs, and supplements) are you taking?
- Do you have any drug allergies or sensitivities?
- What other medical or surgical problems do you have?
- Have you seen another doctor for this problem? If so, what sort of testing was done, and what was recommended? Are those records available?
- What is your family's medical history?
- Do you smoke?
- How much alcohol do you drink?
- Do you use any illegal drugs?
- What are the sources of stress in your life?

HEART HEALTH CHECKLIST:
WHAT YOU SHOULD ASK YOUR DOCTOR

Be sure to bring a list of concerns with you when you visit your doctor. Try to be as specific as possible. This will help your doctor give you the best care possible and make the most of the time allotted for your visit.

- What is my blood pressure? Is that number optimal for me?
- What does my lipid profile (including HDL, LDL, and tri-glycerides) show? What should my numbers be?
- What is my blood glucose (sugar)?
- Is my weight in a healthy range? If not, how can I lose weight safely?
- What should I expect my medications to do for me? Are there common side effects I should know about?
- How can I reduce my need for medications?
- What is my risk for heart disease? How can I lower my risk?
- Here are the symptoms and problems that I am experiencing. What should be done to evaluate them?

KNOW YOUR RISK FACTORS

Although heart disease is the number-one cause of death for both men and women in the United States, some of us are at greater risk than others.

Major Conventional Risk Factors

- high blood pressure (hypertension)
- diabetes
- abnormal blood lipids (including cholesterol and triglycerides)
- tobacco use
- obesity
- lack of regular exercise
- age (over 45 for men; over 55 for women)
- family history of heart disease (in men under 50 or women under 60)

Other factors may also accelerate your risk for heart disease, including diet, inflammation, lack of sleep, stress, pollution, and hormonal changes.

What's Your Risk?

There are a number of different tools you can use to calculate your heart attack risk. Of course, statistics apply to the general population and can't predict what will happen to a particular individual. In addition, if your risk factors are controlled, then the likelihood of a heart attack or stroke is much lower.

If you already have cardiovascular disease or if you are diabetic, you are automatically considered to be at high risk, and your 10-year risk of a heart attack exceeds 20 percent.

If you don't have cardiovascular disease and are not diabetic, you can calculate your Framingham Risk Score by plugging in your age, gender, cholesterol numbers, blood pressure, and smoking status at hp2010.nhlbihin.net/atpiii/calculator.asp. Researchers originally developed this score using data from the Framingham Heart Study, which followed thousands of residents of Framingham, Massachusetts. It will give you a good statistical estimate of your 10-year risk for heart disease.

The Primary Cardiovascular Risk Calculator from the U.K. is more detailed: It incorporates body size, ethnicity, family history, and information from your electrocardiogram. You can find it at patient .co.uk/doctor/Primary-Cardiovascular-Risk-Calculator.htm.

Neither of these calculators takes diet or lifestyle into account, since these are very hard to measure. Nevertheless, a heart-smart diet, regular exercise, and stress management are essential for heart health.

GLOSSARY

ANGINA Pain or discomfort caused by a narrowed or blocked heart artery that may be felt in the chest, back, arms, neck, jaw, or upper abdomen

ANTIOXIDANT A substance that counteracts and neutralizes free radicals, preventing damage to the cells of the body

ATHEROSCLEROSIS Cholesterol deposits, or plaque, in the arteries, including those that feed the heart, brain, other vital organs, and limbs

ATRIAL FIBRILLATION An irregular and disorganized rhythm that starts in the top chambers (*atria*) of the heart, sometimes associated with the formation of blood clots inside the heart

BASAL METABOLIC RATE (BMR) The amount of energy, in calories, that the body burns at rest

BODY MASS INDEX An indicator of body fat calculated using body weight and height (see pages 19 and 346)

CARBOHYDRATE A food classification that includes sugars, starches, and fiber, mainly from plant sources

CARDIOVASCULAR DISEASE Any form of disease affecting the heart or the blood vessels, including coronary artery disease, stroke, heart valve disease, and peripheral vascular disease

CHOLESTEROL A substance produced by the liver and obtained through the diet that is essential for normal hormone production and healthy cell membranes

   HDL cholesterol (also known as "good cholesterol") Helps to transport cholesterol from the arteries and other tissues to the liver so it can be removed from the body

   LDL cholesterol (also known as "bad cholesterol") Transports cholesterol from the liver and into the blood vessels

CONGESTIVE HEART FAILURE A condition generally caused by weakness or stiffness of the heart, characterized by shortness of breath due to fluid buildup in the lungs, and often associated with swelling in the legs

CORONARY ARTERY DISEASE A disease of the blood vessels that supply the heart, usually due to cholesterol buildup, sometimes referred to as coronary heart disease

C-REACTIVE PROTEIN (CRP) A protein that increases in the body in response to inflammation, and that is associated with a higher risk for heart disease

DIABETES A condition in which the body either doesn't make enough of the hormone insulin (which regulates blood sugar) or isn't able to effectively use the insulin it manufactures

FAT Our most caloric source of energy, found in animal foods and some plant foods

> *Monounsaturated fat* A heart-healthy type of fat, sometimes referred to as omega-9, found in olive oil, canola oil, nuts, and avocados

> *Polyunsaturated fat* Includes heart-healthy omega-3 (found in cold-water fish, flaxseed oil, and walnuts) and omega-6 (found in most vegetable oils)

> *Saturated fat* Linked to heart disease risk, examples include fats from animal sources, especially red meat and dairy, and from tropical oils such as palm and coconut

> *Trans fats* Chemically modified fats, also known as partially hydrogenated oils, that increase heart disease risk

FREE RADICALS Highly reactive substances that make LDL cholesterol more dangerous and can cause harmful reactions that damage cells and arteries

GLYCEMIC INDEX A number that measures how fast a carbohydrate-based food is likely to raise blood glucose, or sugar, levels

GLYCEMIC LOAD A number that takes into account both the glycemic index and the typical amount of food per serving

HEART ATTACK Injury or death of a segment of the heart muscle caused by a sudden blockage of a heart artery

HYPERTENSION High blood pressure

ISOFLAVONES Antioxidant chemicals that occur naturally in plants and bear certain similarities to our own estrogen

PERIPHERAL VASCULAR DISEASE Atherosclerosis (cholesterol buildup) in the blood vessels supplying the limbs and abdominal organs

PLAQUE Another term for atherosclerosis, or cholesterol buildup

PROTEIN Long strings of amino acids abundant in meat, poultry, fish, dairy foods, and soy

STROKE A sudden blockage of the blood supply to the brain, usually caused by a clot triggered by an unstable cholesterol plaque, but that also may be the result of a clot that traveled from the heart to the brain or of bleeding in the brain

SUPPLEMENTS Vitamins, minerals, plant products, amino acids, and extracts from certain animal organs and glands that are sold without a prescription and are not regulated by the U.S. Food and Drug Administration

TRIGLYCERIDES A form of fat that circulates in the bloodstream and is also used by the body for fat storage

REFERENCES

MY GOAL IN writing this book was to include the most up-to-date information possible on heart health and prevention. To do so, I reviewed literally hundreds of scientific studies and analyses from scores of peer-reviewed journals. Though by no means an exhaustive list of resources, I relied heavily on the following publications:

- *The American Journal of Clinical Nutrition*
- *Annals of Internal Medicine*
- *Archives of Internal Medicine*
- *British Journal of Nutrition*
- *British Medical Journal*
- *Circulation*
- *The Journal of Nutrition*
- *Journal of the American College of Cardiology*
- *The Journal of the American Medical Association*
- *The Lancet*
- *Nature*
- *The New England Journal of Medicine*
- *Stroke*

We all owe a debt of gratitude to the hundreds of thousands of people who have participated in medical research. Many of the reports I reviewed for this book were offshoots of the following long-term clinical studies:

- Adventist Mortality Study
- Framingham Heart Study

- Health Professional Follow-Up Study
- Iowa Women's Health Study
- Kuopio Ischaemic Heart Disease Risk Factor Study
- NIH-AARP Diet and Health Study
- Nurses' Health Study
- Physicians' Health Study
- Seven Countries Study
- Women's Health Initiative
- Women's Health Study

Other important resources include:

Ornish, D. M. (1996). *Dr. Dean Ornish's Program for Reversing Heart Disease: The Only System Scientifically Proven to Reverse Heart Disease Without Drugs or Surgery.* New York: Ivy Books.

Stedman's Medical Dictionary for the Health Professions and Nursing, Seventh Edition (2011). Baltimore, MD: Lippincott, Williams & Wilkins.

Webster's New World Medical Dictionary, Third Edition (2008). Hoboken, NJ: Wiley.

Willcox, B. J., D. C. Willcox, and M. Suzuki (2001). *The Okinawa Program: How the World's Longest-Lived People Achieve Everlasting Health—And How You Can, Too.* New York: Three Rivers Press.

ACKNOWLEDGMENTS

THIS BOOK WOULD not have been possible without my patients, who inspire me to learn something new every day. I am indebted to my cardiology mentors, Dr. Michael Crawford, Dr. Jonathan Abrams, and the late Dr. Bruce Shively. As a cardiologist, I am fortunate to work with a superb group of physicians, nurses, and staff at Legacy Heart Center, my home away from home. Their support means the world to me.

I am grateful for the encouragement and patience of my literary agent, Linda Konner, who kept me motivated and optimistic. Matthew Lore, president of The Experiment, believed in my message and gave me the opportunity to create this book. Thank you also to my wonderful editors, Iris Bass and Karen Giangreco, who inspired, encouraged, and coached me to create a book that I can truly be proud of.

And finally, my deepest thanks and love to Gary Cooper. Without your unwavering confidence in me, I could never have made this book a reality.

INDEX

and toxins in fish, 83, 85, 86
chitosan, 279, 295
chocolate, 97, 104–5, 106
cholesterol
    and diet, 32–33, 99
    and exercise, 162
    and fatty acids, 71
    and fiber, 65
    and fish oil, 284
    and garlic, 292
    and heart disease, 116
    on high-carb, low-fat diet, 109–10
    in Mediterranean diet, 117, 118
    overview, 26, 27, 33–34, 213, 214
    supplements for reducing, 288–96
    total cholesterol count, 32
    and trans fats, 75
    See also HDL cholesterol; LDL
        cholesterol
cholesterol-related medications
    bile acid sequestrants, 222
    ezetimibe, 222
    fibrates, 219–20
    niacin, 220–21
    overview, 214–15
    prescription omega-3, 223
    statins, 40, 215–19, 223–24, 297
Cholestin, 292, 293
chromium picolinate, 279, 301, 305
cocaine, 158, 159, 160
cocoa (drink), 143
coenzyme Q10 (CoQ10), 279, 296–98, 300
coffee, 139–41, 144
common sense, 173, 174, 186
complementary medicine, 312–16
congestive heart failure, 14, 102, 146,
    228–29, 333
cooking with heat, 180–81
coronary balloon angioplasty, 261
coronary calcium score, 30
cortisol, 190–91, 192–93
COX-2 inhibitors, 274
cranberries, 94, 95
cravings for foods, 21–22
C-reactive protein (CRP)
    and aspirin, 241
    from cooking with high heat, 181
    and fiber, 65
    and inflammation, 39, 40, 41
    and oral contraceptives, 321
    overview, 39–41
    and periodontal disease, 176
    and saturated fats, 73
    and statin drugs, 216
    and trans fats, 75
creatine, 279, 297, 309, 310
creatine phosphokinase (CPK), 219
Crete, Greece, 116
CRP. See C-reactive protein
CVD. See cardiovascular disease

dairy products, 67, 74, 257, 341
decaffeinated coffee, 141
deep venous thrombosis (DVT), 320–21,
    324
dehydroepiandrosterone (DHEA), 328,
    332
dementia
    and alcohol, 146
    and Ginkgo biloba, 298
    from HRT, 324
    and loneliness, 177, 178
    and statin drugs, 216
    and type D personality, 198
    See also mental clarity
dental health, 176
depression, 198–99
DHEA (dehydroepiandrosterone), 328,
    332
diabetes
    complications, 227, 228–30
    diabetic ketoacidosis, 112
    diagnosing, 227–28
    and diet, 110, 120
    factors leading to, 141, 146, 153, 219,
        258–59
    and glycemic load, 57–58
    and insulin, 57–58, 146, 224–25, 229,
        230–35, 301
    and LDL cholesterol, 28
    and magnesium, 270
    medications, 230–35
    and niacin, 220
    nuts as deterrent, 87

resveratrol, 147, 149
rhabdomyolysis, 218–19, 293

saccharin, 131
salatrim, 135
saturated fats, 69, 72–74, 78–79, 87
seizure disorders and aspartame, 132, 133
selenium, 250, 258–59
Seven Countries Study, 115–16, 120–21
shark, 83
Siberian ginseng, 301
sleep apnea, 185
sleeping, 183–86, 194
smoking. *See* tobacco
snacks and snacking, 16–17, 21, 59, 74, 185, 342
social costs of obesity, 13
sodas, 49, 129–31, 133–34, 143, 341
sodium, 97, 100–104
soft drinks, 49, 129–31, 133–34, 143, 341
soluble fiber, 64–65
soy, 89–93, 96
soybean oil, 89
soy isoflavones, 90–91, 282, 287–88
soy milk, 93–94
soy yogurt, 94
spirituality, 182–83
spirulina, 306
starches, 56
statin drugs, 40, 215–19, 223–24, 297
stevia, 134
strawberries, 94, 95
stress
    controlling, 188–89, 313
    effects of, 187–88, 189–90
    managing stress, 193–94
    overview, 199–200
    and personality type, 195–98
    science of stress, 190–93
strokes, 14–15, 152, 153. *See also* heart attacks and strokes
sucralose, 133
sudden cardiac death, 81
sugar alcohols, 134–35
sugars, 55–56, 129–30, 130–31
sugar substitutes, 131–35
sulfonylureas, 231

supplements
    amino acids and their derivatives, 306–10
    for cholesterol reduction, 288–96
    for energy and weight loss, 300–306
    fish oil, 35, 283
    fruit and vegetable concentrates, 310–11
    for heart and brain protection, 296–300
    herbs and herbal medications, 276–78
    isoflavone supplements vs. soy in diet, 92
    labels for, 275–76
    for menopause, 329
    misinformation and mislabeling, 276–77
    multivitamin supplement, 271
    omega-3s, 85, 283–87
    overview, 272–72, 278–82, 311
    soy isoflavones, 90–91, 282, 287–88
    testosterone precursors, 333
    See also minerals; vitamins
surgical interventions for obesity, 23
sweet potatoes, 61
Swiss study on caffeine, 140
swordfish, 83

takotsubo cardiomyopathy (broken heart syndrome), 189–90
tea, 141–43, 144
teeth, caring for, 176
television, watching, 17, 339–40, 342, 343
testosterone, 319, 332–33, 335
texturized vegetable protein (TVP), 94
thiazolidinediones (TZDs), 232
thyroid gland and flaxseed oil, 124
tilefish, 83
tobacco
    addiction to, 150–51
    and alcohol, 148
    and children, 340
    and cholesterol levels, 32
    and diabetes, 235
    effects on smoker, 152–53, 188
    and free radicals, 252
    and inflammation in the body, 31
    and oral contraceptives, 320
    overview, 4, 157–58

ABOUT THE AUTHOR

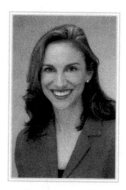

SARAH SAMAAN, MD, FACC, a Vanderbilt University Medical School graduate, is a board-certified cardiologist with additional board certifications in echocardiography and nuclear cardiology, and a Fellow of the American College of Cardiology. Dr. Samaan practices cardiology full-time, caring for patients with a wide range of cardiovascular conditions. She considers heart disease prevention the cornerstone of her medical practice and works passionately to educate her patients with the message that heart disease prevention should be a lifelong pursuit.

For the past six years, *Texas Monthly* magazine has named Dr. Samaan a "Texas Super Doctor." She has also been listed as one of "America's Top Physicians" by Consumers' Research Council of America. In 2005, she was profiled in *Medicine Men*, a book celebrating notable Texas physicians. Dr. Samaan practices cardiology at Legacy Heart Center in Plano, Texas, and at Baylor Heart Hospital, where she is codirector of the Women's Cardiovascular Institute. Away from work, Dr. Samaan's passion is horses. She enjoys dressage and cross-country jumping, and stays fit with a regimen of running, yoga, and Pilates.